PUBLIC HEALTH: PRACTICES, METHODS AND POLICIES

PUBLIC HEALTH THEMES IN GRENADA AND THE CARIBBEAN REGION

PUBLIC HEALTH: PRACTICES, METHODS AND POLICIES

JOAV MERRICK - SERIES EDITOR

MEDICAL DIRECTOR, HEALTH SERVICES, DIVISION FOR INTELLECTUAL AND DEVELOPMENTAL DISABILITIES, MINISTRY OF SOCIAL AFFAIRS AND SOCIAL SERVICES, JERUSALEM, ISRAEL

Public Health Themes in Grenada and the Caribbean Region
Joav Merrick and Lindonne Glasgow (Editors)
2020. ISBN: 978-1-53618-118-0 (Hardcover)
2020. ISBN. 978-1-53618-119-7 (e-book)

Advances in Chinese Children, Adolescent and Family Research
Ariel Tenenbaum, Daniel T.L. Shek, Moon YM Law and Joav Merrick (Editors)
2020. ISBN: 978-1-53617-870-8 (Hardcover)
2020. ISBN. 978-1-53617-871-5 (e-book)

Child Environmental Health Disparities: Looking at the Present and Facing the Future
I. Leslie Rubin and Joav Merrick (Editors)
2020. ISBN: 978-1-53617-823-4 (Hardcover)
2020. ISBN. 978-1-53617-824-1 (e-book)

Positive Youth Development: Digital Game-Based Learning
Ty Lee, Daniel T.L. Shek, Sarah Sw Lee, and Joav Merrick (Editors)
2020. ISBN: 978-1-53617-795-4 (Hardcover)
2020. ISBN. 978-1-53617-796-1 (e-book)

Service Leadership Education in an Era of Service Economy
Daniel TL Shek, Xiaoqin Zhu, and Joav Merrick (Editors)
2020. ISBN: 978-1-53617-514-1 (Hardcover)
2020. ISBN: 978-1-53617-515-8 (e-book)

Parenting and Family Life in a Chinese Society
Daniel TL Shek, Moon YM Law, Joav Merrick (Editors)
2020. ISBN: 978-1-53616-705-4 (Softcover)
2020. ISBN: 978-1-53616-706-1 (e-book)

Public Health: Topics, Themes and Trends
Satesh Bidaisee, Sadik Uddin Emmanuel Keku, Joav Merrick (Editors)
2020. ISBN: 978-1-53616-655-2 (Softcover)
2020. ISBN: 978-1-53616-656-9

Public Health: Environment and Child Health in a Changing World
I. Leslie Rubin and Joav Merrick (Editors)
2019. ISBN: 978-1-53615-394-1 (Hardcover)
2019. ISBN: 978-1-53615395-8 (e-book)

Service Leadership: Tools to Assess Knowledge, Attitude and Behavior
Daniel TL Shek, Xiaoqin Zhu, Li Lin and Joav Merrick (Editors)
2019. ISBN: 978-1-53614-852-7 (Hardcover)
2019. ISBN: 978-1-53614-853-4 (e-book)

Public Health Yearbook 2017
Joav Merrick (Editor)
2018. ISBN: 978-1-53613-792-7 (Hardcover)
2018. ISBN: 978-1-53613-793-4 (e-book)

Resilience and Health: A Potent Dynamic
I Leslie Rubin and Joav Merrick (Editors)
2018. ISBN: 978-1-53613-412-4 (Hardcover)
2018. ISBN: 978-1-53613-413-1 (e-book)

Medical History: Some Perspectives Second Edition
Donald E. Greydanus and Joav Merrick, (Editors)
2018. ISBN: 978-1-53613-319-6 (Hardcover)
2018. ISBN: 978-1-53613-320-2 (e-book)

University Students: Promotion of Holistic Development in Hong Kong
Daniel TL Shek, Lu Yu and Joav Merrick (Editors)
2017. ISBN: 978-1-53612-535-1 (Hardcover)
2017. ISBN: 978-1-53612-537-5 (e-book)

Alzheimer's Disease:
Awareness among Young Adults
Ronald Chow, Drew Hollenberg, Michael Borean and Joav Merrick (Editors)
2017. ISBN: 978-1-53612-456-9 (Softcover)
2017. ISBN: 978-1-53612-457-6 (e-book)

Service Leadership Education for University Students
Daniel TL Shek, Po Chung, Li Lin and Joav Merrick (Editors)
2017. ISBN: 978-1-53611-949-7 (Hardcover)
2017. ISBN: 978-1-53611-969-5 (e-book)

Leadership: Promoting Leadership and Intrapersonal Development in University Students
Daniel TL Shek, Cecilia MS Ma and Joav Merrick (Editors)
2017. ISBN: 978-1-53611-950-3 (Hardcover)
2017. ISBN: 978-1-53611-970-1 (e-book)

Caribbean Adolescents:
Misuse and Abuse of Alcohol
Cecilia Hegamin-Younger and Joav Merrick (Editors)
2017. ISBN: 978-1-63485-880-9 (Hardcover)
2016. ISBN: 978-1-63485-894-6 (e-book)

Public Health: An Ecological Framework for Child Environmental Health Interventions
I. Leslie Rubin and Joav Merrick (Editors)
2017. ISBN: 978-1-53610-700-5 (Hardcover)
2017. ISBN: 978-1-53610-714-2 (e-book)

Diabetes Mellitus:
A Medical History Journey
Donald E. Greydanus and Joav Merrick
2016. ISBN: 978-1-53610-094-5 (Softcover)
2016. ISBN: 978-1-53610-103-4 (e-book)

Education in Hong Kong: Service Leadership for University Students
Daniel TL Shek, Cecilia MS Ma, Li Lin and Joav Merrick (Editors)
2016. ISBN: 978-1-63484-928-9 (Hardcover)
2016. ISBN: 978-1-63484-960-9 (e-book)

Environmental Health Disparities: Costs and Benefits of Breaking the Cycle
I. Leslie Rubin and Joav Merrick (Editors)
2016. ISBN: 978-1-63484-211-2 (Hardcover)
2016. ISBN: 978-1-63484-212-9 (e-book)

Higher Education in Hong Kong: Nurturing Students to be Caring Service Leaders
Daniel TL Shek, Andrew MH Siu, Hildie Leung and Joav Merrick (Editors)
2016. ISBN: 978-1-63484-980-7 (Hardcover)
2016. ISBN: 978-1-63485-009-4 (e-book)

Measles: Epidemiology and Control of Measles in the Gweru Urban District in Zimbabwe
Tawanda Marufu, Seter Siziya, Mazyanga L. Mazaba and Joav Merrick (Editors)
2016. ISBN: 978-1-63485-559-4 (Hardcover)
2016. ISBN: 978-1-63485-573-0 (e-book)

Medical History: Some Perspectives
Donald E. Greydanus and Joav Merrick
2016. ISBN: 978-1-63484-747-6 (Hardcover)
2016. ISBN: 978-1-63484-849-7 (e-book)

Public Health: Some International Aspects
Joav Merrick (Editor)
2016. ISBN: 978-1-63484-612-7 (Hardcover)
2016. ISBN: 978-1-63484-630-1 (e-book)

Public Health: International Aspects on Environment and Health
I. Leslie Rubin and Joav Merrick (Editors)
2016. ISBN: 978-1-63484-834-3 (Hardcover)
2016. ISBN: 978-1-63484-849-7 (e-book)

Smoking and Adolescence: International Public Health Experiences
Mazyanga L. Mazaba, Seter Siziya and Joav Merrick (Editors)
2016. ISBN: 978-1-63484-311-9 (Hardcover)
2016. ISBN: 978-1-63484-312-6 (e-book)

Arbovirus: Public Health Experience from Zambia
Seter Siziya, Mazyanga L. Mazaba, and Joav Merrick (Editors)
2015. ISBN: 978-1-63463-601-8 (Hardcover)
2015. ISBN: 978-1-63463-618-6 (e-book)

Health Issues in Diverse Cultures
Cecilia Obeng, Samuel Gyasi Obeng and Joav Merrick (Editors)
2015. ISBN: 978-1-63463-613-1 (Hardcover)
2015. ISBN: 978-1-63463-619-3 (e-book)

Public Health, Social Work and Health Inequalities
Bruce D. Friedman and Joav Merrick (Editors)
2015. ISBN: 978-1-63482-838-3 (Hardcover)
2015. ISBN: 978-1-63482-850-5 (e-book)

Patient Dumping: Background, Protections, and the Mentally Ill
Tabitha E. Rivers (Editor)
2015. ISBN: 978-1-63483-726-2 (Hardcover)
2015. ISBN: 978-1-63483-727-9 (e-book)

Tomorrow's Leaders: Service Leadership and Holistic Development in Chinese University Students
Daniel TL Shek, Andrew MH Siu and Joav Merrick (Editors)
2015. ISBN: 978-1-63321-880-2 (Hardcover)
2014. ISBN: 978-1-63321-943-4 (e-book)

Environment and Public Health: Environmental Health, Law and International Perspectives
I. Leslie Rubin and Joav Merrick (Editors)
2014. ISBN: 978-1-63463-167-9 (Hardcover)
2014. ISBN: 978-1-63463-189-1 (e-book)

PUBLIC HEALTH: PRACTICES, METHODS AND POLICIES

PUBLIC HEALTH THEMES IN GRENADA AND THE CARIBBEAN REGION

JOAV MERRICK
AND
LINDONNE GLASGOW
EDITORS

nova
Medicine & Health
New York

Library of Congress Cataloging-in-Publication Data

ISBN: 978-1-53618-118-0

Published by Nova Science Publishers, Inc. † New York

Contents

INTRODUCTION

In: Public Health Themes in Grenada … ISBN: 978-1-53618-118-0
Editors: J. Merrick and L. Glasgow

Chapter 1

PUBLIC HEALTH THEMES: GRENADA AND THE CARIBBEAN REGION

Lindonne Glasgow[1,*], MSPH, DrPH
and Joav Merrick[2-5], MD, MMedSci, DMSc
[1]Department of Public Health and Preventive Medicine,
St George's University, St George's, Grenada, West Indies
[2]National Institute of Child Health and Human Development,
Jerusalem, Israel
[3]Department of Pediatrics, Mt Scopus Campus,
Hadassah Hebrew University Medical Center, Jerusalem, Israel
[4]Kentucky Children's Hospital, University of Kentucky,
Lexington, Kentucky, United States
[5]Center for Healthy Development, School of Public Health,
Georgia State University, Atlanta, United States

[*] Correspondence: Dr. Lindonne Glasgow, Assistant Professor, Department of Public Health and Preventive Medicine, St George's University, PO Box 7, True Blue, St George's, Grenada, West Indies. Email: lglasgow@sgu.com.

Abstract

Over the past decade, the Caribbean governments have turned their attention to tackling the rising prevalence of non-communicable chronic diseases, in particular, hypertension, diabetes and cancer. The emergence and rising prevalence of these lifestyle diseases are suggestive of a correlation with the cultural transformation that overtook the region. In the first quarter of 2020, the region's health landscape turned another corner with the emergence of the COVID-19 pandemic, demanding urgent public health and clinical interventions to aadress an infectious disease. Improving the health status of Caribbean populations is at the forefront of the agenda of the regional public health institutions and, in producing this book, we provide support for evidenced-based public health practice in the Caribbean region. We hope readers find the issue informative to understanding the public health situation in the Caribbean and will motivate affirmative action to improve public health.

Introduction

This book is a collection of research and reviews that reflect pertinent public health themes in countries in the Caribbean region. Those themes precipitated from recent research and the insights of the authors who actively engaged with the regional and local public health systems. Many studies have been published, albeit, never before was a production made, bringing an array of public health themes together in the literature to readily provide a comprehensive overview of public health successes and challenges in Caribbean countries. The motivation to write this book came from the expressed yearning to have a fuller understanding of the direction in which public health activities may be focused to improve health and wellness of the Caribbean peoples. Sharing the results and recommendations in this book is especially valuable within the context of the limited resources that is available in the region for a wide range of studies to generate evidence related to public health. This limitation in the region hinders proportional response to significant events.

The information in this book is valuable for many audiences, including public health practitioners, health planners, and policymakers. Incorporating the content in academic settings is a positive step towards developing a conscientious and well-informed next-generation workforce. In this issue, we highlight reviews of the regional public health systems and country-based research findings and recommendations. Readers can deduce information about health status and public health needs in the region. Apart from contributing to inform capacity building, the results and recommendations presented by the authors provide directions to guide in the development of affirmative actions to improve the responsiveness of the regional public health systems. The themes in this book highlight the need for collaboration of the local and regional agencies to mobilize for action and to be more effective in the responses.

The efforts of Caribbean governments and public health institutions to address vulnerabilities and risks, in particular, for non-communicable chronic diseases, are well recognized. This book highlights the current pertinence and complexities of this issue in the region. Readers have an opportunity to make judgments about progress in addressing the problems in respective countries as well as to extrapolate results to predict the situation regarding non-communicable diseases in a broader sphere. At the same time, in the current period of the COVID-19 pandemic, greater emphasis is needed to manage and tackle infectious diseases. Health practitioners, planners, and policymakers may do well to apply the findings and recommendations in strategizing to improve the health and well-being of the Caribbean people. The themes also highlight the need for ongoing research to deepen understanding about health in the region.

We extend special thanks to the authors and reviewers for their contributions to this edition. Thanks to the faculty at St. George's University (SGU) in Grenada and the staff at the Caribbean Public Health Agency (CARPHA) in Trinidad. Improving the health status of Caribbean populations is at the forefront of the agenda of the regional public health institutions and, in producing this book, we provide support for evidence-based public health practice in the region. We hope readers find the issue informative to understanding public health in the Caribbean region and that the information will be transformed into affirmative actions to improve the health and well being of the peoples.

SECTION ONE: PUBLIC HEALTH THEMES

In: Public Health Themes in Grenada ... ISBN: 978-1-53618-118-0
Editors: J. Merrick and L. Glasgow

Chapter 2

RESPONDING TO COVID-19 IN THE CARIBBEAN THROUGH THE NOVEL TOURISM AND HEALTH PROGRAM IN THE CARIBBEAN

Lisa Indar[1,*], PhD, MSc, MPhil, Ornella Cyrus[2], IMPH, EPH, Frieda Mohammed[1], BSC, Cecilia Lesueur[3], MSc and Jonathan Edwin[1], MPH

[1]Surveillance, Disease Prevention and Control,
Caribbean Public Health Agency, St Clair, Trinidad and Tobago
[2]Regional Tourism and Health Program,
Caribbean Public Health Agency, St Clair, Trinidad and Tobago
[3]École des Hautes Études en Santé Publique, Paris, France

ABSTRACT

The health of Caribbean economies is closely related to the health of its travel and tourism industry, given that the Caribbean is the most tourism-

* Correspondence: Dr. Lisa Indar, PhD, MSc, MPhil, Assistant Director, Surveillance, Disease Prevention and Control Caribbean Public Health Agency, 16-17 Jamaica Boulevard, Federation Park, St Clair. Trinidad and Tobago. Email: indarlis@carpha.org.

dependent region in the world. The global spread of the novel coronavirus pandemic (COVID-19) was propelled by travel and is threatening the health security of the region while, at the same time, disrupting tourism and reducing revenues in Caribbean economies. The Caribbean Public Health Agency's Regional Tourism and Health/Travellers Health Program is an innovative program that is addressing the health, safety, and environmental sanitation threats to tourism, with the aim of strengthening regional and national health systems and enhancing the health of visitors and locals. This unique program adopts a multi-prong (real-time early warning and response tourism and health information system (THiS), regional guidelines, food safety and environmental sanitation training, hospitality health safety and environmental standards, policy), and multi-sectoral (regional and international health and tourism partners) approach for implementation. The program has built capacity and equipped countries with regional tools that support preparedness and response to public health threats like COVID-19. This is the first integrated program of its kind, setting an international precedent for improving sustainable tourism and regional health security.

Introduction

The United Nations Sustainable Development Goals are the blueprint for achieving a better and more sustainable future for all. Goal 3 calls for ensuring healthy lives and promoting well-being at all ages and Goal 9 requires building resilient infrastructure, promote sustainable industrialization, and foster innovation (1). The Regional Tourism and Health/Travellers Health Program (THP) was established to promote regional health security and sustainable development throughout the region. This paper describes how the THP is supporting the preparedness and response to the novel coronavirus outbreak, declared a pandemic on March 11, 2020.

Background

The Caribbean region is one of the world's most prominent travel destinations, famous for its tropical weather, crystal blue waters, white-sand beaches, and vibrant culture. These features make the region an attractive destination to foreigners, particularly those seeking to escape colder climates. The tourism industry is crucial for Caribbean economies as it a primary revenue source. According to the World Travel and Tourism Council's (WTTC), tourism is a principal source of employment, foreign currency and economic growth in the Caribbean, accounting for approximately 2.5 million jobs or 15.5% of total employment contributing to 5.8% (US $9.2 billion) to region's Gross Domestic Product (GDP) (2), illustrating the dependency of the Caribbean region on the tourism industry.

Caribbean tourism is vulnerable to many external factors, health being one of them. Due to its tropical climate, the region is highly vulnerable to outbreaks associated such as Chikungunya, Malaria, Dengue, and Zika. Negative health publications against an island or unmanaged epidemics can seriously harm the inflow of tourists and tarnish the reputation of Caribbean tourism destinations. Without a market, the Caribbean economy suffers from a fall in tourism generated revenue.

REGIONAL TOURISM AND HEALTH PROGRAM

The Regional Tourism and Health/Travelers Health Program (THP) is a novel, innovative, multi-sectoral, multifaceted program that aims to strengthen regional and national health systems by addressing the health, safety and environmental sanitation (HSE) threats to tourism, and thereby enhance the health and safety of visitors and locals, regional health security, and the quality, reputation, and sustainability of Caribbean tourism (website: http://carpha.org/What-We-Do/Tourism-and-Health-Programme).

The program is being executed by the Caribbean Public Health Agency (CARPHA), the Caribbean's sole public health agency responsible for preventing disease, promoting and protecting health, in collaboration with the Caribbean Hotel and Tourism Association (CHTA), the Caribbean Tourism Organization (CTO) and countries. The program is improving countries' capacities to provide cost-effective, quality health, food safety and environmental sanitation (HSE) solutions to the HSE threats impacting on sustainable tourism in the Caribbean through real-time, early alert and response monitoring systems for tourism-based health issues; training and certification, HSE standards, and multi-sectoral regional and international partnerships. Countries gain enhanced capacity to mitigate against HSE threats to sustainable tourism. This integrated, multi-sectoral program is the first Caribbean-wide and global effort of its kind, setting an international precedent for improving sustainable tourism. The program is timely as new threats to health and travel in the region emerge.

The Caribbean depends on visitor arrivals more than any other region in the world, with over 55M visitors in 2019 (3). High and increasing numbers of visitors to the Caribbean region increase the health, safety, and security risks to local populations. Travel/tourism-related illnesses are not only a health and security risk but contribute to reputational damage and economic instability in Caribbean economies. This is evident through the introduction and spread of new and re-emerging diseases, such as SARs, H1NI, chikungunya, zika, norovirus, measles, and now, the novel coronavirus (COVID-19) pandemic, by visitor populations. The health of Caribbean economies is thus closely related to the health of its travel and tourism industry, given that the Caribbean is the most tourism-dependent region in the world.

However, even though more people visit the Caribbean than reside, current health monitoring surveillance systems are primarily based on the local population, and there is no ongoing visitor tourism-based surveillance and response system. There is also inadequate food and environmental sanitation training for the tourism sector, lack of cumulative HSE standards and certifying system, and a marked lack of integration between tourism and health stakeholders to address health in tourism in the Caribbean region. These gaps have all contributed to the spread of disease outbreaks, food safety, and environmental sanitation issues in the region; and without adequate information management systems, standards and training, these HSE threats can become a severe tourism crisis. These risks and the importance of the tourism industry in the Caribbean region highlight the need for a system to monitor both traveler's and resident's health, provide rapid dissemination of real-time information, and respond quickly to prevent and control outbreaks. It is within this context that CARPHA established a Regional Tourism and Health Program in 2014, with funding received from the International Development Bank in 2016 to execute.

The THP is strengthening countries' capacity to prepare for and respond to public health threats like COVID-19, which can transcend national boundaries and negatively affect access to goods and services, through the following regional public health goods which have the potential to strengthen regional health security:

1) Tourism and Health Information System
2) Regional Guidelines for a harmonized response to travel-related public health issues occurring among visitors to the Caribbean arriving by sea (passenger ships) and air (accommodations).
3) Advanced Food Safety, Environmental Sanitation capacity building, and certification.
4) Hospitality Health Safety and Environmental standards
5) Partnerships, Mandates, and Policy

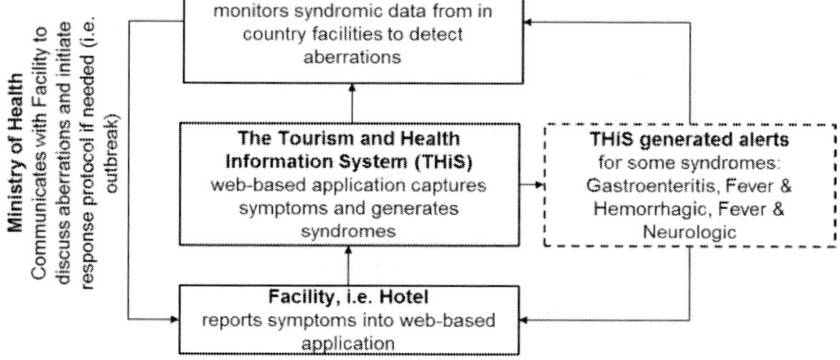

Figure 1. Primary surveillance pathway for the THiS web app.

Each of these components is discussed below and linked to possible COVID-19 preparedness and response actions.

Components

The Tourism and Health Information System (THiS) is a web-based application for syndromic surveillance of populations in tourist accommodations (website: http://www.this.carpha.org). This real-time, early warning system is confidential and only accessible by national authorities. It is currently being implemented in hotels and guest houses in eight countries (Bahamas, Barbados, Belize, Guyana, Jamaica, Trinidad and Tobago, Bermuda, Turks and Caicos Islands).

The THiS web app was designed to enhance national surveillance systems by monitoring illnesses in tourist accommodations to identify public health threats early. Figure 1 shows a schematic of how the THiS web app integrates into the existing national and regional public health surveillance mechanisms.

Data collection and reporting

Data collection in the THiS web app is conducted by staff from registered tourist accommodations, using an online questionnaire administered to an unwell guest or staff member. Accommodations are also required to confirm the absence of cases by epidemiological week using a "zero case" submission on the web app page. Also, the self-reporting page allows visitors and staff to independently report their illness using an online questionnaire located on the THiS web page: this.carpha.org.

The online questionnaires are similar for reporting by registered facilities and self-reporting. The questionnaire includes short questions that ask the user for necessary demographic information such as age and gender, potential exposure information such as recent travel and home country, and most importantly, which symptoms they are experiencing:

1) diarrhoea (≥ 3 loose or watery stools in past 24 hours)
2) vomiting and/or nausea
3) fever (sudden onset of fever >38.0°C or 100.4°C)
4) cough or sore throat
5) bleeding (gums, nose, blood pooling under skin coughing, stool) not due to physical trauma
6) headache
7) joint or muscle pains
8) eye pain/headache/facial pain,
9) generalized rash,
10) blurred vision or convulsions or altered consciousness

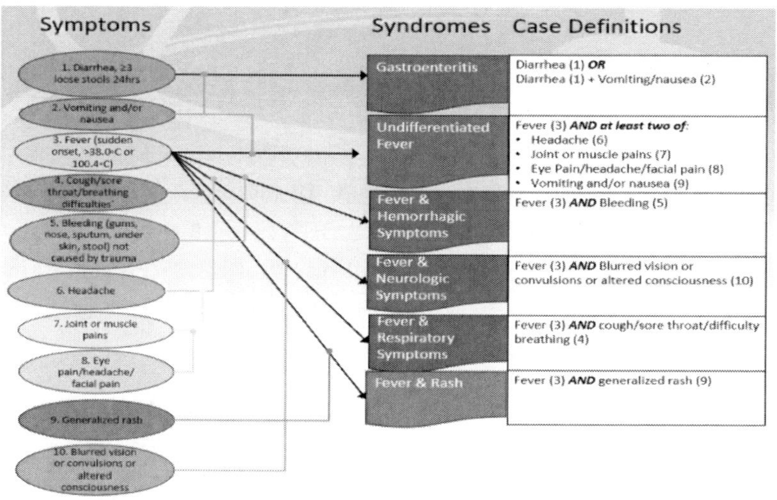

Figure 2. The logic used to generate syndromes from reported symptoms (based on Case Definitions for Syndromes under Regional Surveillance, CARPHA).

Responses to these symptoms are analyzed in the system to generate (see Figure 2) potential syndromes for each case:

1) Gastroenteritis
2) Undifferentiated fever
3) Fever and hemorrhagic symptoms
4) Fever and neurologic symptoms

5) Fever and respiratory symptoms
6) Fever and rash

Data analytics

Data analytics are executed on the inputs from each facility on the THiS web app. The dashboard provides interactive data visualizations and allows the user to slice the information to view cases among guests vs. staff, by facility (for national users only), by country (for regional users only), and for all users by gender, age, and time (weeks vs. months vs. year) facility and national level—for MOH users), and time (case counts by day, week, month, or year). Access is limited to hotel management (i.e., hotel manager, health and safety manager), who would be persons engaging with public health staff at the MOH in the event of a potential public health issue such as an outbreak. At the Ministry of Health, access is given to users determined by the countries health focal point and typically includes an epidemiologist, surveillance officer, and/or Chief Medical Officer (CMO) or Environmental Health Officer. At CARPHA, access is limited to the THP epidemiologist and Project Coordinator.

Regional guidelines

Two sets of regional surveillance guidelines were developed:

- Regional guidelines for managing issues of public health significance on passenger ships coming to the Caribbean (Caribbean Vessel Surveillance System (CVSS)), and
- Regional guidelines for managing issues of public health significance in stay-over arrivals (Tourist Accommodation-Based Surveillance) in the Caribbean

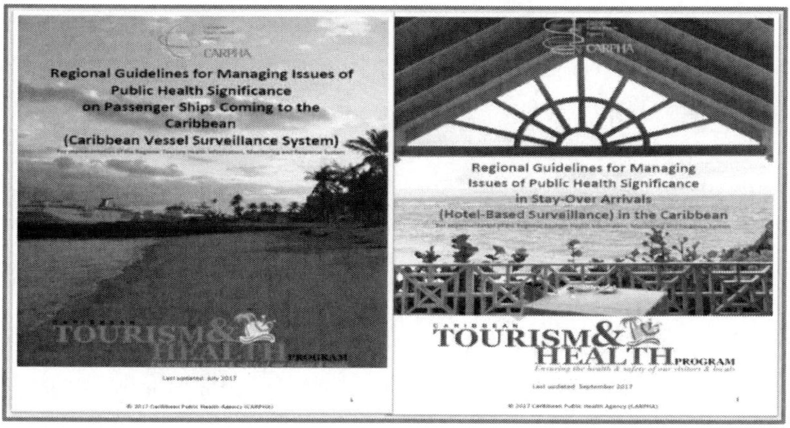

Figure 3. Regional Guidelines.

These guidelines, collectively called the "Regional guidelines" (see Figure 3), were developed to provide instructive guidelines for harmonized scientific response to travel-related public health issues occurring among persons aboard passenger ships and those in stay-over arrivals (tourist accommodations) in the Caribbean.

A key challenge in the tourism-dependent Caribbean countries is the marked variation and lack of standardization in the surveillance and response to travel-related public issues occurring among visitors arriving by sea and those in stay-over arrivals. Although the core competencies and protocols for investigating and reporting public health emergencies on passenger ships in the Caribbean are described in the 2005 International Health Regulations (IHR), how these are implemented vary by country, since each country is sovereign. The commonality of tourism-based illnesses, nearby borders, and frequent travel (both intra-regional and international) in the Caribbean necessitates the need for uniform and harmonized surveillance and response to travel-related public health events. This harmonized approach aims to avoid the introduction of new diseases, mitigate the spread of illnesses, and protect the health and security of visitors and locals.

CARPHA, as the Caribbean authority for public health surveillance, developed the Guidelines for harmonized surveillance and response to travel-related public health illnesses to prevent and mitigate public health events on passenger ships and in stay-over arrivals in the Caribbean region. It will support countries in carrying out public health action to manage issues of public health importance in a timely and coordinated fashion and thus protect the health and security of visitors and locals. It will also allow for the collection of surveillance data to establish baselines for outbreak detection and strengthen national surveillance

The Guidelines are based on the IHR (2005), the World Health Organization (WHO) management of public health events onboard ships (2016) and other documents developed over a 3-year period involving country and agency consultations; and in close collaboration with the Cruise Lines International Association (CLIA) and CDC Vessel Sanitation Program (VSP). It was presented to the 33rd COHSOD, endorsed at the 2018 CARICOM CMOs meeting, and supported at the 2018 Regional Tourism & Health Stakeholder workshop (13 agencies, 14 countries).

Advanced food safety and environmental sanitation training

Food safety affects the health, wealth, and reputation of countries. Diarrheal illness resulting from contaminated food or water (FBD) is the most common health problem faced by visitors to the Caribbean. In the last 15 years, the Caribbean has experienced an increase in the number of large and costly visitor-based outbreaks of illness, with negative impacts on the tourism industry. From 2010-2016, over 250 outbreaks of gastroenteritis (GE) from 23 countries were reported to the CARPHA, 15% occurring in hotels/resorts, and accounting for over 25,000 cases. One outbreak in 2012 resulted in over 800 ill persons, hotel closure, and a 20% decline in arrivals. Investigations of FBD outbreaks have repeatedly demonstrated that they were costly, yet preventable. The root causes of these illnesses were traced to inconsistent attention to existing food and environmental safety standards, inadequately trained staff, and a lack of an effective monitoring and reporting system. Reducing the incidence of FBD is, therefore, a continuing challenge to the Caribbean hospitality industry. The most effective tools for preventing foodborne and other illnesses are science-based food safety management, education, and training.

The THP provides advanced food safety and certification train the trainer course for health and hospitality stakeholders This training is done by certified regional experts, using the globally recognized SERVSAFE food safety material uniquely infused with the Caribbean experience based on CARPHA's illnesses investigations of public health threats. SERV Safe is the internationally recommended comprehensive capacity-building proficiency course, using practical science-based knowledge and skills. It builds countries' capacities in the areas of advanced food safety, illness causation and prevention, outbreak response, and environmental sanitation (see Figure 4). It will also allow for globally recognized certification through the internationally recognized USA National Restaurant Association Educational Foundation (SERV Safe).

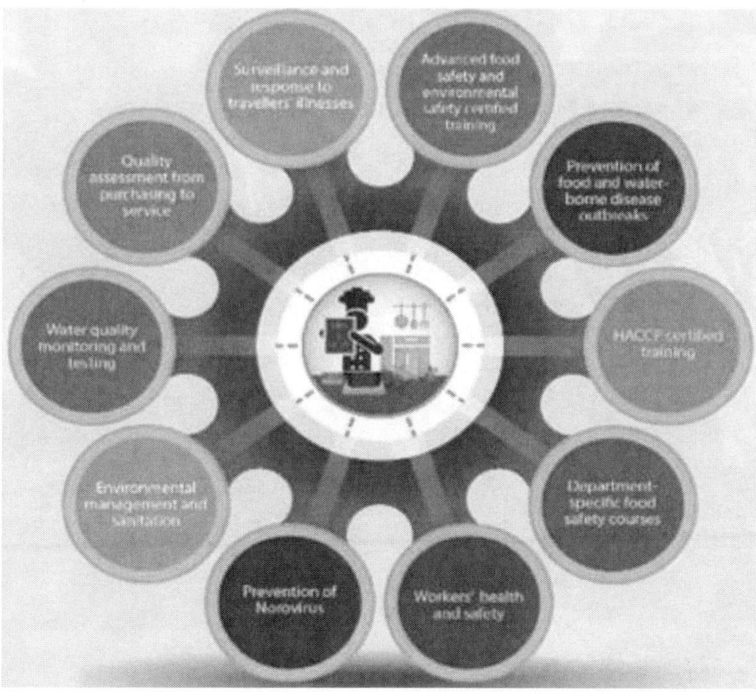

Figure 4. Topics covered in Advanced Food Safety and Environmental Sanitation Training.

Hospitality health safety and environmental (HSE) standards

Seven Caribbean-wide health safety and environmental (HSE) "clean and green" hospitality standards have been developed to improve health, safety, and environmental quality in the hospitality sector. These standards were developed under the authority of the CARICOM Regional Organization for Standards and Quality (CROSQ) through CARPHA THP. These are now being submitted for approval as the CARICOM Regional Hospitality Standards to the CARICOM Council for Trade and Economic Development (COTED):

1) Energy management and efficiency
2) Food safety and sanitation for the tourism industry
3) Environmental management systems for the tourism industry – Guidelines
4) Integrated pest management for the tourism industry
5) Sewage treatment and management for the tourism industry
6) Solid waste management for the tourism industry
7) Water treatment, management and efficiency for the tourism industry

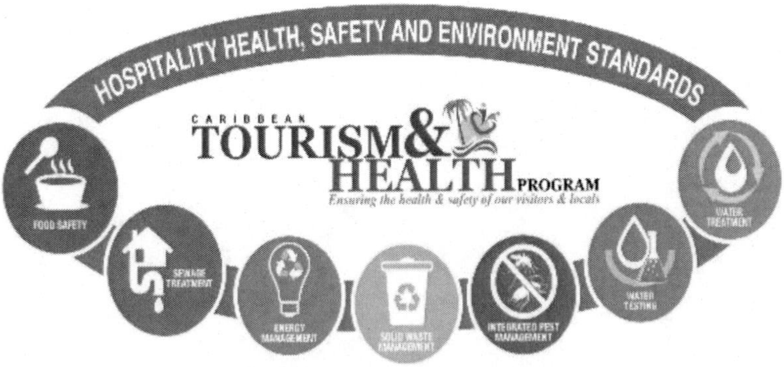

Figure 5. Hospitality health safety and environmental (HSE) standards.

The adoption and implementation of these standards by the Caribbean tourism industry will significantly reduce the adverse impact of HSE issues, which in turn would increase the contribution of the sector to the economic well-being of the region. Implementing these standards will be the comparative advantage, as it would protect the region's fragile environment and lead to a safer and better-quality environmental product, and a standards-based certified destination, which increases the comparative advantage of Caribbean tourism. Substantial benefits are possible if these standards are adopted and referenced in legislation/regulation that can be made sufficiently similar across the Caribbean Region. One such benefit is a substantial improvement in health food safety and environmental sanitary conditions in the hospitality sector throughout the region. The implementation of the standards would be recognized by the Association of British Travellers (ABTA) and other tour operators. Certified facilities would also be published on CTO, CHTA, CARPHA websites.

Partnerships, mandates, and policy

The THP developed a Regional THP Policy Framework to mandate the reporting of tourism/visitor illnesses to national authorities from the hospitality sector for the successful implementation and sustainability of the THP. The regional THP Policy Framework aims at ensuring an enabling environment for optimal implementation of the THP and its components. The Regional THP Policy Framework is a critical tool in the drive to secure the Caribbean Region's health security. Implementation of the Policy provides a basis for creating a sense of urgency among hospitality sector partners and travelers to reduce the risk posed to people in the Caribbean by communicable disease outbreaks and public health emergencies, through early detection and a strengthened rapid response.

- In 2017, the 33rd CARICOM Council of Health Ministers (COHSOD) mandated CARPHA through the THP to prepare a draft tourism/traveler's health policy for improving regional health security.

- During 2018-2019, through a consultative process, the Travellers Health Policy Framework was developed
- On September 29, 2019, the Regional Travellers Health Policy Framework was approved at the 37th COHSOD

Partnership

The THP involves the implementation of a new non-traditional health information and monitoring system (i.e., tourism/visitor-based illnesses), new clients/data users (private sector hotels, cruise ships, visitors), and new partners (Ministry of Tourism, tourism authorities, tourism agencies). In this regard, a critical factor for successful implementation and sustainability of the program is global and regional recognition, partnership development, and endorsement from international public and private health and tourism agencies. The THP, starting with an MOU between CTO and CHTA, is building multi-sectoral, multi-agency partnerships with regional and international health and tourism stakeholders to address travel-related public health threats in a rapid and well-coordinated manner for seamless information flow and response to traveler's illness across regional and international borders Other key partners to date include CROSQ, VSP, Public Health Agency Canada (PHAC), and Public Health England (PHE) and Cruise Lines International Association (CLIA), Association of British Traveler (ABTA).

Discussion

Surveillance is critical for protecting and improving improve population health. In particular, during a pandemic such as COVID-19, public health officials must be able to rely on a system that produces real-time and accurate data on the outbreak, collected and monitored over time, directly from the communities, so that they can rapidly identify and implement the most effective interventions. In a region such as the Caribbean, consisting of small islands developing countries and territories, where tourists/travelers outnumber residents, there is a crucial need for a surveillance system that goes beyond national public health surveillance platforms. The Tourism and Health Information System (THiS) web app meets this requirement by monitoring illnesses among visitors and staff in tourist accommodations, in real-time. From January 2017-February 2020, the THiS was successfully implemented in 254 hospitality accommodations in eight countries (Bahamas, Barbados, Belize, Guyana, Jamaica, Trinidad, Tobago, Turks and Caicos Islands). Before its establishment, no system was in place to compile disease data on this population. The systems can detect aberrations in patterns of illness among travelers, which is even more important if they originate from multiple nations or regions. The strength of the platform is also that the visitors themselves are considered as part of the surveillance system. Being able to collect these data in the context of the COVID-19 pandemic cannot be overstated. It allows reporting of more comprehensive and timely data about the outbreak to public health officials.

Pre COVID-19, the THiS has been instrumental in identifying important clusters of illness that that would not have been reported through current national systems, resulting in a rapid action to prevent further spread. This innovative travel/tourism syndromic surveillance crucial during this COVID-19 pandemic for strengthening existing core national health surveillance systems of tourism-dependent Caribbean economies to collect real-time data for early alerts and triggering a rapid coordinated response. CARPHA is promoting the reporting of illnesses, including suspected cases of coronavirus, on THiS both by hospitality accommodation sand self-reporting, as a proactive COVID-19 surveillance measure. This pandemic is a reminder that our first line of defense starts with people. We must consistently protect ourselves so that we are more prepared.

Advanced food safety training

There is no evidence that food or food packaging is directly involved in the transmission of COVID-19 (4). Unlike foodborne gastrointestinal viruses that can make people ill through contaminated food, SARS-CoV-2, which causes COVID-19, is a virus that causes respiratory illness. The main transmission occurs from person-to-person, either between people who are in close contact with one another or through respiratory droplets produced when an infected person coughs or sneezes (5). However, a person can also contract COVID-19 by directly touching surfaces that have "cough or sneeze" droplets from an infected person, and then touching their mouth, nose, or eyes. For that reason, it is more critical for food handlers to follow the four key steps of food safety: clean, separate, cook, and chill (4). The advanced food safety and environmental sanitation training contributes to COVID-19 prevention by building capacity and reinforcing behaviors that help avoid coming in contact with the virus (and pathogens in general): frequent washing and sanitizing of all food contact surfaces and utensils, frequent hand washing and glove changes before and after preparing food, frequent cleaning and sanitizing counters and condiment containers. To date, almost 600 health and hospitality workers were trained in the eight implementing countries, providing a solid platform of knowledge and training for proper hand hygiene, cleaning and sanitizing, and other behaviors to prevent COVID-19. Implementing and or reinforcing the food safety and environmental sanitation programs is essential to maintaining a hygienic and safe environment, keeping the risk of infectious diseases and COVID19 outbreak low and customers and staff healthy.

Hospitality health safety and environmental (HSE) standards

According to WHO, "the provision of safe water, sanitation, and hygienic conditions are essential to protecting human health during all infectious disease outbreaks" (6). Although the risk of contracting COVID-19 from the feces of a person is low and there is no evidence about the survival of the virus in water or sewage, implementation of the Caribbean-wide Health, Safety and Environmental "clean and green" Standards will further contribute to preventing transmission of communicable diseases, including the COVID-19 pandemic. In particular, the HSE standards encompass different components that are relevant to mitigate the spread of the virus: within the Food Safety and Sanitation component, frequent and proper hand hygiene is one of the key measures to prevent contamination and transmission and disinfection will facilitate more rapid die-off of the virus. These HSE standards constitute a critical component of a set of preventive interventions to enhance not only the region's capacity to respond to the public health threats, but also to support the region's drive towards achieving quality and sustainability and to remain competitive in this rapidly growing global tourism trade.

Response to COVID-19 through THP

Regional guidelines

The COVID-19 pandemic is causing worldwide disruption and challenge for response in countries. Responding to this pandemic and other emerging and re-emerging infectious diseases in the tourism-dependent, small island developing states like the Caribbean region requires a strong, harmonized coordinated regional approach, given the proximity and interconnection between the islands, their limited and varying capacity to quarantine to respond (test, isolate, treat, and contact tracing). CARPHA is leading the regional health response to COVID-19, in keeping with its Intergovernmental Agreement (IGA) mandate from CARICOM and recommendations from COHSOD- Health working group on regional coordination for management. As such, CARPHA convened the Regional Coordinating mechanism for Health Security (RCM-HS), consisting of Member States, regional and international agencies, to work with its partners and countries, towards a harmonized regional response.

Tourism and health information system (THiS)

The web-based application, THiS, allows monitoring and provision of alerts in real-time on the health of guests and staff members. In particular, when indicating the symptoms the tourist(s) or staff member(s) are experiencing, fever, cough/sore throat/difficulty breathing, diarrhea (6-8) – known symptoms of COVID-19 – can be captured as well as information on recent travel history. Those symptoms can trigger an immediate response following the Regional Guidelines for Managing Issues of Public Health Significance in Stay-Over Arrivals in the Caribbean. Time is of the essence in the fight against the virus. Being able to detect and respond immediately to potential new COVID-19 outbreaks but also assess the impact of the measures taken on the trends of illness reported, can buy the world precious time to contain the spread.

Multisectoral partnerships

Public health emergency preparedness and response aim to minimize the risks posed by communicable diseases and mitigate their impacts. Sharing and aligning activities in public health emergency preparedness adds value to efforts of single countries to strengthen their capacities and ensure coordinated, effective support with cross-border health threats. Responsibility for the preparedness and the response lies not only with public health agencies but involves every level of government, the private sector, non-governmental organizations, and individuals. In particular, tourism is currently one of the most affected sectors by the COVID-19 crisis as it is based on interaction amongst people. Guiding the tourism sector's response requires strong public-private intersectoral partnerships at national and regional levels between tourism, health, and environment stakeholders. This is the only way to support a rapid and well-coordinated approach to managing the pandemic – and this is what the Tourism and Health Program has executed since its inception. In response to the crisis, regular webinars were convened with CHTA, CTO members, and regional Ministers of

Tourism to provide technical guidance to the hospitality sector for mitigating the spread of the virus throughout the region.

COVID-19 Situation reports, travel brief, and travel advisory providing a consolidated view of the health situation in the Caribbean are communicated every two days to countries, regional agencies (CARICOM, CDEMA, IMPACs) international development partners (World Bank, IDB, EU, ECDC, CARICOM, CHTA, and others). Guidelines for travelers, hotels and guesthouses, food and beverage industry, conveyances, front line workers, Ports of Entry in the region have also been developed with support from the THP and disseminated to promote a coordinated response. CARPHA THP, CHTA, CTO, and Global Tourism Resilience and Crisis Management Centre (GTRCMC) also established the COVID-19 Caribbean Tourism Task Force to formalize their efforts and harmonized the regional messaging.

CONCLUSION

In conclusion, the ongoing COVID-19 pandemic is causing worldwide disruption. It demonstrates that for new and emerging public threats, it is critical to capture and monitor the variables that drive illness occurrence in real-time, for informing strategies to tackle emerging and re-emerging infectious diseases. This requires a well-coordinated multi-sectoral response. In particular, the dependence of the Caribbean islands on tourism, the high volume of people traveling to the islands, and the speed of international travel, heightens the public health challenges for the region. The novel regional Tourism and Health Program, through its multi-prong components and multi-sectoral partnerships, is supporting the regional fight against COVID-19. Efforts are already being made to expand this transdisciplinary approach to more countries regionally.

ACKNOWLEDGMENT

The authors would like to acknowledge the IDB for funding the implementation of the THP.

REFERENCES

[1] United Nations. About the Sustainable Development Goals 2020. URL: https://www.un.org/sustainabledevelopment/sustainable-development-goals/.

[2] World Travel and Tourism Council. Tourism is a principal source of employment, foreign currency and economic growth in the Caribbean. (WTTC), 2013. URL: http://www.wttc.org/site_media/uploads/downloads/caribbean2014.pdf.

[3] Caribbean Tourism Organization (CTO) Annual statistical report 2019 URL: https://www.onecaribbean.org/buy-cto-tourism-statistics/annual-statistical-report/.

[4] US Food and Drug Administration. Food Safety and the Coronavirus disease 2019 (COVID-19). 2020. URL: https://www.fda.gov/food/food-safety-during-emergencies/food-safety-and-coronavirus-disease-2019-covid-19.

[5] Centers for Disease Control and Prevention. Coronavirus disease 2019. How it spreads. 2020. URL: https://www.cdc.gov/coronavirus/2019-ncov/prepare/transmission.html.

[6] World Health Organization. Water, sanitation, hygiene and waste management for the COVID-19 virus 2020. URL: https://www.who.int/publications-detail/water-sanitation-hygiene-and-waste-management-for-covid-19.

[7] Centers for Disease Control and Prevention. Coronavirus disease 2019. Symptoms and testing. 2020. URL: https://www.cdc.gov/coronavirus/2019-ncov/symptoms-testing/symptoms.html.

[8] Song Y, Liu P, Shi XL, Chu YL, Zhang J, Xia J, et al. SARS-CoV-2 induced diarrhoea as onset symptom in patient with COVID-19. Gut 2020 Mar 05. doi: 10.1136/gutjnl-2020-320891.

In: Public Health Themes in Grenada … ISBN: 978-1-53618-118-0
Editors: J. Merrick and L. Glasgow © 2020 Nova Science Publishers, Inc.

Chapter 3

WHITE PAPER ON VAPING: ELECTRONIC CIGARETTES USE – A CASE FOR RESTRICTIVE POLICIES IN GRENADA, WEST INDIES

Christine Richards, MPH, PhD, Lindonne Glasgow, MSPH, DrPH, Satesh Bidaisee, DVM, MSPH, EdD, Prakash Ramdass, MD, MPH, Tolulope Oladimeji, MD, MPH, Marios Loukas, MD, PhD and Emmanuel Keku*, MD, MA, MSPH

School of Medicine, Department of Public Health and Preventive Medicine, St George's University, Grenada, West Indies

* Correspondence: Emmanuel Keku, , Professor, School of Medicine, Department of Public Health and Preventive Medicine, St George's University, St George, Grenada, West Indies. Email: ekeku@sgu.edu.

Abstract

The use of electronic cigarettes (e-cigarettes) or the practice of vaping has emerged as a global public health concern. If this practice remains unchecked, all the gains due to public health efforts to reduce smoking of combustible cigarettes and thus reduce morbidity and mortality from tobacco-related deaths will be reversed. While e-cigarettes were initially introduced as a smoking cessation strategy, sufficient evidence for this has not been forthcoming. In fact, the use of e-cigarettes has produced more negative health outcomes than positive ones, as evidenced in the recent morbidity and mortality related EVALI. While this is more evident in developed countries, governments of low- and middle-income countries such as Grenada, need to protect youth and young adults from initiating and/or continuing use of these potentially harmful products. Many countries, as well as states in the United States, have implemented some level of restrictive policies on the use of e-cigarettes based on the available evidence of harm caused by these products. It is proposed that the same interventions that have worked for smoking of combustible cigarettes reduction should be applied to e-cigarettes.

Introduction

Within the decade, the practice of vaping, including the use of electronic cigarettes (e-cigarettes), has increased globally. Due to its significantly reduced cost per month when compared with regular cigarette smoking, e-cigarettes usage has become increasingly prevalent in high-income countries than in low- and middle-income countries. Vaping or e-cigarettes has been marketed as a strategy for smoking cessation tool. The advertisement strategy claimed that the tapering of nicotine delivery devices is more effective for quitting regular cigarette smoking without concerns about the adverse effects of combustible by-products. Studies have documented and demonstrated nicotine addictiveness through regular cigarette smoking among adults and teenagers.

The evidence of adverse effects of e-cigarettes on health is not clear. In the latter part of 2019, a brand of e-cigarette was linked to lung injuries and deaths among young people as a result of inhaling vitamin E acetate. However, for public health and preventive medicine experts, the concern is evident. Nicotine is highly addictive, and the increased use of nicotine-containing e-cigarettes among teenagers, youths, and adults will lead to greater nicotine dependence. Few studies have reported that vaping solutions and their emissions could contain more than nicotine but also aerosolized products (propylene glycol) and other contaminants which could lead to potential health hazards to e-cigarette users and non-users (passive users). Though using e-cigarette may decrease exposure to the risks associated with conventional cigarette use, the health effects of nicotine and aerosol exposures from e-cigarettes are not at present fully understood. Vaping aerosols and products are dangerous for passive users or non-users in environments with reduced ventilation or to those with disease comorbidities and compromised health conditions. A recently published manuscript (December 2019) in the American Journal of Preventive Medicine reported the first longitudinal analysis of the association between vaping and lung disease.

The research investigators followed e-cigarette users for three years and found that they had a 1.3-times higher risk of developing respiratory disease than people who did not use any tobacco product. Cigarette smokers had a 2.5-times higher risk, and those who both smoked regular cigarettes and vaped had a 3.3-times higher risk of developing respiratory disease (1). Though the data from this study showed that using e-cigarettes appeared to show the minimal risk of developing respiratory disease, the three years follow-up is not a long time to follow vapers. It's also likely that many people who entered the study as smokers had likely started that habit much earlier, hence allowing risks to accumulate. In terms of the biological effects of e-cigarettes, it's likely that following e-cigarette users for 10 to 20 years will produce similar effects of risks associated with regular cigarettes smoking or worse. In light of this new publication that established an independent risk factor for respiratory disease among e-cigarettes users and dual users (e-cigarettes and regular cigarettes smoking), the latter being the most popular, we are proposing a more aggressive ban of e-cigarettes in Grenada. Further studies are needed to fully establish the adverse effects of e-cigarettes on developing respiratory diseases. Nonetheless, until these studies are available, and since the health hazards and safety of vaping to users, non-users, and passive users are not completely understood, it is important to ban vaping or e-cigarettes use in Grenada. Grenada is a middle-income country and has no policy on e-cigarettes or vaping usage. The St. George's University is also located in Grenada. Most of the enrolled students are from the United States of America, and the probability of possessing vaping products and the use of e-cigarettes is high among these students. Policies are needed to be developed for the students at St George's University, and other institutions in Grenada. Presently, very few Caribbean countries such as Barbados, Jamaica, and Trinidad have policies that address e-cigarette or vaping. Specifically, in Jamaica, "Nicotine-containing e-cigarettes are classified as medicinal products under the Food and Drugs Act. As such, they must be registered before they can be imported (no approval has been granted for these products to date). The Food and Drugs Act prohibits the sale, distribution, importation, or manufacture of a drug that is not registered with the Ministry of Health. A tobacco control regulation prohibits the use of electronic nicotine delivery systems (ENDS) in public places and on public transportation." In Barbados, the Parliament in Barbados passed legislation on February 2, 2017 to ban smoking and vaping in public areas and to prohibit sales of vaping products to minors. On that date, the Minister of Health, Hon. John Boyce, concluded that the dangers that are associated with e-cigarettes are the same as the with combustible cigarettes. "The Health Service Amendment Bill 2017, which classifies e-cigarettes as electronic smoking devices, extends the prohibition on smoking to e-cigarettes."

In Trinidad and Tobago, "According to Chapter 30:04 #18 (Prohibition on toys or candy cigarettes) (1) No person shall (a) import or manufacture; or (b) sell, display for sale, distribute or supply, any sweets, snacks, toys or other non-tobacco items or objects in the form of tobacco products, or which imitate tobacco products. This act is to regulate tobacco products. Electronic Vaporizers or Electronic Cigarettes that do not contain tobacco or produces smoke." The Chapter 30:04 # 18 to e-cigarettes was designed to stop the importation of toy and candy that resembles traditional cigarettes. This act has resulted in debates and possibly not enforced. Countries that have banned e-cigarettes use include Argentina, Brazil, Brunei, Cambodia,

Indonesia, Jordan, Oman, Qatar, Singapore, Taiwan, Thailand, United Arab Emirates, Uruguay, and Venezuela (2). The experts at St. George's University, School of Medicine, Grenada, West Indies have concerns with the usage of e-cigarettes or vaping and recommends the following proposed solutions for consideration in order to protect the public from the health hazards that are associated with e-cigarettes or vaping in Grenada.

Develop and add an amendment to legislation to ban importation, sale, and practice of vaping associated products in Grenada

E-cigarette devices and the practice of vaping are relatively new to Grenada and, as such, are not considered under existing legislation to enforce regulation of its use. Vaping products are currently marketed as consumer goods, however, with reference to existing laws; it is an offense to sell nicotine vaping products to young people under age 18. The recommended amendment should include vape devices and e-liquids. The Drug Abuse (Prevention and Control) Act was not designed for vaping and does not include safety standards on what can be sold. Moreover, flavoring used in vaping products are regulated under respective Food Standards and are not a part of the drug regulatory provisions. Options for consideration are:

1) In the absence of any specific legal framework for regulating vaping and its products, the government should draft and legislate vaping-specific laws and regulations as an amendment to existing legislation.
2) Primary and secondary schools, higher-educational institutions, and individual businesses can make their own policies and rules around vaping that include penalties such as fines for first and second violations and dismissal with persistent or chronic violations.

Establish health education and promotion against vaping as a practice and substances used for vaping

Health education and promotion efforts against vaping are a component towards prevention and control, which will complement a legislative agenda to include vaping within existing laws. Education and promotion campaign should focus on e-cigarettes/vapes and combustible cigarettes. Awareness campaigns should be designed to reach youth directly through a variety of channels:

a) Online and social media advertisements on platforms popular with youth (e.g., Snapchat, Spotify, Instagram).
b) Web page and Instagram account where youth can seek more information and resources.
c) Through organizations such as schools and community-based organizations with posters, fact clings, and a handout.

Establish policy and legal interventions against vaping at primary and secondary schools, higher educational institutions, and individual businesses in Grenada. Review and strengthen current school health policy, which relates to tobacco and cigarette smoking to include vaping. Themes to include are

a) Educate: E-cigarettes and other vaping products are often not easily recognizable. Educating staff about these products and about the school's policy to address them is an important part of a strategy to reduce student use.
b) Know more about vaping use: Collecting data on types of vaping products students are using and where they obtain vaping products can help inform education efforts and decisions about school health policies. Sample surveillance questions about vaping use, as well as

questions about how students obtain vaping products, perceptions of harm, locations of use, are included.

c) Share resources for quitting vaping: While the use of vaping on school grounds is not regulated, that doesn't mean they are not current vaping users. It is important to support persons who use vaping products by providing them resources to address their own nicotine addiction.
d) Know more about resources in your community: Work with student groups to provide support, education, and connections to resources to address issues of vaping use in their community.

ELECTRONIC CIGARETTES

The use of electronic cigarettes (e-cigarettes), also known as electronic nicotine delivery systems (ENDS) or the practice of vaping has emerged as a global public health concern. While this is more evident in developed countries, governments of low- and middle-income countries such as Grenada, need to protect youth and young adults from initiating and/or continuing use of these potentially harmful products. The US Surgeon General landmark report of 1964 linked smoking cigarettes to the development of lung cancer and heart disease. Following this report, a number of interventions, targeting the advertising, sale, and use of cigarettes, were successfully implemented and proven to be effective in reducing smoking rates (3). However, the use of e-cigarettes, which was introduced as a potential cessation device and an alternative cigarette product, is threatening to reverse the successes of these interventions. To prevent this from occurring, governments need to take preventive measures. The most effective strategies involve examining best practices and evidence-based solutions that can be tailored to the local context and implemented. In this paper, we present evidence to make a case for the prohibition of some sort and/or restrictive policies in Grenada.

THE E-CIGARETTE DEVICE: BASIC STRUCTURE

Vaping is the practice of inhaling heated and aerosolized constituents of e-cigarettes liquids. The design of e-cigarette devices has changed over time. The change in size, shape, and style has evolved into an efficient nicotine delivery machinery capable of delivering greater concentration and volume of nicotine than older versions. The documented versions of these nicotine delivery devices are delineated into four generations (4).

Common to these designs through all the generations is a battery, liquid that can be turned into vapor, an electrical heating system, and a tank (which serves as a reservoir for the liquid). These innovations are generally classified into two categories; open and closed. The open system is designed such that the components can be replaced; also, it has a system that serves as liquid storage (tank). The closed type has a less flexible design, devoid of the tank, and doesn't offer the option for part replacement. A classical representation of these designs is illustrated in Figure 1 below, showing the various essential components of an e-cigarette (5).

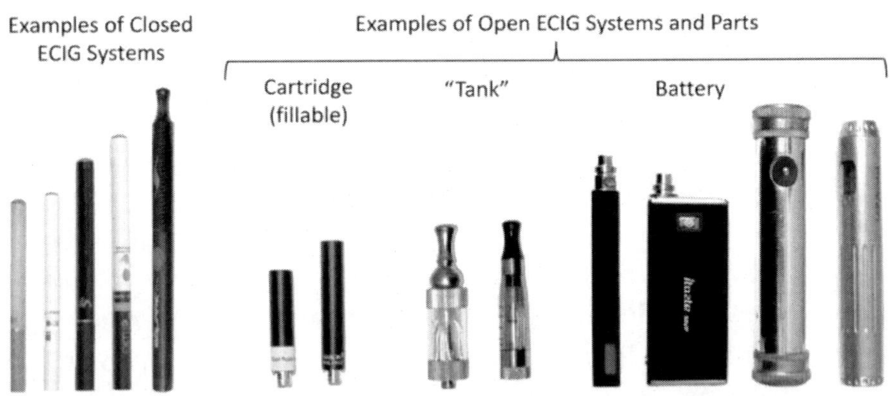

Figure 1. Basic components of closed and open e-cigarettes, adapted from, Electronic cigarettes: what are they and what do they do? (5).

THE E-CIGARETTE DEVICE: HOW IT WORKS

E-cigarette devices comprise of a battery, a reservoir for holding a solution that usually contains nicotine, a heating element or a vaporizer, and a mouthpiece through which the user puffs. The user puffs on it but does not light it, and it does not produce smoke. The solution, which typically uses glycol or glycerine as a solvent for the nicotine and flavoring chemicals, is heated into an aerosol that is inhaled by the user (6). The solution can also contain other harmful products such as volatile organic compounds (VOCs), nicotine, carcinogens, heavy metals, flavorings such as diacetyl; a chemical linked to a serious lung disease, and ultrafine particles that can be inhaled deeply into the lungs. Nicotine is highly addictive, toxic to the developing fetus, and harms brain development of adolescents. Peripartum, fetal, and developmental adverse effects of nicotine are well documented (7, 8).

The increased use of e-cigarette by female adolescents and women of childbearing age also raises concerns about the effects of e-cigarette during pregnancy and the safety of the fetus. Pregnant traditional smokers are making a switch to vaping because of the perceived lower risk noncombustible cigarette offers (9). Bystanders can also breathe in this aerosol when the user exhales into the air, causing irritation of the upper airways and eyes and effects from nicotine, including palpitations and an increase of the systolic blood pressure (10). As e-cigarettes have increased in popularity, their designs, due to a lack of standardization, have also become more diverse (11). They come in many different shapes and sizes, resembling regular cigarettes, cigars, or pipes, pens, USB sticks, and other everyday items. The larger devices such as tank systems, or "mods," do not resemble other tobacco products (4). The implications of these new delivery devices are that the level of nicotine and other chemicals inhaled by the user varies, thereby increasing the potential risk to the user. Moreover, there is the potential for e-cigarette devices to be used as illicit drug use delivery systems. Evidence shows e-cigarettes have been used to vape substances such as cannabis, methylenedioxy-methamphetamines, synthetic cannabinoids, methamphetamines, cocaine, heroin, and fentanyl (12). The first device of what is currently used today was developed by Lik Hon, a

Chinese pharmacist (13), and the original design has since evolved into the variety of e-cigarette devices that currently exist. This novelty was introduced into the Chinese market in 2004 and used as a potential cessation device or an alternative cigarette product (14). The product was later introduced into the US market in the mid-2000s and quickly expanded into a variety of brands and flavors. The practice of vaping was promoted to assist smokers in quitting as it aimed to reduce and/or eliminate smoking withdrawal symptoms and cravings (15). However, few robust studies have found e-cigarette use to be more effective than other traditional strategies. A recent Randomized Control Trial, which examined the effectiveness of e-cigarettes versus nicotine replacement therapy as a smoking cessation strategy, found e-cigarettes to be more effective when accompanied by behavioral support (16). On the other hand, evidence in support of the effectiveness of this intervention is inconclusive, as noted in several systematic reviews (17). What has been found is that e-cigarettes reduce harm, in that exposure to poisonous and carcinogenic substances present in combustible cigarettes are reduced, thereby reducing adverse health outcomes. Nevertheless, while intended to be less harmful, the use of e-cigarettes has produced numerous biological effects resulting in injury and death. More rigorous studies are therefore needed to determine the effectiveness of e-cigarettes on harm reduction and quitting behavior. Furthermore, a study that compared the effect of co-use of traditional cigarettes with e-cigarette observed a quadruple increase in cigarette smoking compared to individuals who only smoked traditional cigarettes (18). This result alludes to the body of academic evidence that questions the beneficial effect of vaping as an alternative to traditional smoking.

The recent trend in increasing prevalence, globally, is a cause for concern because there are reasons to believe that the public health gain from a decline in smoking tobacco could be reversed with the alarming rate of use of e-cigarette. In 2019, the prevalence of self-reported current e-cigarette use was high among US high school and middle school students, at 27.5% and 10.5%, respectively (19). During 2017–2018, current e-cigarette use increased by 78% among high school students (from 11.7% to 20.8%), in 2011, it was 1.5%. Among middle school students, current e-cigarette use increased from 0.6% in 2011 (60,000 students) to 4.9% (570,000 students) in 2018 (20). This increase in prevalence is also observed globally. In Canada, it was observed that 15.4% (4.6 million) reported the use of an e-cigarette. In 2017, 14.6 million Canadians who are 15 years and older had tried an e-cigarette, which translated to an appreciable increase from about 13% (3.9 million) in 2015 (21). Among Korean youth use of e-cigarettes increased from 0.5% in 2008 to 9.4% in 2011 (22); while in England among youth, the use of e-cigarette increased from 22% in 2014 to 25% in 2016 (23). In Trinidad, in a study among young adults 18-40, the prevalence was 24.6%, and of that, 16.9% had never smoked tobacco (24). These trends are worrisome, and use has recently been linked to deaths in the US. According to the US Centres for Disease Control and Prevention (CDC), as of November 20, 2019, 2,290 cases of electronic cigarettes, or vaping, product use-associated lung injury (EVALI) has been reported, including 47 deaths. Vitamin E acetate, an additive in some tetrahydrocannabinol (THC) containing products, was found in all analyzed bronchoalveolar lavage (BAL) fluid samples of patients. THC is the psychoactive mind-altering compound of marijuana that produces the "high." However, it is unclear whether other chemicals are also causing the lung injury and, for this reason, the CDC has advised persons to refrain from the use of all e-cigarettes or vaping products (25, 26). Among youth and young adults, the use of e-cigarettes has also been shown to increase the likelihood of smoking combustible-cigarettes (27). Some researchers believe that the unabated acceptance of vaping further perpetuates smoking habit and could serve as a portal for some tobacco naïve adolescents.

Furthermore, while the association of e-cigarette use and long-term health effects are unclear, evidence shows that e-cigarette use increases heart rate, increases cough and wheeze in adolescents, can induce acute endothelial dysfunction and oxidative stress of tissues. Potential pathological effects of vaping also include the development of pulmonary diseases such as COPD, cardiovascular diseases, neurodegenerative disorders such as Alzheimer's disease and cancer (28, 29). More importantly, use of e-cigarettes can increase the number of youth and young adults who are exposed to nicotine, increase the likelihood that former smokers will again become addicted to nicotine, encourage non-smokers to start smoking conventional cigarettes and other burned tobacco products and sustain nicotine addiction instead of quitting completely (30, 31).

While there is no data on e-cigarette use among youth and young adults in Grenada, a survey conducted among secondary school students in 2013 showed that the prevalence of lifetime use of combustible cigarettes is high, although it decreased from 37% in 2005 and 2007 to 27% in 2013. Overall, there was also a decrease in the prevalence of past-year use and current use of combustible cigarettes (32). With access to e-cigarettes, these statistics can quickly be reversed.

DETERMINANTS/CONTRIBUTING FACTORS AND CHALLENGES

The use of e-cigarettes has been viewed by many users as a safe alternative to the use of combustible cigarettes. With a few brands being advertised as nicotine-free, consumers may regard e-cigarette use as a safe practice and one that may even contribute to lower nicotine craving. E-cigarettes are popularly used in many countries, including the US, UK, and Canada. The majority of e-cigarettes, however, contain nicotine (33) and, without making a deliberate choice to select non-nicotine products, the substance and its by-products are consumed by users, unawares. To date, the USFDA has not issued any advisory endorsing e-cigarettes as a quit aid.

Consumers may also fail to understand other risks associated with the use of e-cigarettes. In addition to nicotine, e-cigarettes also contain carcinogenic metals, such as cadmium, chromium, lead, manganese, and nickel that are added to e-liquids (34). Although considered safer than combustible cigarettes (35), within the last five years, the evidence has also been mounting from research and epidemiological surveillance on the health effects of solvents, flavorants, and toxicants used in e-liquids. Compared to combustible cigarette, e-cigarette affords a more discrete use, and there is less disapproval of its use by the wider public. Although the electronic nicotine delivery systems (ENDS) are perceived and marketed as a safer alternative to traditional tobacco smoking; the anti-tobacco campaigns have largely succeeded in creating awareness about the dangers of second-hand smoke for bystanders from the use of combustible cigarettes. A similar second-hand smoke effect occurs among bystanders in close proximity to e-cigarette users. Increased levels of nicotine, tobacco-specific nitrosamines (TSNAs), propylene glycol, and copper were found in the exhaled breath of bystanders in a study, mediated by ventilation, size of the room, and behavior of the user (36). When heated, the volatile particulates in e-cigarettes are quickly dispersed in the air, exposing non-uses to the toxic chemicals.

Age

The teenage years are important for brain development, which continues into adulthood. At that stage, young people are also most susceptible to addictions and organ damage from drug use (37). This stage of development is usually characterized by risky behaviors that provide a sense of maturity and social acceptance for youth. Little regard is given for the implications of exposure to hazardous substances, such as drugs and alcohol, on future physical and mental health. E-cigarettes are popularly used by young people in the United States; a trend that signifies the potential for steady increase in the number of new users (38). Between 2014-2018, e-cigarette use increased 160% among youth in the US (39). The United States Surgeon General has continually warned of the use of tobacco products and other drugs during youth and young adulthood, which leads to habitual use in adulthood (40). The copycat mentality perceived among young people in Caribbean countries towards the trends in the United States, in particular, favors an introduction and increase in the use of e-cigarettes in Grenada.

Apart from peer pressure, availability of the devices, alluring advertisements, attractive flavors, and the perception of a safe alternative appeal to young people. E-cigarette marketing projects vaping as glamourous and enchanting; this advertising style downplays and disguises the lethal effects of vaping to unwary teenagers and adolescents. The products and messages are packaged to appeal to the younger population as a harmless alternative method of recreation. The goal is to normalize the lifestyle of alternative nicotine consumption among teenagers and adolescents. Statistics show that there has been some degree of successes recorded by the vaping marketing industries, evident by the teeming and surging numbers of teenagers adopting vaping as a form of nicotine intake. Regulation of this industry has been described as a major part of several national strategies aimed at reducing the level of exposure of younger populations to these marketing strategies (41).

The perceived absence of stigmatization typically associated with the use of combustible smoking products may serve as an encouragement for the use of e-cigarettes. Nicotine is highly addictive and causes a plethora of problems in young people, including problems with cognition and attention, reduced impulse control, mood disorders, and physical damage to the brain and lungs (40). These effects can contribute to a significant increase in morbidity and mortality in the youth and early adult population. With the emergence of concrete evidence of the dangers of smoking, public health agencies have ramped up campaigns against the practice over the years and were successful in securing support for banning or restricting the use of tobacco products in several countries. The Government of Grenada and governments and other small island states should consider the epidemiological and financial burdens that may emerge should e-cigarette use become widespread in these countries. Huge social and economic burdens may also be placed on young people, their families, and the wider Grenadian community to address any emerging epidemic related to the use of e-cigarettes. This burden will also extend to the state level, as the health care system in small island states quickly become stretched when confronted with new challenges.

Social norms

The social acceptance of e-cigarette compared to combustible cigarette is discussed above. E-cigarette use is likely to be more popular among people who reside in communities and/or households where the practice is also acceptable. Young people usually obtain the devices from family members and friends (38). In a study in four states in the US, young people reported that their families were aware of their use of e-cigarettes, and they also received positive messages about the use of the devices (38). The media has also publicized celebrities using e-cigarettes. Not only is the practice acceptable in many societies, but provisions are also made for smoking and e-cigarette use in highly patronized areas, such as in airports, universities (schools), and restaurants. Such provisions may project the impression that smoking and e-cigarettes use is "normal," although confined to designated spaces. In August 2016, the FDA issued a Final Rule to regulate the manufacture and sale of e-cigarette in the US (42) and, by 2019, 98 countries had national or federal laws regulating manufacture, sale, and use of e-cigarettes (43). Currently, there is no move towards prohibiting the importation and sale of e-cigarettes in Grenada. In order to follow the course of countries that have banned or prohibited the use of e-cigarettes to protect public health, the legal and policy provisions in Grenada need to be revised. The narrow focus of several laws and policies also need to be addressed to put Grenada in a more opportune position to respond to the new products that are constantly available on the market.

Cost and availability

High taxation has been used as a mechanism to control the purchase and use of combustible cigarettes. In most cases, e-cigarettes do not attract the same high taxes that may deter sale. The Ministry of Health in Grenada has not produced any documentation on the local sale of the device and accessories nor the extent to which those are used on the island, although there are observations of e-cigarettes being used by tourists, international students, and other visitors. There may soon be a market in Grenada for the devices and refills. Should the products become available in markets in Grenada, other residents will also have access. Applying the precautionary principle or prevention measures may be most prudent and relevant to protect the health of Grenadians.

Other drug use

Recently, the CDC reported that some brands of e-cigarettes also contain the marijuana compound tetrahydrocannabinol (THC) (44), which is one of the main chemicals that produce physical effects when the leaves and other parts of the plant are used in smoking. Marijuana use and sale are illegal in Grenada. The use of e-cigarette, however, remains a legal and easy way to access and consume THC. In Canada, a study found that e-cigarette use was significantly associated with marijuana use among young people (45). Another study in the US found that adults who used both marijuana and alcohol had increased odds of e-cigarette use (46). The CDC also found that almost 90% of patients in two states in the US who developed lung injury reported they used vaping products with THC within three months before the study (44).

The CDC warned consumers of fake THC used in some e-cigarette brands and which also heighten the risk for damage to the lungs and other organs (44). The study in 2013 among students in secondary schools in Grenada indicated that a relatively high number of young people had smoked combustible cigarette or marijuana in their lifetime and/or used alcohol (20). Alcohol and marijuana can be gateway drugs to the use of e-cigarettes (46). In another study, the reverse trend was also found; e-cigarette use was associated with subsequent use of other drugs (33, 47). Young people may experience several years of healthy life lost and high social and economic burdens associated with chronic diseases from the use of e-cigarettes. Similar to the situation in the US during the opium crisis, the health care system in Grenada may also become stretched to deal with a new challenge.

PROPOSED SOLUTIONS

The same interventions that have worked for youth smoking reduction are recommended to be applied to e-cigarettes. The approach, therefore, should be multipronged. In the US, seven states have taken action to ban or restrict the use of e-cigarettes (48). According to a recent WHO survey, the sale of ENDS with nicotine is banned in 13 of 59 countries in which there are regulations. However, the majority of the 13 report availability of ENDS through illicit trade and cross border internet sales (49). The WHO, therefore, advises countries to consider the following when designing a regulatory strategy for ENDS (a) impede ENDS promotion to and uptake by non-smokers, pregnant women, and youth; (b) minimize potential health risks to ENDS users and non-users;(c) prohibit unproven health claims from being made about ENDS; and (d) protect existing tobacco-control efforts from commercial and other vested interests of the tobacco industry (49). Based on the WHO guidelines, the following are recommendations for Grenada:

Amendment to legislation to regulate importation and sale practice of vaping associated products

The recommendation is for vaping and its tobacco-based products to be listed for regulation under the Drug Abuse (Prevention and Control) Act No. 7 of 1992, Amended, January 2002, Amended by SRO 16 of 2011. E-cigarette devices and the practice of vaping are relatively new to Grenada and, as such, are not considered under existing legislation to enforce regulation of its use. Vaping products are currently marketed as consumer goods, however, with reference to existing laws; it is an offense to sell nicotine vaping products to young people under age 18. There are no legal restrictions on where people can vape, although the Drug Abuse Act which makes provisions for the demarcation of smoking free spaces. The recommended amendment should include vape devices and e-liquids to be regulated under respective and comparable laws.

The Drug Abuse (Prevention and Control) Act was not designed for vaping and does not include safety standards on what can be sold. Moreover, flavorings used in vaping products are regulated under respective Food Standards and are not a part of the drug regulatory provisions. Options for consideration are:

1) In the absence of any specific legal framework for regulating vaping and its products, the government should draft and legislate vaping-specific laws and regulations as an amendment to existing legislation.
2) Institutions and individual businesses can also make their own policies and rules around vaping, which is the only current measure for them to decide where persons can vape.

Any proposed legislative and policy initiatives should consider the following:

a) Provide protection from environmental (second-hand) smoke and vapor by prohibiting smoking and vaping of tobacco, nicotine or related products except in the established outdoor designated smoking areas and prohibiting all smoking and vaping;
b) Foster health and wellness by restricting the consumption, promotion, advertising and sale of smoking and vaping related products;
c) Recognize the permitted burning of traditional medicines during Traditional Aboriginal Ceremonies;
d) Communicate restrictions on smoking, vaping, and use of tobacco, nicotine, and cannabis.

Health education and promotion against vaping as a practice and substances used for vaping

Health education and promotion efforts against vaping is another component towards prevention and control, which will complement a legislative agenda to include vaping within existing laws. Education and Promotion campaign should focus on e-cigarettes/vapes and combustible cigarettes. These are different products that pose the same dangers. A public information campaign to raise awareness among school-aged youth about the dangers of e-cigarettes/vapes is critical towards informing healthy behaviors. Reference is made to a campaign by the CDC as resources available to schools and community-based organizations, and ideas for utilizing the resources (50, 51). Awareness campaigns should be designed to reach youth directly through a variety of channels:

a) Online and social media advertisements on platforms popular with youth (e.g., Snapchat, Spotify, Instagram).
b) Web page and Instagram account where youth can seek more information and resources.
c) Through organizations such as schools and community-based organizations with posters, fact clings, and a handout.

The CDC recommends use of organizational resources for these campaigns. Some examples include:

a) Reinforce adult education about the topic. The youth campaign and materials are a great way to reinforce educating parents/guardians and staff in organizations about e-cigarettes. Adults may not be up to date with information regarding vaping and should be considered for a presentation with basic information about e-cigarettes.
b) Hang campaign posters. The Vapes and Cigarettes: Different Products. Same Dangers posters were created to deliver messaging to youth. Consider hanging them throughout schools where they are visible. Ideas for placement include bathrooms, locker rooms, classrooms, counselor's office, nurse's office, coach's office, bulletin boards, hallways, lunchroom walls, concession stands at school events, and meeting rooms.
c) Hang fact clings. Each of the four main facts on the campaign poster is printed as small "clings" that adhere to windows, mirrors, doors,

and other surfaces. Because young people reported during the campaign focus groups that school bathrooms are often a favored vaping location, the clings were developed with school bathrooms in mind—but they can be used in other areas of the organization's building as well.

d) Distribute the campaign handout. A two-sided handout or fact sheet contains more facts about the dangers of vaping/using e-cigarettes. The handout expands upon the four main facts in the poster and fact clings and provides resources for youth.

Examples of Schools Based Awareness Campaigns include CATCH My Breath program. CATCH (Coordinated Approach to Child Health) is a school-based initiative which uses relevant, youth-friendly lesson plans. CATCH a youth e-cigarette prevention program targeting ages 11-18. The program uses a Tobacco Prevention Toolkit for teachers with in-classroom units and lesson plans on e-cigarettes, tobacco, and nicotine. The toolkit includes PowerPoints, discussion guides, worksheets, and activities. ASPIRE is also a free, bilingual, online tool that helps middle and high school teens learn about being tobacco-free, and smokescreen is a Smoking Prevention Videogame – play2PREVENT (52, 53).

Policy and legal interventions against vaping

Review and strengthen current school health policy which relates to tobacco and cigarette smoking to include vaping. Themes to include are:

a) Educate: E-cigarettes and other vaping products are often not easily recognizable. Educating staff about these products and about the school's policy to address them is an important part of the strategy to reduce student use.

b) Know more about vaping use: Collecting data on types of vaping products students are using and where they obtain vaping products can help inform education efforts and decisions about school health policies. Sample surveillance questions about vaping use, as well as questions about how students obtain vaping products, perceptions of harm, locations of use, are included.

c) Share resources for quitting vaping: While the use of vaping on school grounds is not regulated, that doesn't mean they are not current vaping users. It is important to support persons who use vaping products by providing them resources to address their own nicotine addiction.

d) Know more about resources in your community: Work with student groups to provide support, education, and connections to resources to address issues of vaping use in their community.

BENEFITS

Support for smoke and tobacco-free policies in public spaces continue to be implemented over the last several years as the benefits of preventing second-hand smoke and reducing primary use of cigarettes is well documented. The advent of vaping and its associated adverse health effects have also led to current efforts to support policies that prohibit vaping in public spaces. Additionally, the numbers of higher education institutions with comprehensive smoke or tobacco-free policies are now extending their regulations towards vaping in an effort to prevent the adverse effects of vaping. Working to prevent vaping use among youth is especially important because 99 percent of vaping use starts at a young age. Similarly, citizen groups and professional organizations of healthcare providers have started advocating for the adoption of prohibiting vaping practices and vaping products out of an abundance of precaution towards preventing the established burdens associated with vaping exposure. Four particular benefits of prohibiting vaping practice and products for Grenada are:

Decline in use

The lessons learned from the increase in smoke and tobacco-free policies have led to a decline in the number of persons who smoke cigarettes. Data describing the downward trends in cigarette use was also reported for other tobacco products, including e-cigarettes, hookah, little cigars, and traditional cigars. The expectation is for the practice of vaping to also be reduced through the implementation of policing prohibiting vaping together with an anti-vaping campaign.

Health promotion

Additional benefits are also derived besides helping to reduce vaping use through education. Changing attitudes towards other substance use and eliminating second-hand exposure make it easier for users to quit. From a health behavior and health promotion perspective, a vaping free policy presents opportunities to educate persons about other health-related issues and the benefits of a health-seeking lifestyle.

Clean environment

A policy prohibiting vaping will benefit the environment through reduced emission in the air, reduced litter, and reduction in the risk of fire. The policy on vaping prohibition will also reduce maintenance costs associated with cleaning and restoring spaces affected by vaping use and litter.

Professional preparation

Policies aimed at reducing practices such as vaping also prepare persons to be functional for the workforce and other professional settings. An increasing number of worksites are prohibiting tobacco and other substance use, including through vaping. Smokers/vapers have a harder time getting hired and the chances of getting a job are reduced for unemployed job seekers who smoke/vape.

Reduced healthcare cost from managing adverse health effects

In 2019, vaping has become a public health priority after accidents of sudden lung diseases reported in the US and UK. Active research is currently underway to find out more negative side effects of vaping, but it will be a while before results are available. Vaping side effects can be from short-term, minor issues to something so severe affecting multiple organ systems in the body. From a cost perspective, per capita, health care costs for smokers are higher than those of non-smokers. For example, smoking is the largest single cause of preventable illness and premature death within the UK and places a significant financial burden each year. When applied to projected costs associated with vaping, the scale of use and effects is not comparable, but the cost of treating effects is considerable and increasing. The financial impact of vaping, like smoking, extends to businesses and its workforce productivity; smoking/vaping breaks are said to cost billions of dollars per year, and increased absenteeism is estimated in the billions. There is also a reduced life expectancy and decreasing the country's workforce and its productivity.

CONCLUSION

The use of electronic cigarettes (e-cigarettes) or the practice of vaping has emerged as a global public health concern. If this practice remains unchecked, all the gains due to public health efforts to reduce smoking of combustible cigarettes and thus reduce morbidity and mortality from tobacco-related deaths will be reversed. While e-cigarettes were initially introduced as a smoking cessation strategy, sufficient evidence for this has not been forthcoming. In fact, the use of e-cigarettes has produced more negative health outcomes than positive ones, as evidenced in the recent morbidity and mortality related EVALI. While this is more evident in developed countries, governments of low- and middle-income countries such as Grenada, need to protect youth and young adults from initiating and/or continuing use of these potentially harmful products. Many countries, as well as states in the US, have implemented some level of restrictive policies on the use of e-cigarettes based on the available evidence of harm caused by these products. It is proposed that the same interventions that have worked for smoking of combustible cigarettes reduction should be applied to e-cigarettes. With the reported high prevalence of conventional cigarette smoking among secondary school students in Grenada, the recommendation is for vaping and its tobacco-based products to be listed for regulation under the Drug Abuse (Prevention and Control) Act No. 7 of 1992, Amended, January 2002, Amended by SRO 16 of 2011. Health education and promotion against vaping is another component of the effort towards prevention and control, which will complement a legislative agenda to include vaping within existing laws. Also, there should be a review and strengthening of current school health policies that relate to tobacco and cigarette smoking to include vaping. Benefits of prohibiting vaping practice and products for Grenada are health promotion with a decline in the use and associated reduction in healthcare costs, cleaner environment and promoting health seeking behavior, and professional conduct among youth and young adults.

ACKNOWLEDGMENTS

The White Paper Team Experts, St George's University, School of Medicine, St George, Grenada, West Indies:

Marios Loukas, MD, PhD, Dean of Basic Sciences and Chair (Department of Anatomy)

School of Medicine

Christine Richards, PhD, MPH, Chair

Department of Public Health and Preventive Medicine

Satesh Bidaisee, DVM, MSPH, EdD, Associate Dean of Graduate Studies

Department of Public Health and Preventive Medicine

Lindonne Glasgow, MPH, DrPH, Deputy Chair

Department of Public Health and Preventive Medicine

Prakash Ramdass, MD, MPH, Track Director, Epidemiology

Department of Public Health and Preventive Medicine

Oladimeji Tolulope Tunde, MD.

Department of Pathophysiology

Emmanuel Keku, MD, MA, MSPH, Track Director, Preventive Medicine (MD/MPH)

Department of Public Health and Preventive Medicine

REFERENCES

[1] Bhatta DN, Glantz SA. Association of e-cigarette use with respiratory disease among adults: A longitudinal analysis. Am J Prev Med 2020;58(2):182–90.

[2] Which countries ban E-cigarettes? Ecigarette Reviewed, 2015. URL: https://ecigarettereviewed.com/which-countries-ban-e-cigarettes.

[3] Commar A, Prasad VK, Tursan d'Espaignet E, Wolfenden L, WHO global report on trends in prevalence of tobacco smoking 2000-2025. Geneva: World Health Organization, 2018.

[4] US Department of Health and Human Services. E-cigarette use among youth and young adults: A report of the Surgeon General. Rockville, MD: DHHS, 2012.

[5] Breland A, Soule E, Lopez A, Ramôa C, El-Hellani A, Eissenberg T. Electronic cigarettes: What are they and what do they do? Ann NY Acad Sci 2017;1394(1):5–30.

[6] E-cigarette use among youth and young adults A report. URL: https://www.cdc.gov/tobacco/data_statistics/sgr/e-cigarettes/pdfs/2016_sgr_entire_report_508.pdf.

[7] Bruin JE, Gerstein HC, Holloway AC. Long-term consequences of fetal and neonatal nicotine exposure: A critical review. Toxicol Sci 2010;116(2):364–74.

[8] George L, Granath F, Johansson ALV, Annerén G, Cnattingius S. Environmental tobacco smoke and risk of spontaneous abortion. Epidemiology 2006;17(5):500–5.

[9] Suter MA, Mastrobattista J, Sachs M, Aagaard K. Is there evidence for potential harm of electronic cigarette use in pregnancy? Birth Defects Res A Clin Mol Teratol 2015;103(3):186–95.

[10] Visser WF, Klerx WN, Cremers HWJM, Ramlal R, Schwillens PL, Talhout R. The health risks of electronic cigarette use to bystanders. Int J Environ Res Public Health 2019;16(9). pii: E1525. Doi.10.3390/ijerph16091525.

[11] Brown CJ, Cheng JM. Electronic cigarettes: Product characterisation and design considerations. Tob Control 2014;23(suppl 2):ii4–10.

[12] Breitbarth AK, Morgan J, Jones AL. E-cigarettes: An unintended illicit drug delivery system. Drug Alcohol Depend 2018;192:98–111.

[13] Hon L. Electronic cigarette, 2015. URL: https://patents.google.com/patent/US20150034103A1/en.

[14] Sanford Z, Goebel LJ. E-cigarettes: An up to date review and discussion of the controversy. W V Med J 2014;110(4):10-5.

[15] Bhalerao A, Sivandzade F, Archie SR, Cucullo L. Public health policies on e-cigarettes. Curr Cardiol Rep 2019;21(10):111.

[16] Hajek P, Phillips-Waller A, Przulj D, Pesola F, Myers Smith K, Bisal N, et al. A randomized trial of e-cigarettes versus nicotine-replacement therapy. N Engl J Med 2019;380(7):629–37.

[17] Malas M, van der Tempel J, Schwartz R, Minichiello A, Lightfoot C, Noormohamed A, et al. Electronic cigarettes for smoking cessation: A systematic review. Nicotine Tob Res 2016;18(10):1926–36.

[18] Jorenby DE, Smith SS, Fiore MC, Baker TB. Nicotine levels, withdrawal symptoms, and smoking reduction success in real world use: A comparison of cigarette smokers and dual users of both cigarettes and e-cigarettes. Drug Alcohol Depend 2017;170:93–101.

[19] Cullen KA, Gentzke AS, Sawdey MD, Chang JT, Anic GM, Wang TW, et al. E-cigarette use among youth in the United States, 2019. JAMA 2019;322(21):2095–103.

[20] Cullen KA. Notes from the field: Use of electronic cigarettes and any tobacco product among middle and high school students: United States, 2011–2018. MMWR 2018;67(45):1276-7.

[21] Reid J, Hammond D, Rynard VL, Madill CL, Burkhalter R. Tobacco use in Canada: Patterns and trends. Waterloo, ON: Propel Centre Population Health Impact University of Waterloo, 2017.

[22] Lee S, Grana RA, Glantz SA. Electronic cigarette use among Korean adolescents: A cross-sectional study of market penetration, dual use, and relationship to quit attempts and former smoking. J Adolesc Health 2014;54(6):684–90.

[23] Smoking, drinking and drug use among young people in England, 2016. NHS Digital. URL: https://digital.nhs.uk/data-and-information/publications/statistical/smoking-drinking-and-drug-use-among-young-people-in-england/2016.

[24] Electronic cigarette use among emerging and young West Indian adults. Eur Med J 2017. URL: https://www.emjreviews.com/respiratory/article/electronic-cigarette-use-among-emerging-and-young-west-indian-adults/.

[25] Moritz ED, Zapata LB, Lekiachvili A, Glidden E, Annor FB, Werner AK, et al. Update: characteristics of patients in a national outbreak of e-cigarette, or vaping,

product use–associated lung injuries — United States, October 2019. MMWR 2019;68(43):985–9.

[26] Centers for Disease Control and Prevention. Outbreak of lung injury associated with the use of e-cigarette, or vaping products. URL: https://www.cdc.gov/tobacco/basic_information/e-cigarettes/severe-lung-disease.html.

[27] Chaffee BW, Watkins SL, Glantz SA. Electronic Cigarette use and progression from experimentation to established smoking. Pediatrics 2018;141(4). URL: https://pediatrics.aappublications.org/cocnt/141/4/e20173594.

[28] Cai H, Wang C. Graphical review: The redox dark side of e-cigarettes; exposure to oxidants and public health concerns. Redox Biol 2017;13:402–6.

[29] Rubinstein ML, Delucchi K, Benowitz NL, Ramo DE. Adolescent exposure to toxic volatile organic chemicals from e-cigarettes. Pediatrics 2018;141(4):e20173557.

[30] US Surgeon General. Get the facts on e-cigarettes. Know the risks: E-cigarettes and young people. URL: https://e-cigarettes.surgeongeneral.gov/getthefacts.html.

[31] Vogel EA, Cho J, McConnell RS, Barrington-Trimis JL, Leventhal AM. Prevalence of electronic cigarette dependence among youth and its association with future use. JAMA Netw Open 2020;3(2):e1921513–e1921513.

[32] Third secondary schools drugs revalance survey. URL: https://www.gov.gd/egov/pdf/ncodc/docs/final-third-secondary-schools-drugs-revalance-survey.pdf.

[33] National Institutes of Health. Vaping devices (electronic cigarettes), 2019. URL: https://www.drugabuse.gov/publications/drugfacts/vaping-devices-electronic-cigarettes.

[34] Hess CA, Olmedo P, Navas-Acien A, Goessler W, Cohen JE, Rule AM. E-cigarettes as a source of toxic and potentially carcinogenic metals. Environ Res 2017;152:221–5.

[35] Rubinstein ML, Delucchi K, Benowitz NL, Ramo DE. Adolescent exposure to toxic volatile organic chemicals from e-cigarettes. Pediatrics 2018;141(4):e20173557.

[36] Visser WF, Klerx WN, Cremers HWJM, Ramlal R, Schwillens PL, Talhout R. The health risks of electronic cigarette use to bystanders. Int J Environ Res Public Health 2019;16(9):1525.

[37] DiFranza JR. Initial symptoms of nicotine dependence in adolescents. Tob Control 2000;9(3):313–9.

[38] Alexander JP, Williams P, Lee YO. Youth who use e-cigarettes regularly: A qualitative study of behavior, attitudes, and familial norms. Prev Med Rep 2019;13:93–7.

[39] York York State Department of Health. Bureau of Chronic Disease Evaluation and Research. Electronic cigarette use by youth increased 160% New York State Youth Tobacco Survey 2000-2018. URL: https://www.health.ny.gov/prevention/tobacco_control/reports/statshots/volume12/n1_electronic_sig_use_increase.pdf.

[40] US Department of Health and Human Services. Preventing tobacco use among youth and young adults: A report of the surgeon general. Surgeon General's Report, 2016. Rockville, MD: DHHS, 2016.

[41] Gostin LO, Glasner AY. E-cigarettes, vaping, and youth. JAMA 2014;312(6):595–6.

[42] Barraza LF, Weidenaar KE, Cook LT, Logue AR, Halpern MT. Regulations and policies regarding e-cigarettes. Cancer 2017;123(16):3007–14.

[43] Shih C-S, Etter J-F. Stakeholders' views on e-cigarette legislation: A qualitative study in Taiwan. Front Public Health 2019;7:354.

[44] Ghinai I, Pray IW, Navon L, O'Laughlin K, Saathoff-Huber L, Hoots B, et al. E-cigarette product use, or vaping, among persons with ssociated lung injury — Illinois and Wisconsin, April–September 2019. MMWR 2019;68(39):865–9.

[45] Mehra VM, Keethakumar A, Bohr YM, Abdullah P, Tamim H. The association between alcohol, marijuana, illegal drug use and current use of E-cigarette among youth and young adults in Canada: results from Canadian Tobacco, Alcohol and Drugs Survey 2017. BMC Public Health 2019;19(1):1208.

[46] Bluestein M, Kelder S, Perry CL, Pérez A. Exploring associations between the use of alcohol and marijuana with e-cigarette use in a U.S.A. nationally representative sample of young adults. Int J Health Sci 2019;13(1):30–9.

[47] Bold KW, Kong G, Camenga DR, Simon P, Cavallo DA, Morean ME, et al. Trajectories of E-Cigarette and Conventional Cigarette Use Among Youth. Pediatrics 2018;141(1):e20171832.

[48] Rense S. 7 States have banned vapes ao far. Is all of America next? Esquire 2019 Dec 6. URL: https://www.esquire.com/lifestyle/health/a29067489/which-states-banned-flavored-e-cigarettes-vaping-juuls/.

[49] Conference of the parties to the WHO framework concention on tobacco control. Moscow 2014 Oct 13-18. URL: http://apps.who.int/gb/fctc/PDF/cop6/FCTC_COP6_10-en.pdf?ua=1.

[50] Centers for Disease Control and Prevention. Smoking and tobacco use. Electronic cigarettes. URL: https://www.cdc.gov/tobacco/basic_information/e-cigarettes/index.htm.

[51] Get the facts. Make smoking history. URL: http://makesmokinghistory.org/dangers-of-vaping/facts/.

[52] Electronic cigarette dangers and information: Vape prevention program. CATCH. URL: https://catchinfo.org/modules/e-cigarettes/.

[53] The real cost of vaping. URL: https://www.scholastic.com/youthvapingrisks/.

In: Public Health Themes in Grenada ... ISBN: 978-1-53618-118-0
Editors: J. Merrick and L. Glasgow

Chapter 4

PROTECTING HEALTH SECURITY IN THE CARIBBEAN: A COORDINATED REGIONAL RESPONSE TO THE NOVEL CORONAVIRUS DISEASE (COVID-19) AND OTHER GLOBAL PUBLIC HEALTH THREATS

Stephanie Fletcher-Lartey[1,*], PhD, Lisa Indar[1], PhD, Tamu Davidson[1], MD, Gabriel Gonzalez Escobar[1], PhD and Joy St John[2,3], MBBS, MPH

[1]Surveillance, Disease Prevention and Control, Caribbean Public Health Agency, [2]Caribbean Public Health Agency and [3]Co-Chair of the Virgin United Climate Accelerator Board

[*] Correspondence: Dr Stephanie Fletcher-Lartey, Consultant, Health Information, Communicable Diseases and Emergency Response, CARPHA, Port of Spain, Trinidad and Tobago. Email: stephjewels100@yahoo.com.au

Abstract

Small island developing states like those of the Caribbean Region need strong Regional Coordination of Health Security to mitigate the impact of emerging and re-emerging infectious diseases. The importance of countries working together to achieve functional cooperation and ensure a strong emphasis is placed on Regional Health Security is especially evident with the Caribbean's response to the pandemic of novel coronavirus disease (COVID-19). The aim of this chapter is to describe health security in the Caribbean region and how this has been addressed in the context of a coordinated regional response to the coronavirus disease epidemic. The Caribbean Community (CARICOM) Member States were among the last countries in the world to see an introduction of the COVID-19 infection. The health security efforts of multiple CARICOM regional institutions and stakeholders saw a level of coordination to achieve increased vigilance, early detection of importation of the novel coronavirus and the provision of additional critical care resources to deal with the rapid increase of illness which has come to characterize the progression of disease in affected countries around the world. While it is still early days in the COVID-19 pandemic, the Regional Coordinating Mechanism for Health Security has continued to be the mechanism by which CARPHA has gained agreement on policy and operational issues among the multiple stakeholders determining a more cohesive and transparent method for Health Sector action in CARICOM.

Introduction

The Caribbean consists of many small island developing states, which makes them extremely vulnerable to public health emergencies and disasters (hurricanes, floods, earthquakes). This is due to several factors, including variability in their capacity to respond to public health threats, geographical vulnerabilities to disasters, limited resources for health sector response and surge (human, financial, infrastructural), capacity. Traditionally the CARICOM Member States have individually only been able to respond to a moderate degree of threat. The porous borders and interconnectedness of countries through travel and trade further increases the risk from health threats (1). The Caribbean also boasts one of the highest numbers of travelers per population worldwide. However, whilst tourism is the key economic driver for the region and is adversely impacted by emergencies and disasters, the high number of travelers per population increases the health, safety, and security risks to the local populations. This has been evident through the introduction and spread of several new and re-emerging diseases (2), as exemplified by outbreaks of Norovirus, H1NI, Chikungunya, Zika, and the current novel coronavirus (COVID-19).

Over the past five years, the Caribbean region has been negatively impacted by repeated outbreaks of new and emerging infectious diseases that have tested the regional health security capacity. The emergence of mosquito-borne diseases Chikungunya and Zika (3); H1N1, and the preparedness for the possible introduction of Ebola are more recent events that have required the building of internal and regional capacity for emergency response and have highlighted the need for boosting regional health security. The Caribbean has been impacted by multiple hurricanes over the past years. In 2017, Hurricanes Irma and Maria devastated several of the Member States. According to one report, Hurricane Irma's impact from insured losses was estimated at around $2 billion in 2019 (4). The collective experiences gained across multiple sectors from many years of preparing for responding to public health emergencies and natural disasters have contributed to building resilience and adaptive capacity of the Caribbean people to the impacts of disasters.

Public health emergencies and disasters have the potential to adversely affect the health of the population. Hence public health systems must play an integral role in preparing communities to respond to and recover from hazard impacts. The public health consequences of disasters and emergencies can be far reaching. During the initial response, the people and communities that are impacted must rely on local community resources and then on external support. As a result, all local, national and regional emergency response stakeholders must be prepared to coordinate, cooperate, and collaborate with cross-sectoral partners and organizations at all governmental levels when emergencies occur, regardless of the type, scale, or severity.

The novel coronavirus disease outbreak in late 2019/early 2020 occurred following recent outbreaks, including Chikungunya and Zika, in multiple countries across the Caribbean region. Outbreak preparedness activities, as well as activities aimed at building core capacities for the IHR (2005) by health sector stakeholders, should have provided the foundation to build regional cooperation to any new and emerging health threat.

The COVID-19 pandemic initially created international anxiety because of its novelty, coupled with extensive media coverage, and a plethora of fake news and misinformation. The ease of modern-day global travel meant that people from the original and subsequent epicenters traveled freely to several parts of the globe. The importance of travel in the movement of infected people from one geographical area to the other has been evident in the current COVID-19 pandemic. The heightened risk of importation of cases facilitated by tourism travel has been an important consideration for the island nations and the regional governance mechanisms of the Caribbean.

Some of the health issues observed in the region, including a combination of the increased burden of non-communicable diseases (NCDs), and injuries, new, emerging and endemic infectious diseases, and an aging population, will increase the vulnerability of populations and health systems in Member States (4, 5). A significant proportion of Caribbean people have underlying health conditions that place them in the high-risk categories for severe outcomes from COVID-19. Health security measures must consider the NCD issues and prepare to mitigate the risk to the most vulnerable population.

The Caribbean Community (CARICOM), the regional body for governance, has established various institutions and mechanisms in partnership with regional stakeholders and international development partners to safeguard the health security of the region. The Caribbean Public Health Agency (CARPHA) as the sole regional public health agency, is leading the regional health response to COVID-19, in keeping with its Intergovernmental Agreement (IGA) mandate from Heads of CARICOM Government and recommendations from Council for Human and Social Development (COHSOD) - Health working group on regional coordination for the management of COVID-19.

The aim of this chapter is to describe the health security situation in the Caribbean region and how the Security Cluster of CARICOM has been mobilized to provide the foundation of a coordinated regional response to the Pandemic of COVID-19 disease. The paper also highlights the leading role of the CARPHA, in the CARICOM regional health response to COVID-19 and the importance of strong partnerships with non-Health sectors in achieving functional cooperation for regional health security.

HEALTH SECURITY IN THE CARIBBEAN

The World Health Organization defines global public health security (6) as the activities required to minimize the danger and impact of acute public health events that endanger the collective health of populations living across geographical regions and international boundaries. The goal of global public health security is to demonstrate how collective international public health action can build a safer future for humanity. Many of the lessons learned from the West African Ebola Outbreak have catalyzed actions that have enabled faster and more effective response to outbreaks and emergencies (7). The Health Security Interface is the point where two systems - the public health sector and the security sector meet and interact in a variety of situations. Some examples where the health security interface occurs are: outbreak response operations in non-permissive environments, such as highly politicized contexts, conflicts, and wars; deliberate events, including the intentional use of chemical or biological agents in order to cause harm; Issues related to mass gatherings, such as major sporting events, festivals, and regular religious migrations; and activities that may arise in the course of a natural disease outbreak.

The interconnectedness of the globe is now facilitated by the ease of travel from one end to the other by aircraft, and infectious disease threats can now spread much faster across geographical regions. The travel industry is vulnerable to public health emergencies and, in the context of the COVID-19 outbreak, the impact on travel is well noted. The updated and expanded

International Health Regulations (2005) provides the legislative framework to enable international collaboration for public health emergencies of international concern. It also facilitates the mobilization of essential resources for effective and timely implementation of actions and, at the country level, requires national core capacity in disease detection. In the last five years up to 2017, WHO reported that more than 1100 epidemic events were verified worldwide; 48 of these in the region of the Americas (8). Securing the health of the Caribbean surpasses keeping residents safe but extends to the millions of tourists and other visitors that travel to the Caribbean region each year. Implementing systems to eliminate, prevent, and control the spread of infectious diseases is essential for regional health security.

Regional Health Security in the Caribbean describes the capacities required for CARICOM Member States to prepare for and respond to public health threats, issues, and concerns that transcend national boundaries and potentially impact on economic and political stability, trade, tourism, and access to goods. The Caribbean region has a long history of cooperation for health, evidenced by the establishment of various regional organizations from as far back as the 1940s (9, 10). While multiple efforts have targeted health security over the years, various activities have been carried out in the region in the last six years as part of efforts to bolster regional capacity and coordinated regional response.

The Caribbean Public Health Agency (CARPHA), is the sole public health agency of the Caribbean and commenced operations on Jan 1, 2013, with the aim of delivering the functions of five previous regional health institutions (Caribbean Epidemiology Centre, Caribbean Environmental Health Institute, Caribbean Food and Nutrition Institute, Caribbean Health Research Council, and Caribbean Regional Drug Testing Laboratory) through one platform for greater synergy and cost-effectiveness and as the principal institutional expression of the Caribbean Cooperation in Health (11). CARPHA provides public health surveillance, emergency response, laboratory, information, research, training, and policy development services that benefit a diverse population of 17 million people in 26 English, French, Spanish and Dutch-speaking member states and territories.

As the regional public health agency, CARPHA plays a pivotal role in defining the scope of health risks associated with many emergencies, including those associated with the natural occurrence of highly infectious diseases, such as COVID-19. In health emergencies, CARPHA serves as a key leader in the regional health response, working closely with other regional and international agencies, to design protective strategies, to instruct health professionals about preventive or treatment interventions and to provide guidelines and technical input to inform the health sector and mechanisms involved in the health security interface. Mechanisms at CARPHA for supporting and coordinating regional health security include:

- CARPHA's Medical Microbiology Laboratory (CMML) which includes a biosecurity level 3 (BSL 3), that serves as the CARICOM regional reference laboratory.
- Health Information, Communicable Diseases and Emergency Response (HCE) Unit, well equipped with qualified epidemiologists, and other technical experts experienced in addressing public health emergency and response.
- Incident Management Team: multi-skilled team consisting of experienced scientists ranging from epidemiologists, laboratorians, risk communicators, behavioral scientists, non-communicable diseases, and other public health experts. This team is activated, once an emergency is verified, to provide real-time daily response to CARPHA member states.
- Regional travelers/tourism and health program (THP) that addresses health, safety, and environmental issues impacting on tourism through an integrated approach and works closely with regional and international tourism sector partners for health security. This unique program adopts a multiprong (surveillance, guidelines, standards, capacity building, policy) and multisectoral (partnerships with CLIA, WTO, VSP Travelers Health: PHE, CDC, PHAC, WHO) approach for implementation and endorsement from Ministers of Health and Tourism across the region. The THP provides a real-time

Early Warning and Response Travel Health Information Monitoring (THiS; website http://this.carpha.org) that can serve as a proactive measure to help fight the importation and spread of this novel viral illness. Facilities housing stay over arrivals, such as hotels and guesthouses can register to report illness confidentially, and visitors can also self-report. The system will provide information to help identity and confidentially manage early warning COVID-19 symptoms reported by employees and guests in a rapid manner.

- Medicines Quality Control and Surveillance Department (MCQSD) forms part of the robust mechanisms for regulating medicines in CARICOM, in close collaboration with Member States, the CARPHA/PAHO Caribbean Regulatory System (CRS) and other partners such as PAHO/WHO. In heath emergencies, they monitor the effectiveness, safety of medicines in use and on the market.
- Environmental Health and Sustainable Development (EHS) Department of CARPHA supports the Caribbean's sustainable development agenda by playing a lead role in key areas related to environmental management for optimal public health. There is a full-service microbiological and analytical laboratory that is accredited to ISO 17025 and provides environmental analyses, including water quality monitoring, plant, soil and tissue analyses, microbiological food testing, indoor environmental quality monitoring, and noise testing. Some of the areas where EHS supports Member States include monitoring, alert and outbreak response for communicable diseases, conducting Environment Impact Assessments (EIAs), and environmental auditing services led by certified ISO 14001 lead auditors.

In response to the Ebola emergency in West Africa in 2014, CARICOM Heads of Government at their Seventeenth Special Meeting in Port of Spain, Trinidad and Tobago in 2014 called for the establishment of a Regional Coordination Mechanism on Ebola (RCME) with a ten-point plan of action. Recognizing the vulnerability of the region and the likelihood of future health threats, this RCME was then extended into the Regional Coordination

Mechanism for Health Security (RCM-HS) to help counter any risk to regional health security from new and emerging threats. In recognition of the issue inherent in a region of very small, highly vulnerable and inter-connected countries and territories coupled with the political and economic integration movement, a regional approach to health security was considered necessary.

The RCM-HS provides oversight of the coordinated planning and implementation of the regional response to public health threats and emergencies with a focus on strengthening the capacity of member states, including those capacities related to the revised International Health Regulations (2005). The members of the RCM-HS are the Caribbean Public Health Agency (CARPHA) (Chair), Caribbean Community (CARICOM), Organisation of Eastern Caribbean States (OECS), CARICOM Implementation Agency for Crime and Security (IMPACS), Caribbean Disaster Emergency Management Agency (CDEMA), Pan American Health Organization/World Health Organization (PAHO/WHO), and selected Member States based on their lead roles in CARICOM. In 2017, participants from CARPHA Member States, regional and international organizations came together in Trinidad and Tobago to discuss the implementation of a Regional roadmap for health security.

Caribbean Regional governments have recognized that the Global Health Security Agenda complements the WHO IHR and has the ability to accelerate compliance through a multi-stakeholder approach. The CARICOM Council for Human and Social Development (COHSOD) agreed that the development of a five-year Roadmap for CARICOM would assist the regional governments in accelerating their national IHR compliance. The mechanism recognized that the region must focus on means of leveraging existing regional capacities, prioritize the importance of Regional Health Security at the political levels to garner continued support and develop means of sustainable financing through mechanisms such as the Stop the Epidemic There and Here (SETH) Fund.

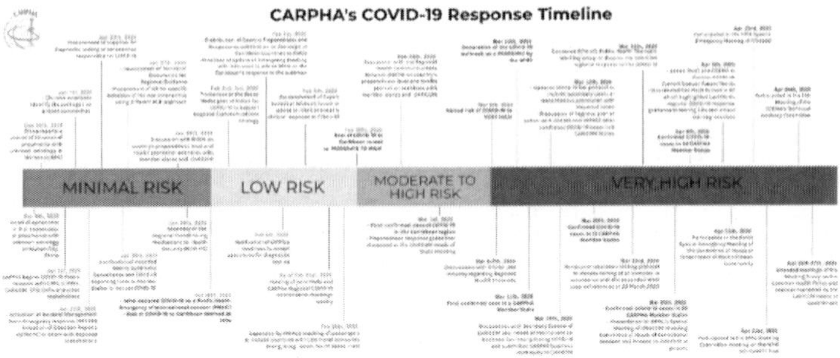

Figure 1. Timeline of CARPHA's key actions carried out in the context of COVID-19 preparedness and response.

A COORDINATED REGIONAL RESPONSE TO COVID-19

The coronavirus disease (COVID-19) outbreak was first reported in December 2019. The newly identified SARS-COV-2 virus, which was first detected in Wuhan City, China, with suspected links to an animal source, has rapidly spread from person to person. On January 30, 2020 the Director-General of the World Health Organization (WHO) declared the outbreak of a novel coronavirus disease (COVID-19) to be a Public Health Emergency of International Concern. Whilst the outbreak originated in China, in just over three months, the virus rapidly spread to more than 197 countries affecting more than 400,000 persons, as of March 25, 2020. On March 11, 2020 WHO characterized the outbreak to be a pandemic considering the 13-fold increase in COVID-19 cases outside of China with a tripling of the number of affected countries within the previous two weeks. The concerns associated with the rapid spread include the severity of disease and the disturbing lack of action observed in some countries. These, along with other factors, are expected to result in an increase in the number of cases and deaths in affected countries.

Within a few weeks, the numbers of cases reported from China and countries reporting imported cases made it evident that the outbreak was spreading globally quite fast. It became obvious that it would only be a matter of time before an outbreak of great magnitude would impact the Caribbean. Early epidemiological assessments revealed that the elderly, those with chronic diseases, and smokers are among the high-risk groups for poorer outcomes (12, 13). In the Caribbean context, there is a high prevalence of these risk factors, among others. The Caribbean region has one of the oldest populations in the world. Non-communicable diseases are the leading causes of morbidity and mortality in many countries in the region (4, 5).

According to the WHO, the public health security of all countries depends on the capacity of each to act effectively and contribute to the security of all. The early actions of China to quarantine people and restrict movements have been described as beneficial to the containment of the COVID-19 outbreak in China and delayed the spread of disease to other regions of the world. According to the Director General of WHO in a Statement on March 5, 2020 a collective, coordinated and comprehensive approach that engages the entire machinery of government is what is necessary to push back this COVID-19 epidemic (14).

Recognizing the vulnerability of the region and in keeping with its mandate, CARPHA sought an early audience with key experts in infectious disease internationally in January, 2020 prior to the spread of the disease outside of Wuhan. The advice obtained was acted upon to inform the initial health preparedness and response actions to the outbreak in the region.

Multi-sectoral response

CARPHA has been coordinating the CARICOM regional health response, conducting regular update meetings with Member States and partners including tourism partners, producing situation reports every two working days, performing tests on suspected cases from its Member States, enhancing its syndromic surveillance to capture suspected COVID-19 cases, developing technical guidelines including those on sampling, laboratory testing, ports of entry, algorithms for response, management of cases on ships, aircrafts, hotels and their staff, infection prevention and control, health sector response plan; regional communications plans, convening expert groups and participating in CARICOM Heads of Government meetings.

The Regional Coordinating Mechanism for Health Security was activated on January 29, 2020 as a means of bringing order and coherence to the responses of the Health and non-Health sectors as this outbreak evolved. Support for the RCM-HS was garnered from the highest level of regional governance. The CARICOM Council of Human and Social Development convened two Emergency Meetings and the CARICOM Heads of Government convened an emergency meeting of Heads of Government to discuss COVID-19 response and establish guidance for the region, including guidelines for cruise ships and other conveyances.

In keeping with CARICOM recommendations, various key actions were taken across multiple sectors, including:

- Coordination with the national Ministries of Health and Disaster Preparedness Offices
- Participation in national emergency preparedness planning processes
- Receiving training on critical areas such as: infection prevention and control

Health sector

As a leading health agency, CARPHA took early actions to activate its Incident Management Team for Emergency Response and worked closely with regional and international health partners to define the response needed to this health threat and provide timely advice and assistance to its Member States. As the outbreak emerged, CARPHA convened multiple meetings to provide updates and information to assess the level of readiness and provide support for preparedness and response planning. CARPHA provided technical support and a plethora of technical guidance in keeping with international standards and best practice to ensure as uniform a response as possible across the region.

For COVID -19, CARPHA's Medical Microbiology Laboratory (CMML) is the regional reference laboratory and primary testing site initially, while internal capacity was subsequently built in various CARICOM countries by PAHO to enable testing for COVID-19, including Barbados, Suriname, Guyana, Dominica, Jamaica, Belize, Bahamas, and Haiti. Other countries in the region with capacity for testing included Martinique, French Guiana, Curacao, Aruba, St Martin, and the British territories of Cayman Islands, and Bermuda.

Another area where the strength of regional coordination was evident was in the actions of the Regional Security System facilitating the prompt transportation of samples to be tested at the CARPHA CMML from Member States and the adjustments made by the host country, Trinidad and Tobago, to expedite the clearance of samples by their Customs Department.

Most Caribbean countries have national emergency response plans and designated health emergency coordination structures in place. The last critical outbreak of similar nature in the region would have been Influenza H1N1 in 2009. Countries were advised to use the window of opportunity created by the delay in the importation of cases to the region, to review, update and adapt their pandemic influenza response plans for COVID-19, implement the necessary structures and legislative frameworks, ensure staff was trained and regular exercises carried out to prepare for an epidemic response. A decision was made by the COHSOD working group that a coordinated regional approach would be needed should the epidemic become escalated to a pandemic. CARPHA was tasked to develop a Health Sector Pandemic Response Plan for COVID-19 in this regard for a consistent approach among Member States. Figure 1 outlines the timeline of key actions carried out in the region in the context of COVID-19 response.

CARICOM reaffirmed CARPHA's responsibility and adopted their recommended Regional Approach to the Coronavirus – COVID-19 at the 31st Inter-Sessional Meeting of the Conference of Heads of Government of CARICOM 18-19 February 2020. In recognition of the rapid spread of the disease both at the epi-center and subsequently globally, CARPHA asked Member States to step up their preparedness and response actions as a matter of urgency.

A summary of other key actions recommended in the preparedness phase for the health sector includes:

- Public health authorities providing information to travelers to reduce the general risk of acute respiratory infections, via health practitioners, travel health clinics, travel agencies, conveyance operators, and at Points of Entry.
- Revision of stockpiles of medical equipment and logistical support tools.
- Revision of the list of medical and response personnel with adequate training and identification of staff with prior experience with the diagnosis and management of severe acute respiratory infection (SARS) and Influenza H1N1 cases.
- Member States should incorporate planning for health crisis responses into national disaster risk reduction preparedness and response mechanisms and plans.
- Engagement of all relevant stakeholders to identify response capacities and resources for a whole of government response.
- Development of pandemic plans and carry out simulation exercises for all relevant responders, including security forces.
- Implementation of routine measures, train staff, identify appropriate space and stockpile of adequate equipment in place at points of entry for assessing and managing ill travelers detected before travel, onboard conveyances (such as planes and ships) and on arrival at the points of entry.

Tourism sector

The COVID-19 outbreak sent shockwaves through the cruise ship industry, and this was exacerbated by an outbreak aboard a cruise ship that docked and became quarantined at a port in Japan for an extended period of time. By March 13, 2020 there had been 696 cases and seven deaths associated with the ship. Development of disease during cruise ship voyages and the ability of their passengers to disembark at ports of entry continues to be a major challenge across the region. Multiple countries across the region have issued travel advisories, and some have banned travel to and from certain affected countries; the list is changing as the disease spread across regions.

In response, the Cruise Lines International Association (CLIA), the leading voice in the cruise ship industry, initially issued a series of enhanced policies for guests and crew who have recently traveled from or through China, including Hong Kong and Macau (15). On March 8, 2020 the boarding restrictions were extended to South Korea, Iran, and any municipality in Italy subject to lockdown (quarantine) measures by the Italian government (16). Five cruise ships (Diamond Princess, World Dream, Anthem of Seas, Westerdam and Costa Smeralda) have been quarantined after news of possible coronavirus infections emerged. The Diamond Princess in particular, represents the largest concentration of coronavirus cases outside China with 634 infections and two deaths. Another cruise ship, the Grand Princess, had been quarantined off the US coast with 21 people that have tested positive for coronavirus (17). Several cruise operators have either canceled or changed their itineraries as countries across the world implement travel restrictions to curb the disease spread (18).

Airline travel has also been impacted globally, with multiple airlines canceling flights on multiple routes. In the Caribbean region, the regional carrier, Caribbean Airlines implemented measures to ensure their readiness in case of any eventualities, although none of their destinations had travel bans imposed. They also were permitting travelers on Caribbean Airlines with connections to or from mainland China, Iran, Italy, Japan, South Korea, and Singapore to rebook the Caribbean Airlines travel segment without change fees, subject to conditions (19).

In recognition of the significant contribution of the travel and tourism industry to the financial health and wealth of the region, CARICOM Heads and COHSOD - Health working group on regional coordination for the management of the virus, mandated CARPHA to lead the development of various regional guidelines for the management of cases on cruise ships, aircrafts, hotels, and among hotel staff.

Other organizations, such as the Global Tourism Resilience and Crisis Management Centre (GTRCMC), are working closely with CARPHA as the regional health lead in the GTRCMC, to promote a multisectoral coordinated response with academia, private and public health care providers, and tourism agencies for protecting Caribbean travel and tourism during the global coronavirus global crisis. During the response, the Head of the GTRCMC called upon the global travel and tourism industry to play a pivotal role in shaping global response efforts, with a focus on preventing exposure beyond the currently affected areas as well as to isolate infected persons from uninfected populations" (20).

CARPHA is also working with the Caribbean Tourism Organization (CTO), the region's tourism development agency, and the Caribbean Hotel and Tourism Association (CHTA) with which it shares an MOU to enhance the health and safety of tourism and protect the tourism product. In keeping with their mandate of sustainable tourism, they facilitate the sustainability of tourism in the region through liaising with their partners, members, and stakeholders and providing technical advice on important issues e.g., standards development; the execution of projects on issues such as climate change, disaster risk management, energy efficiency (21).

Recognizing that tourism is the lifeblood of the Caribbean region and the essential need to safeguard the health and safety of residents and visitors to mitigate the impact of the COVID-19 threat to the region; and further recognizing the importance of building upon the collaborative efforts which are already underway, and the need to pool organizational resources to do so. On March 4, 2020 CARPHA, CHTA, GTRCMC formalize their efforts and messaging through the establishment of the COVID-19 Caribbean Tourism Task Force (CCTTF). The organizations acknowledged concerns about the high level of misunderstanding about the virus, which has elevated the panic level globally and resulted in the dissemination of a high level of misinformation. The CCTTF aim is to focus on sharing accurate information; strengthening monitoring at airports, sea ports, and hotels and accommodations; improving coordination among stakeholder organizations and locally between tourism and health officials; sharing best practices; training and education; and conducting tourism impact research. This agreement allows for rapid cross-sectional movement of resources, planning, targeted response, and messaging in response to this emergency. Other tourism specific response actions that were recommended include:

- Ensuring an inventory of the tourism properties with preparedness action plans and supporting plan development and testing
- Ensuring knowledge of protocols for management of illness among staff and guests
- Ensuring a protocol for reporting any illness to the Ministry of Health is in place
- CTO/CHTA work with CARPHA for Regional Level Training and Communications

Immigration, customs and security sectors

The Caribbean Community (CARICOM) Implementation Agency for Crime and Security (IMPACS) was established by the Conference of Heads of Government in July 2006, as the implementation arm of a new Regional Architecture to manage CARICOM's action agenda on crime and security (22). IMPACS played a significant role in the RCM-HS primarily through their Joint Regional Communications Centre (JRCC), that has responsibility for the operations and management of the Advance Passenger Information System (APIS), which screens approximately forty (40) Million passengers annually, specifically those entering, and traveling within the CARICOM Region by air and sea ports (23). The information provided from APIS enabled countries to effectively monitor passengers arriving from high-risk settings, in the early stages of the outbreak.

In addition, immigration and customs departments were advised to take various sector-specific actions; viz:

- Provision of national protocols for personal protective equipment (PPE) use by Immigration and Customs personnel
- Receiving training on critical areas such as: infection prevention and control and handling of specimens or reagents for testing of

COVID-19; strengthening passenger surveillance; and granting practice for cruise ships
- Participate in national emergency preparedness planning processes

The Security Sector engaged in various sector-specific actions, including:

- Ensuring the Security of Government Ministers and Key Officials as identified by the Cabinet
- Ensuring areas requiring additional security are identified as requested by Ministries of Health, e.g., quarantine or isolation centers, the main government stores of PPE, specialized health equipment and medicines, and the supply chain.

The Caribbean Disaster Emergency Management Agency

The Caribbean Disaster Emergency Management Agency (CDEMA) is a regional inter-governmental agency for disaster management in the Caribbean Community (CARICOM). The agency operates based on the principles of Comprehensive Disaster Management (CDM): an integrated and proactive approach to disaster management and seeks to reduce the risk and loss associated with natural and technological hazards and the effects of climate change to enhance regional sustainable development (24). Through its Regional Response Mechanism (RRM) - a network of CDEMA Participating States (PSs), national, regional and international disaster stakeholders through which external response and relief operations in support of an impacted CDEMA Participating State (PS) are coordinated, CDEMA is recognized as the leader in regional disaster management. During the COVID-19 response, CDEMA's role was to identify the combined resources available and appropriately match these to the needs of the impacted state(s), and effectively coordinate a response in the context of a global health threat (25).

Recognizing the wide-scale impact of COVID-19 across multiple sectors and the need for a coordinated response from whole of government, in addition to the key actions taken across multiple sectors, specific actions recommended for those in the private and education sectors included:

Private sector

- Determining critical processes for maintaining operations of the Businesses
- Determining numbers and persons for maintaining operations
- Development of alternate working arrangements e.g., telework

Education sector

- Establishment of reporting protocols for illness in staff and students
- Determining critical levels of staff required to keep schools open
- Ensuring parents receive instructions re reporting illness
- Ensuring that for institutions with residential facilities/health stations, there are guidelines for managing illness, quarantine, and reporting illness to the Ministry of Health for staff and students.

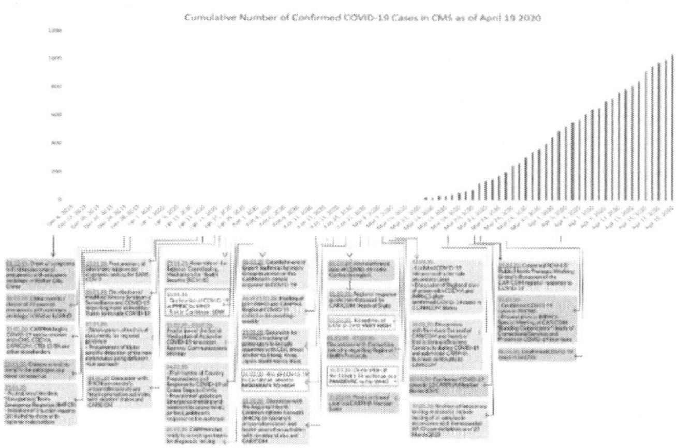

Figure 2. Timeline of Regional Actions and initial imported cases of COVID 19 to CARICOM Member States up to April 19, 2020

CONCLUSION

Caribbean Countries have rallied together to mount a regional response to the COVID-19 pandemic. Preparedness efforts in the region may have contributed to delayed importation of cases and afforded countries in the region time to shore up their health sectors and enabled a more robust whole of government response. The heightened level of vigilance not only at the country level, but across regional health security systems, is evidence of the early recognition of the risks of importation of cases on the health and wellbeing of the region's population (see Figure 2).

The regional coordination efforts, including the leadership of CARICOM and CARPHA as health lead, brought together a wide range of stakeholders and resulted in a coordinated approach to regional health security. The regional response was based on the utilization of existing networks and support systems for health security that saw cohesion and rapid response among key stakeholders. The ability to mobilize regional partners and their respective resources are based on these existing relationships between and within agencies and systems that facilitated ease of understanding amongst the various players.

Notwithstanding there were gaps in the regional response, some of which were influenced by the general lack of knowledge and understanding of the effect of the novel virus on human health, the lack of epidemiological evidence to inform response and the fragility of the CARICOM region to a new and emerging health threat. While there is no scientific evidence of whether the measures implemented by Member States were effective to delay the importation of cases to the region, the earliest confirmed cases imported to the region were exposed outside of the region in areas where containment measures had failed.

The COVID-19 outbreak provided an opportunity to test the regional mechanisms for health security. The early response, support from regional Heads of Government, and the subsequent level of preparedness revealed that there is strong regional capacity for health security, despite the gaps identified in some areas. The Regional Coordinating Mechanism for Health security should continue to assess the internal capacity of its members and devise more cohesive and transparent methods for collaboration between members.

Acknowledgment

The authors would like to acknowledge and appreciate the staff of the Caribbean Public Health Agency and those of the various partners and members of the Regional Coordinating Mechanism for Heath Security for their hard work, resilience and devotion during the COVID-19 pandemic. A special thanks to Dr. Sastee Kissoodan, Behavioral Science Intern in the Surveillance Disease Prevention and Control Department for her contributions to developing the figures included in this paper. We would also like to acknowledge staff in CARPHA Member States who have ensured that the recommendations and actions have been implemented.

Declaration of Conflict of Interest

The authors declare that they do not have any conflicts of interest with respect to this paper.

References

[1] Rhiney K. Geographies of Caribbean vulnerability in a changing climate: issues and trends. Geography Compass 2015;9(3):97-114.

[2] Colón-González FJ, Peres CA, Steiner São Bernardo C, Hunter PR, Lake IR. After the epidemic: Zika virus projections for Latin America and the Caribbean. PLoS Negl Trop Dis 2017;11(11):e0006007.

[3] Van Bortel W, Dorleans F, Rosine J, Blateau A, Rousset D, Matheus S, et al. Chikungunya outbreak in the Caribbean region, December 2013 to March 2014, and the significance for Europe. Euro Surveill 2014;19(13):20759.

[4] Insurance Information Institute. Facts and statistics: Hurricanes13 March 2020. URL: https://www.iii.org/fact-statistic/facts-statistics-hurricanes.

[5] Glassman A, Gaziano TA, Bouillon Buendia CP, Guanais de Aguiar FC. Confronting the chronic disease burden in Latin America and the Caribbean. Health Aff 2010;29(12):2142-8.
[6] Organization WH. Health Security 2020. URL: https://www.who.int/health-security/en/.
[7] Chan DM. Ten years in public health, 2007–2017. Geneva: World Health Organization, 2017.
[8] World Health Organization. The world health report 2007: A safer future: global public health security in the 21st century. Geneva: World Health Organization, 2007.
[9] Alleyne G, Sealey K. [Cooperación Caribeña en materia de salud]. Integr Latinoam 1991;16(164):13-20.
[10] Carrillo Roa A, Santana JPd. Regional integration and south-south cooperation in health in Latin America and the Caribbean. Rev Panam Salud Publica 2012;32:368-75.
[11] Hospedales CJ. Caribbean public health: achievements and future challenges. Lancet Public Health. 2019;4(7):e324.
[12] World Health Organization. Clinical management of severe acute respiratory infection when novel coronavirus (2019-nCoV) infection is suspected: interim guidance, 28 January 2020. Geneva: World Health Organization, 2020.
[13] Zhou F, Yu T, Du R, Fan G, Liu Y, Liu Z, et al. Clinical course and risk factors for mortality of adult inpatients with COVID-19 in Wuhan, China: A retrospective cohort study. Lancet 2020;395(10229):P1054-62.
[14] World Health Organization.. WHO Director-General's opening remarks at the media briefing on COVID-19 - 5 March 20202020 10 March 2020. URL: https://www.who.int/dg/speeches/detail/who-director-general-s-opening-remarks-at-the-media-briefing-on-covid-19---5-march-2020.
[15] Association CLI. Statement on COVID-19. URL: https://cruising.org/news-and-research/press-room/2020/march/clia-covid-19-toolkit.
[16] Cruise Industry News. US State Department. Issues cruise travel warning 2020 Mar 23 March. URL: https://www.cruiseindustrynews.com/cruise-news/22559-u-s-state-dept-issues-cruise-travel-warning.html.
[17] Al-Arshani S. Passengers on the Grand Princess said they found out 21 people on the ship tested positive for coronavirus from the news. URL: https://www.businessinsider.com.au/cruise-ship-passengers-not-told-21-people-had-new-coronavirus-2020-3.
[18] Vara V. Cautious sails: Coronavirus (Covid-19) measures and impact on the cruise industry. Ship Technol. 2020 Mar 23. URL: https://www.ship-technology.com/features/coronavirus-outbreak-2019-ncov-impact-cruise-operators-measures-tourism/.
[19] Parsanlal N. Caribbean Airlines gears up for COVID-192020. URL: http://www.looptt.com/content/caribbean-airlines-gears-covid-19.

[20] Global Tourism Resilience and Management Center. Multisectoral coordination for protecting Caribbean travel and tourism for novel Coronavirus (COVID-19). URL: http://gtrcmc.org/news/multisectoral-coordination-protecting-caribbean-travel-and-tourism-novel-coronavirus

[21] Caribbean Tourism Organization. Our work 2020. The CTO's mission is to provide to and through its members, the services and information needed for the development of sustainable tourism for the economic and social benefit of the Caribbean people. URL: https://www.onecaribbean.org/our-work/.

[22] CARICOM IMPACS. Caribbean Community for Crime and Security 2020. URL: https://www.caricomimpacs.org/aboutus.

[23] CARICOM IMPACS. Joint Regional Communication Centre 2020. URL: https://www.caricomimpacs.org/subagencies.

[24] Caribbean Disaster Emergency Management Agency. About us. URL: https://www.cdema.org/about-us.

[25] Caribbean Disaster Emergency Management Agency. Regional response mechanism (RRM). URL: https://www.cdema.org/rrm.

In: Public Health Themes in Grenada … ISBN: 978-1-53618-118-0
Editors: J. Merrick and L. Glasgow

Chapter 5

RAINWATER HARVESTING WATER QUALITY PARAMETERS RELEVANT TO THE CARIBBEAN REGION: A SHORT OVERVIEW

Adrian Cashman[1,*], CEng, BSc(Eng), MSc(EEEM), DIC, PhD, MCIWEM
and Clive Carpenter[2], BSc(Hons), MSc, FGS, CGeol, MCIWEM, CWEM, EurGeol, AMAE
[1]AKWATIX Water Resources Management, Barbados, Formerly Centre for Resource Management and Environmental Studies, University of the West Indies, Barbados and [2]Head of Water Resources GWP,
Consultants LLP, Oxfordshire, UK

* Correspondence: Dr. Adrian Cashman, AKWATIX Water Resources Management, Ashford Plantation, St. John, Barbados, West Indies. Email: adrian.c.cashman@gmail.com.

Abstract

Harvesting rainwater for domestic use has been practiced for millennia and in recent historical times in the Caribbean. It is increasingly being put forward as a climate adaptation strategy. However, if it is to be promoted, due consideration has to be given by authorities to water quality. Although there is much literature on rainwater harvesting, the absence of specific regulatory responsibility for domestic rainwater harvesting means that there are few definitive guidelines for monitoring and testing. This short chapter aims to contribute to a better understanding of which water quality parameters might be of interest. This, though, needs to be coupled with a systematic approach to water safety assessment and planning.

Introduction

Rainwater harvesting, as a source of domestic water use, has been practiced around the world for millennia (1). In recent times it has been increasingly put forward as a resilience and adaptation response to climate change and climate variability (2), and a water security response in the aftermath of extreme events when formal water systems might be compromised to a greater or lesser extent. The technicalities around the sizing, design, and configuration of systems for harvesting rainwater are relatively straight forward and understood. However, as more attention is given to rainwater harvesting as a climate adaptation intervention, what might be called the 'governance aspects' are coming under increasing scrutiny. These include the relationship with public health and questions of responsibility for ensuring appropriate water quality if authorities encourage the adoption of rainwater harvesting. A key part would be understanding what water quality parameters might be appropriate for the different potential uses of harvested rainwater.

This paper is a brief overview of water quality aspects that have been associated with domestic rainwater harvesting systems (DRWHS). It is based on a literature review of some 60 published reports, guidance documents, and peer-reviewed journal articles. The focus of the review is to indicate the water quality issues that have been associated with DRWHS and, in particular, those that have been identified as having a potential impact on water safety and human health. It should be stated that there is a great deal of literature available on the quality of harvested rainwater and there is a high degree of consensus around which are the most important aspects potentially affecting human health. Another important point is that many of the studies reported in journal articles are concerned with a particular water quality aspect peculiar to a set of environmental conditions that are seldom widely replicable. An example of such a study is reported by Báez et al. (3), which considered the chemical composition of rainwater collected in Mexico City. One of the purposes of the study was to determine the extent to which the atmospheric pollution present in Mexico City affected rainwater quality. Given its focus, the study looked at an extensive range of parameters. A similar study, also in Mexico City, considered rainwater used to provide drinking water fountains on a university campus. Such studies are informative as they consider the role and impact of atmospheric conditions, albeit under circumstances that are unlikely to be replicated in the Caribbean.

It is also apparent from the review that water quality standards are an issue. In general, there are no specific water quality standards covering DRWHS. That said, in most instances, it is the World Health Organisation Drinking Water Quality Standards that are used as the benchmark. A further difficulty with the application of appropriate standards is that DRWHS tend to fall outside of the drinking water quality regulatory regime and, as a result, monitoring and testing tend to be carried out on an ad hoc basis. The main focus of concern relates to risks associated with bacteriological contamination and the effects on human health associated with gastrointestinal diseases.

The presented evidence with respect to links between bacteriological contamination of water used for domestic purposes e.g., drinking, washing, cooking, but not outdoor uses and gastrointestinal diseases, is ambiguous. The guidance on use of rainwater tanks produced by the Commonwealth of Australia (4) notes that studies;

> "found no measurable difference in rates of gastrointestinal illness in children who drank rainwater compared to those who drank mains water. However, there are examples of *Campylobacter* and *Salmonella* enteritis associated with rainwater tanks and one example of cryptosporidiosis/ giardiasis associated with an underground tank."

On the other hand, several case studies have linked gastrointestinal illnesses with the consumption of untreated rainwater sources (5). This is supported by evidence from the Caribbean, particularly studies of DRWHS water quality in the Grenadines, West Indies. Ahmed et al. (5) concluded that health risk assessment models should be used to manage and mitigate health risks associated with drinking and non-potable uses of harvested rainwater. In general, though, harvested rainwater, when properly collected, stored, and treated can provide a safe and reliable source of supply.

CONTAMINATION SOURCES AND HEALTH CONCERNS

Following the approach adopted in the "Handbook of rainwater harvesting in the Caribbean" (6), the following section sets out the potential sources of contamination and their associated health risks.

Contamination from Atmospheric Sources

Rainwater, as it starts to fall, is a very pure form of water. However, as it falls, it interacts with pollutants in the air, either reacting with them or absorbing them into raindrops. For example, the atmosphere contains carbon compounds, and their interaction with water gives rise to a weak carbonic acid, which can corrode materials it comes into contact with. However, the concentrations are so low that they pose no threat to human health. The presence of other physical particles and chemical compounds that may be entrained or react with rainwater depends on the activities and sources of pollution that emit or otherwise give rise to them. These do not have to originate in the local vicinity as contaminants can be carried by air currents and winds over considerable distances; the finer the particles, the further they can be transported. Airborne contaminants can either be of geomorphic or anthropogenic origin; Sahara dust, for example, is of geomorphic origin. Anthropogenic activity has substantially increased the concentration of trace metals in the atmosphere as well as manufactured chemicals emitted through industrial processes or other activities such as the burning of fossil fuels and the use of pesticides, insecticides, and fertilizers. Generally, airborne contamination is a problem in developed countries where industrial activity contributes to poor air quality and airborne pollution. Studies, such as those carried out in Mexico City indicate that in urban settings, air pollution is a risk factor that requires monitoring as high concentrations of trace metals have been associated with increased health risks. Agriculture, too, can pose a threat where there is widespread use of chemicals and fertilizers.

In the Caribbean, the main sources of ambient airborne pollution are associated with vehicle and transport emissions, industrial and waste disposal operations. As already mentioned, Sahara dust is a known source of airborne pollution, which varies intra- and inter-annually and has been associated with respiratory difficulties. In the Pacific region, the presence of volcanic ash was noted as a potential risk factor. Wet and dry deposition of the dust particles could be an issue but is unlikely to have any significant water quality impact. Of more concern would be airborne particulates associated with bushfires or of geomorphic origin, mobilize from dry surfaces by wind, particularly during dry periods. With increasing aridity associated with climate change, greater influxes of dust, and mobilization of geomorphic particles (soil and trace elements e.g., magnesium), some consideration of their impact on operation and maintenance procedures should be given. Peters (7), in his study of rainwater harvesting practices in Carriacou noted that poor harvesting practices, particularly with respect to the maintenance of collection surfaces, were correlated with poor water quality.

Contamination during rainwater capture

Catchment contamination can be physical, chemical, or biological. Physical contamination refers to the dry deposition on the catchment surface of airborne particulate matter or the deposition of organic and non-organic matter. The airborne particulate matter has been considered above and would be washed off the surface during rainfall events. Organic matter (biological contamination) refers to vegetation and fecal matter deposited on the rainwater collecting surfaces. The fecal matter could be of either avian or other animal origins and is probably one of the main hazards of concern noted in the literature. Fecal matter is of concern because it is associated in the literature with the transmission of harmful pathogens, such as legionella, cryptosporidium, and giardia lamblia. These are of concern if there is a direct connection to sources of water, but there are other risk factors to consider, such as the time between deposition and entry through flushing. The risk can be significantly reduced by a combination of disinfection and ultrafiltration. In general, most fecal pollution from man and animals occurs at or below ground level, so water collected from raised roof catchments is likely to be of better bacteriological quality than that collected from ground-level catchments. Studies have highlighted the high variability in the presence of contaminants among different systems, their configuration, operation, and maintenance.

Decaying vegetation would affect physical characteristics such as color and taste, and chemical properties such as level of dissolved oxygen as well as chemical and biological reactions (e.g., algal growth). Under certain circumstances, high levels of chlorine used during disinfection interacting with naturally occurring organic material can give rise to the production of harmful by-products; but as the WHO states, "the risks to health from these by-products are extremely small in comparison with the risks associated with inadequate disinfection." Non-organic matter, other than the particulates referred to above, could be materials and items that are on the collection surface, concrete blocks, and discarded items.

Chemical contamination may occur if the catchment surface consists of materials that have a coating that can leach or be dissolved in water that collects on the surface. This could be related to the use of roofing sheets coated with toxic paints (containing lead and other compounds), asphalt coverings, shingles, or other forms of covering. Although the use of lead-based paints has been phased out, there are still roofs that could be painted with them. A further potential hazard noted in the literature is the potential chemical reaction between deposited material and the roofing materials. Research, though, indicates that chemical contamination is not a major concern, while geographic location and type of exposure are more important factors.

Contamination during storage

This is probably the most important part of the linkages between harvested rainwater and humans as it is from storage that water is taken for use and consumption. The quality of stored water depends on factors such as the measures to prevent contamination before it enters storage, the residence time, maintenance practices, and the environmental exposure of the storage vessel. The inclusion of a filtration and disinfection system as part of the system greatly reduces the risk of infection and the use of contaminated water, which would otherwise pose a risk.

A common issue with storage is that it can provide a breeding place for mosquitos, which, although it does not pose a direct health threat through ingestion, puts people at risk of vector-borne diseases transmitted via mosquitoes, such as Dengue, Chikungunya, Zika, Malaria, and other potentially emerging vector-borne diseases. Prevention and control are, therefore, highly important. Traditional vector control measures have included the introduction of predatory fish that feed on mosquito larvae. In addition, other animals need to be excluded from access to the water storage, such as vermin (rodents, other insects), frogs, and toads, as they too can transmit potentially harmful pathogens. Once storage tanks are fitted with properly fitting lids, all openings are screened, and water extracted using a tap or pump, the likelihood of contamination can be reasonably reduced. With control over the introduction of new contamination (through the use of screens and first-flush diverters), any bacteria and other pathogens that are in the tank will eventually die-off, resulting in improvement of the stored water over time.

There are additional risks associated with the use of below-ground cisterns. Poor construction practices could allow seepage through cistern walls. In areas where use is made of septic tanks and soakaways, there is a further risk of contamination via groundwater ingress. Other risks are associated with potential flooding. Polluted floodwaters, particularly when contaminated with human septage, might inundate below-ground cisterns. If this happens then the water would be unusable and have to be drained, and the cistern disinfected.

Whilst above ground storage would not be as susceptible to flooding, exposure to outdoor elements may pose minor risks. For example, stored water temperatures are likely to be higher, and if pathogens are present, such as legionella, then this would provide favorable reproduction conditions.

The message with respect to storage is that minimizing health risks and maintaining good water quality can be achieved through the proper design of a DRWHS, preventing sources of contamination entering the storage together with proper maintenance procedures that prevent the build-up of sediments and conditions for algal growth.

Contamination during maintenance

The last link in the chain where risks to human health may occur is during the cleaning and maintenance of the collection and storage components of the DRWHS. Maintenance tasks include the cleaning and disinfection of collection surfaces, guttering, and piping; desilting, tank cleaning and disinfection; cleaning or replacement of screens, and traps. These are hands-on activities that use cleaning chemicals. Care needs to be exercised that material is not transferred from one part of the system to another or foreign material is introduced, such as on footwear.

WATER QUALITY TESTING

As indicated above, there are not any water quality standards specific to harvested rainwater. The applicable standards are those which would relate to the use of the water, whether for potable or non-potable use. In the absence of national standards for drinking water, the WHO standards have been widely adopted. The problem is not, therefore, an absence of standards but rather of a regulatory regime that addresses and enforces a requisite level of water quality sampling, testing, monitoring, and reporting requirements, and lays down codes of practices governing the installation, operation, and maintenance of DRWHS. Some jurisdictions have developed regulatory regimes, particularly where DRWHS are an important part of the national water supply landscape. Water quality criteria depend on the political and social setting as well as resources and capacity available. Generally, the better off a country, the more developed its regulatory system would be. Examples from the literature of countries that have regulations include; Australia, Bermuda, the United States, US Virgin Islands, United Kingdom, though this is not exhaustive.

Parameters

The following parameters have been mentioned in papers and reports in connection with the testing of the water quality of harvested rainwater. This is an extensive list, and it is unlikely that these would all normally be tested for. In the literature where proposals are made with respect to which parameters to test for, the range is very limited. This probably reflects the understanding of the practical challenges and difficulties involved. Most propose between 4 and 5 parameters, with an emphasis on biological parameters associated with gastrointestinal illnesses.

	Parameter	Comment
	Physical	
X	pH	Frequently mentioned
	Conductivity	Frequently mentioned
	Alkalinity	Mentioned
	Hardness	Probably not necessary
	Turbidity (NTU)	Mentioned
	Temperature	Infrequently mentioned
	Odour	Seldom mentioned
	Colour (Hazen Units)	Seldom mentioned
	Total Dissolved Solids (TDS)	Mentioned
	Total Suspended Solids (TSS)	Mentioned
	Chemical	
	Chemical Oxygen Demand (COD)	Mentioned
	Dissolved Oxygen	Infrequently mentioned
	NO_3 – N Nitrate	Frequently mentioned
	Nitrites	Seldom mentioned
X	NH_4 – N Ammonia	Frequently mentioned
	SO_4 Sulphate	Mentioned
	Cl- Chloride	Mentioned
X	Cl Residual	
	PO_4 Phosphorus	Frequently mentioned
	Pb Lead	Infrequently mentioned
	Fe Iron	Infrequently mentioned
	Al Aluminium	Infrequently mentioned
	Cd Cadmium	Infrequently mentioned
	Zn Zinc	Infrequently mentioned
	Br Bromide (Residual)	Seldom mentioned
	B Boron	Seldom mentioned
	Mg Magnesium	Seldom mentioned
	Na Sodium	Seldom mentioned
	Ni Nickel	Seldom mentioned
	K Potassium	Infrequently mentioned
	Mn Manganese	Seldom mentioned
	Cu Copper	Seldom mentioned
	As Arsenic	Seldom mentioned
	Cr Chromium	Infrequently mentioned
	Se Selenium	Seldom mentioned
	TOC Total Organic Carbon	Infrequently mentioned
	DOC Dissolved Organic Carbon	Infrequently mentioned

	TPC Total Particulate Carbon	Infrequently mentioned
	Biological	
X	TC Total Coliforms	Frequently mentioned
	Faecal Coliforms	Frequently mentioned
X	Escherichia coli (E-coli)	Frequently mentioned
	Enterococci	Not frequently mentioned
	Legionella	Not frequently mentioned
	Giardia lamblia	Not frequently mentioned
	Salmonella	Not frequently mentioned
	Cryptosporidium	Not frequently mentioned
	Camplyobacter	Not frequently mentioned
	Shigella	Not frequently mentioned
	Psuedodomenas	Not frequently mentioned
	Vibrio	Not frequently mentioned
	Mosquito larvae	Mentioned
	Dead animals & faecal droppings	Frequently mentioned
	In a few cases mention was made of testing for viruses and pathogens	

	Mentioned by the UK Environment Agency
	Mentioned by Texas RWH Manual
X	Suggested parameters for testing – taken from the literature

CONCLUSION

Harvested rainwater is used around the world as a source of water for domestic purposes. Under certain circumstances, contact with sources of pollution can result in adverse health outcomes, especially among more vulnerable members of the population. If authorities are going to promote DWRHS as a climate adaptation strategy or a response to the adverse effects of extreme events that disrupt normal supplies, then more attention will have to be paid to the public health dimensions. This paper has aimed to make a contribution to the discussion that has to be had around what an appropriate monitoring and testing regime might look like and which parameters should be considered for inclusion. It is recommended that this has to be part of a process of water safety assessment and planning to ensure that whatever systems are put in place are appropriate, fit for purpose, and responsive to the potential hazard exposure.

ACKNOWLEDGMENTS

This work was carried out as part of the Investment Plan for the Caribbean Regional Track of the Pilot Program for Climate Resilience – Rainwater Harvesting Assessment, Mapping and Manual Development, and Training project and also supported by the Mona Office for Research and Innovation, University of the West Indies, Mona Campus, Climate Investment Funds, Inter-American Development Bank, and the Caribbean Public Health Agency. All opinions expressed are solely those of the author.

RECOMMENDED LITERATURE

- Environment Agency. Harvesting rainwater for domestic uses: an informational guide. Bristol, UK: Environment Agency, 2010.
- Environmental Protection Department. Guidelines for the submission of building development applications to the Environmental Protection Department. Bridgetown, Barbados: Environmental Protection Department, 2015.
- Gispert M, Hernandez M, Climent E, Flores M. Rainwater harvesting as a drinking water option for Mexico City, 2018. doi:10.3390/su10113890.
- Health. Guidance on use of rainwater tanks. Sydney: Commonwealth of Australia, 2011.
- Intven L. Scaling up domestic rainwater harvesting St Cuthbet's Mission, Guyana. Quebec, Canada: McGill University, 2009.
- Kohlitz J, Smith M. Water quality management for domestic rainwater harvesting systems in Fiji. Water Sci Technol 2015;15(1):134-41.

- Mendes C, Afshar B, Kinney K, Barrett M, Kirisits, M. Effect of roof material on water quality for rainwater harvesting systems. Austin, TX: Texas Water Development Board, 2010.
- RAIN. RAIN water quality guidelines. Amsterdam: Rain Foundation, 2008.
- Reijtenbagh R. Minimum design requirements for domestic rainwater-harvesting systems on small volcanic islands in the Eastern Caribbean to prevent related water quality and quantity issues. Delft: Delft University of Technology, 2010.
- Stewart A. Microbial quality of domestic water quality in rural communities of the southern Caribbean. St Augustine, Trinidad: University of the West Indies, Department Life Sciences, 2018.
- Texas Water Development Board. The Texas manual on rainwater harvesting, Third edition. Austin, TX: Texas Water Development Board, 2005.
- Department of Planning and Natural Resources. Water quality standards for waters of the Virgin Islands. Virgin Islands: Department of Planning and Natural Resources, 2015.
- World Meteorological Organization. Planning water quality monitoring systems. Technical Report Series No 3. Geneva: World Meteorological Organization, 2013.

REFERENCES

[1] Yannopoulos S, Antoniou G, Kaiafa-Saropoulou M, Angelakis N. Historical development of rainwater harvesting and use in Hellas: A preliminary review. Water Sci Technol 2017;17:1022-34.

[2] Kahinda J, Taigbenu A, Boroto R. Domestic rainwater harvesting as an adaptation measure to climate change in South Africa. Physics Chem Earth 2010;35(13-14):742-51.

[3] Baez A, Belmont R, Garcia R, Padilla H, Torres M. Chemical composition of rainwater collected at a southwest site of Mexico City, Mexico. Atmospheric Res 2007;86:61-75.

[4] Chubaka C, Whiley H, Edwards J, Ross K. A review of roof harvested rainwater in Australia. J Environ Public Health 2018;2018:6471324. https://doi.org/10.1155/2018/6471324.

[5] Ahmed W, Gardner T, Toze S. Microbiological quality of roof-harvested rainwater and health risks: A review. J Environ Qual 2010;40:1-9.

[6] Caribbean Environmental Health Institute. A handbook on rainwater harvesting in the Caribbean. Castries, St Lucia: Caribbean Environmental Health Institute, 2009.

[7] Peters E. Water quality of rainwater cisterns in the Grenadines. West Indies J Engineering 2011;33(1/2):56-64.

In: Public Health Themes in Grenada … ISBN: 978-1-53618-118-0
Editors: J. Merrick and L. Glasgow © 2020 Nova Science Publishers, Inc.

Chapter 6

BACTERIAL VAGINOSIS IN WOMEN OF REPRODUCTIVE AGES IN LATIN AMERICA AND THE CARIBBEAN: A LITERATURE REVIEW

Attah Timothy Adejoh, BSc, MPH
and Gerard St Cyr*, CPH, MPH, MSci (cand)
Department of Public Health and Preventive Medicine,
St George's University, True Blue, St George's, Grenada

ABSTRACT

The objectives of this chapter are to (i) to summarize the prevalence of bacterial vaginosis (BV) in Latin America and the Caribbean and (ii) review risk factors associated with BV and (iii) review health complications associated with BV. Using key search terms such as bacterial vaginosis, Latin America, and the Caribbean, a combination of

* Correspondence: Mr. Gerard S Cyr,, Instructor, Department of Public Health and Preventive Medicine, St George's University, St George's, Grenada, West Indies. Email: gstcyr@sgu.edu.

1,206 articles from EBSCO and PubMed were assessed for inclusion. Six articles met the inclusion criteria, and were retrieved and used in this review. Columbia had the highest prevalence of BV (39.6%), while Grenada in 2009 had the lowest prevalence (16.1%). Other regions had a prevalence ranging from 21.0-32.0%. In Bogota (Columbia), the most common co-infection was between BV and C. trichomatis 78 (14.0%) followed by BV and Candida 41 cases (7.5%), and occasional sexual relationship, being a sex worker, weekly consuming alcohol, and older ages were significantly associated with BV. Of this, 10% of women who had co-infection in Pacoti (Brasil), BV, and human papillomavirus (HPV) were the most common (14%). In Grenada, the most common co-infection was Candida (3.6%, 95% CI: 2.9-4.5). Parity was significantly associated with cervical pathology (OR = 0.51, 95% CI: 0.31, 0.83, p = 0.007) among women with BV. Studies within the Latin American and Caribbean regions had a low to average prevalence of BV. However, only limited studies have been conducted, and there may be possibilities of increasing patterns within different study populations. Therefore, more population-based studies with scientifically appropriate methodologies should be conducted in order to determine the population-based prevalence, associated risk factors, possible co-infections, and the trend in the prevalence of BV in Latin America and the Caribbean.

INTRODUCTION

Bacterial vaginosis (BV) is a polymicrobial vaginal infection which causes an alteration in the naturally occurring vaginal microbiota, as a result of a reduction in the naturally occurring Lactobacillus and an invasion of aerobic pathogens such as gardnerella vaginalis, G. prevotella, mycoplasma hominis, peptostreptococcus, and bacteroides spp. which rapidly multiplies in the vagina of women of reproductive ages (1-5). Formerly known as Gardnerella vaginitis, the infection derives its name from G. vaginalis; a microbe which was first isolated from the genital of infected females, and was implicated as the causal microbe in 1892 (6, 7). Although the presence of G. vaginalis remains strongly associated with BV, subsequent scientific findings have been able to isolate G. vaginalis from women who are asymptomatic and never end up with BV, thereby disputing the primary role G. vaginalis plays in the identification of BV (8-10). About 50% of women infected with BV are asymptomatic; however, symptoms of BV may include milky discharge from the vagina, which often has a foul smell, and abdominal pain, which could get worse after the menstrual cycle (10).

To diagnose BV, a swab of vaginal discharge of the lateral and posterior vagina wall and assayed for an alkaline pH (>4.5) or clue cells using wet mount microscopy (11, 12). Gram staining and Nugent scoring are widely considered the gold standards for BV. This criteria identifies and estimates the number of Lactobacillus and G. vaginalis, bacteroides, or mobiluncus in each field of a microscope slide and categorizes BV as normal bacterial flora (0-3 morphotypes), intermediate (4-6 morphotypes) and 4-7 morphotypes for the presence of BV (11, 12). Because this assay technique may not be practical in some sites, an alternative known as Amsel's criteria is usually considered as an alternative to the aforementioned techniques. Amsel's criteria identify BV using four key properties such as a fishy odor of vaginal discharge, pH above 4.5, thin homogenous discharge, and = 20% clue cells in saline microscopy (11, 12).

BV is considered one of the most common vaginal infections in women of reproductive ages, with 1 of 3 women getting infected with BV at some time in their life. The etiology is unknown as no clear case definition for the disease has been determined. While previous studies suggest BV to be sexually transmitted, some studies also suggest otherwise (13, 14). However, promiscuity remains a significant risk factor for BV among sexually active women with a greater risk among females who have sex with females, females who have oral sex and unprotected anal sex (15-17). Because this infection may be asymptomatic and poses no direct implications on infected females, it is usually not considered a major public health concern. However, evidence has identified BV as a significant risk factor for pregnancy/birth complications as well as sexually transmitted infections (STIs) such as herpes simplex virus type 2, Chlamydia trachomatis, Neisseria gonorrhoeae, Trichomonas vaginalis, and human immunodeficiency syndrome (HIV) among women of reproductive age. The risk for these infections highlights the significance of BV in causing multiple complications and the need to implement public health actions to control this infection/risk (18, 19). Some of the related birth complications associated with BV are preterm delivery and low birth weight in pregnancy (1, 20).

Preterm birth could result in poor cognitive functioning and other respiratory problems in low birth weight babies (1, 20).

Scientific studies in the United States (2000-2001) and the United Kingdom show a disproportionate distribution of BV among African American and Afro-Caribbean women when compared to other ethnicities, with higher risk amongst women of older ages and/ with multiple sexual partners (20-24). Studies in Africa also identified multiple sexual partners, previous history of spontaneous abortion orthodox religion followers, douching practices, and male circumcision as significant risk factors associated with this infection (20-24). Similar practices may exist among women of reproductive ages in Latin America and the Caribbean, which may elevate the risk and burden of the disease; however, only a few studies have been conducted to generate such findings from Latin America and the Caribbean. A review on the global epidemiology of BV revealed an intermediate prevalence of BV among subpopulations (Afro-Caribbean, African, Hispanic women) in developed countries, which may suggest there are similar trends within these regions (15). Given the undeniable importance of researching and controlling the burden of BV as it relates to other STIs and health complications, it may also be important to understand the level of risk in individual countries to recommend evidence-driven solutions.

Table 1. Studies in countries within Latin America and the Caribbean

Country	Countries where studies were selected
Caribbean	Grenada
Latin America	Brazil, Chile, Colombia, Chile, and Haiti

This study aims to summarize the epidemiology of BV in Latin America and the Caribbean. This review provides an understanding of the current BV epidemiology and will help raise awareness regarding the prevention and control of BV in women of reproductive age (14-49 years) in Latin America and the Caribbean. The objectives are; (i) To summarize the prevalence of BV in studies conducted within Latin America and the Caribbean, (ii) review risk factors associated with BV within the regions (iii) review health complications associated with BV in Latin America and the Caribbean.

OUR STUDY

In August 2016, the St George's University Library was used to conduct a literature search using EBSCO HOST and PubMed, and cited references were evaluated for inclusion. The search terms were bacterial vaginosis, lower genital tract infection, prevalence, women of reproductive age, and 15-54 years. This literature search resulted in 1,206 publications (873 articles from EBSCO, 318 articles from PubMed, and 15 articles from references).

Inclusion and exclusion criteria

All articles in English (or English translation) and free full-text articles published within the past ten years were considered for inclusion. Peer-reviewed articles that were assessed for inclusion provided information on the prevalence and risk factors associated with BV in Latin America and the Caribbean. Publications that used random sampling technique, population-based studies, antenatal/health care based samples, and reproductive health care center studies were preferably included in the review. When studies based on representative samples were not available, other studies conducted on special groups (pregnant women, women attending medical centers for HIV testing), were considered for inclusion. Only studies conducted on women of reproductive age (14-59 years), and studies using retrospective and cross-sectional designs were considered for inclusion in this review.

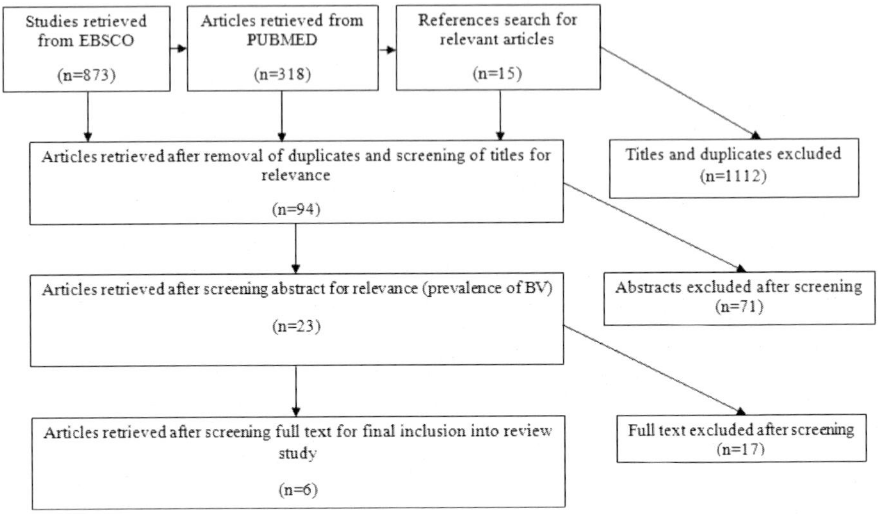

Figure 1. Summary of literature search.

Selection of studies

Figure 1 shows a flow diagram describing the stages of the study selection based on the inclusion and exclusion criteria, which led to the final selection of studies used in this review.

Data extraction

Six peer-reviewed articles from Latin America and the Caribbean were written in English (or English translation) and met the inclusion criteria for selection in the review. For each individual study, the following data were extracted; Age group, study design, country and city of study, study population, diagnostic criteria, sample size, sampling technique, and prevalence of BV. Figure 2 shows a summary of the sample sizes of studies conducted in Latin America and the Caribbean.

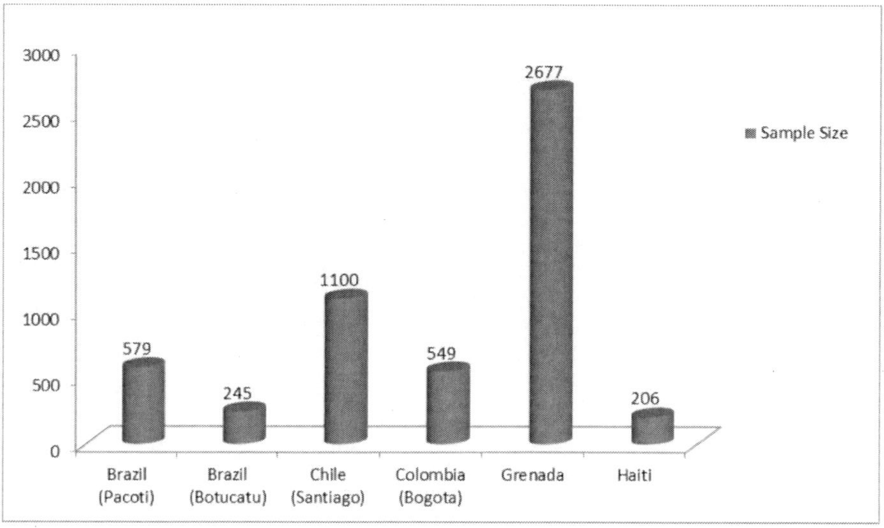

Figure 2. Summary of the sample sizes of students conducted in Latin America and the Caribbean.

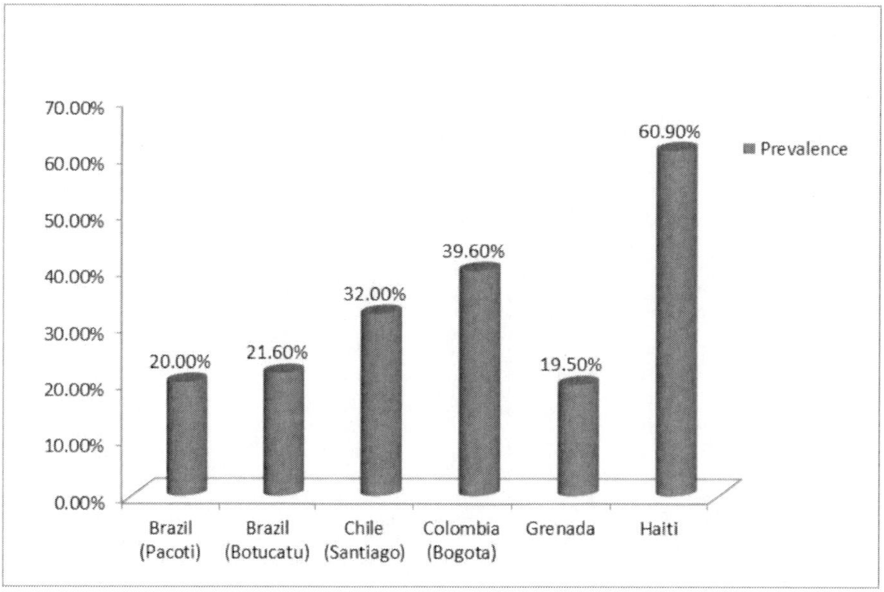

Figure 3. Prevalence of BV in studies conducted in Latin America and the Caribbean.

Table 2. Prevalence of bacterial vaginosis of four countries in the Caribbean and Latin America

Location	Study location, age group and date of study	Study design, Selection process, and Sample size	Diagnostic Procedure	Prevalence of BV % (Number)
Brazil	Pacoti, 12-49 years [26] 2007	Population based cross-sectional study of women of reproductive ages from 7 hamlets of and centre of Pacoti, (579 examined for BV)	Nugent scoring system	20.0 (116)
	Botucatu, 2006-2007[27]	Cross-sectional study of pregnant women (5-40 weeks of gestation) from 8 family health strategy units of primary care services, (245 examined for BV)	Nugent scoring system	21.6 (53)
Chile	Santiago, 16 -54 years 2006[28]	Cross sectional study of 100 randomly selected sexually active women attending Family Planning clinics.	Nugent Scoring System	32
Colombia	Bogota, 14-49 years, Feb-Dec 2010[29]	Cross-sectional study of women with lower genital tract infection at 3 healthcare attention centers, (549 examined for BV)	Nugent scoring system	39.6
Grenada	Grenada, 15-49 years, Jan 2009-Dec 2011[30]	Retrospective study of women of reproductive ages who had pap smear with a reported diagnosis of BV (2677 eligible women with BV within this period)	Pap smear test	19.5
		2009		16.1
		2010		21.0
		2011		21.4
Haiti	Rural Haiti, >18 years, Mar 2013[31]	Cross-sectional systematic sampling of consecutive women complaining of vaginal itching, discharge, pain or lesion associated urinary symptoms, (206 examined for BV)	Amsel criteria	60.9

FINDINGS

Figure 3 summarizes the prevalence of BV in the studies in Latin America and the Caribbean. Table 2 shows the prevalence of BV in the studies. Bogota, Columbia, had the highest prevalence (39.6%) followed by Chile (30.0%) when compared to other regions with prevalence ranging between 16.1%-28.2% (25-31). In Bogota, the largest co-infection was found between BV and C. trichomatis, 78 (14.0%), and BV and Candida, 41 (7.5%) (25). Also, a significant association between STIs and occasional sexual relationship, sex workers, weekly alcohol consumption, and older age was identified (25). In Pacoti, out of 10% of women who had co-infection, BV with HPV was the most common (14%) (23). However, not significant, BV was higher in women in older populations (23). In Grenada, the highest co-infection was found with Candida (3.6%, 95% CI: 2.9-4.5) (26). Parity was significantly associated with cervical pathology (OR = 0.51, 95% CI: 0.31, 0.83, $p = 0.007$) when nulliparous women were compared to women with 2 or more parity in women affected with BV (26). In Botucatu, 66.0% of women infected with BV had symptoms; 35.8% ($p = 00026$) with vaginal odor, and 50.0% with white vaginal discharge. 57.1% of participants who had normal flora had clinical vaginal signs. No significant association was identified with age, ethnicity, marital status, education, parity, or time of sample collection in Botucatu (24). Similarly, in rural Haiti, no risk factors were identified; however, 12.5% of infected women were identified to have increased vaginal discharge (27).

DISCUSSION

As illustrated in Figure 3, the prevalence of BV among women of reproductive ages in studies conducted within Latin America and the Caribbean was between 19.5-60.9%, with an average prevalence of 32.3% (30). Due to the absence of prevalence studies in some countries within the regions, the findings do not provide a generalized estimate of people who have been diagnosed with BV in the past ten years. We can suggest that due to the existence of similar epidemiological, geographical, and data availability characteristics of the countries in these regions, there may also be a similar prevalence of BV in countries where studies are lacking. Therefore, this review may be valuable to inform stakeholders of the possible risks in countries where studies were not conducted.

In order to present a recent review of BV estimates within Latin America and the Caribbean, only peer-reviewed articles conducted within the past ten years were included in this study. Although a literature review was published on the global epidemiology of BV, this review is the first of its kind that looks at the prevalence, risk factors, as well as co-infections or health complications associated with BV in these regions. This is expected to raise awareness on the prevalence of BV within Latin America and the Caribbean and inform advocacy for public health action to mitigate the potential risks of other STIs and health complications.

There are, however, some limitations related to the representativeness, diagnostic assay, and bias in this study. Only studies conducted within the past ten years met the criteria, hence, a small number of articles were eventually included in the review. This, therefore, limits the ability to estimate the prevalence of BV in the wider population. All studies were conducted with convenient samples, which may have introduced selection bias and prevented direct comparison between study populations in the regions. Only six studies were conducted within these regions, and no standard criteria of the study population for the literature search was used, which resulted in the inclusion of different study populations (population-based, married women, antenatal care based, or reproductive health care based) and prevented comparison between groups. Also, different diagnostic criteria were used to diagnose BV in women of reproductive ages, and because these techniques have different specificity and sensitivity as well as other properties, it may also affect the validity and prevent comparison between studies. In order to protect the reliability of the review, comparisons between groups were avoided. Similarly, variation in the prevalence of BV within the regions is consistent with results from other reviews; this suggests that the study is reproducible. However, no conclusion was drawn about the study population based on the studies included in this review.

Although the study conducted in Grenada (30) identified increasing prevalence of BV, yearly data in most countries within the study region has not been generated or readily available. In other cases, the results of the studies were not evaluated to identify prevalence trends. This lack of readily available data at the country level affects the ability to conduct studies with representative samples, resulting in the use of non-representative samples used in prevalence studies. Trend evaluation is often very important in evaluating disease outbreak amongst populations and can indicate whether there is a need for immediate public health action to prevent and control the disease within the population. This evaluation can be achieved by instituting an active surveillance system that captures all cases of BV within the country and as related to other STIs. Surveillance would make data readily available to conduct public health studies and to identify prevalence and risk factors for the disease in order to develop and execute evidence-based public health actions to control BV.

Based on scientific findings, BV infection in women has a high propensity of co-infection with other STIs as well as to lead to other health complications (25). BV infection was found to be strongly associated with HPV, which is also a significant risk factor associated with cervical cancers in females. Although insignificant, BV infection in pregnancy is associated with the risk of low birth weight and preterm delivery. Evidence within the Latin America and Caribbean regions are most likely to be identified in reproductive healthcare and antenatal care facilities. Because this infection is 50% asymptomatic, only individuals who display symptoms for BV and women who are pregnant are likely to be tested for BV and, as a result, BV statistics from these sites may be underreported.

A higher risk of BV in young women of reproductive ages was demonstrated in most studies conducted within these regions except for the study conducted in Pacoti, Brazil. Although the study in Brazil identified increased risks among the older population, the sample was not representative and, therefore, not comparable to other older populations, which may have resulted in the unusual disparity in the prevalence of BV

(26). This shows there is a need for further standardized studies to be conducted across the regions to identify the prevalence of BV among different sub-groups.

Given the various risks from infections, it is important for BV to be included as a priority STI for reporting in Latin American and the Caribbean countries. Epidemiological studies with representative, multi-level, population-based samples should be conducted to accurately determine the prevalence, risk factors, and protective factors associated with BV in women of reproductive ages in these countries. Also, prospective studies should be conducted to determine existing trends in the prevalence of BV risk factors associated with BV and possible BV co-infections that may exist in the regions. A standard diagnostic criterion should be adopted to allow for comparison of findings of the burden of BV. From studies conducted so far in these regions, prevalence of BV is intermediate and may potentially increase with time. It is important to conduct awareness programs in the form of sex education in schools, media campaigns, amongst others, to enhance the knowledge base and increase individual and public health actions to prevent BV among women in Latin American and the Caribbean.

Acknowledgment

My profound thanks to God almighty, who has shown me his mercies and favor. My sincere appreciation goes to Dr. Emmanuel Keku for his relentless mentorship and encouragement during the course of my capstone. Gratitude is also extended to Attah Abraham, Benjamin Ogundele, Janille William, Ghisline Ghessoum, and Elan Amstrong for their moral support during this period. Lastly, to my parents, who have shown me love and have done everything within their power to always provide me with the best. I will never ask for anything more than the blessing of having you both in my life.

REFERENCES

[1] Adam S, Tessa S, Susan R, Caroline M. Bacterial vaginosis and adverse outcomes among full-term infants: a cohort study. BMC Pregnancy Childbirth 2016;16:278.

[2] Forsum U, Holst E, Larsson PG, Vasquez A, Jakobsson T, Mattsby-Baltzer I. Bacterial vaginosis: A microbiological and immunological enigma. APMIS 2005;113:81–90.

[3] Larsson PG, Forsum U. Bacterial vaginosis: A disturbed bacterial flora and treatment enigma. APMIS 2005; 113:305–16.

[4] Wang J. Bacterial vaginosis. Prim Care 2000;7:181-5.

[5] Hillier S, Holmes K, Marrazzo J. Bacterial vaginosis: Sexually transmitted diseases. Clin Infect Dis 2008;16(4)737–68.

[6] Gardner HL, Dukes CD. Haemophilus vaginalis vaginitis: a newly defined specific infection previously classified non-specific vaginitis. Am J Obstet Gynecol 1955;69:962–76.

[7] Srinivasan S, Liu C, Mitchell CM, Fiedler TL, Thomas KK, Agnew KJ, et al. Temporal variability of human vaginal bacteria and relationship with bacterial vaginosis. PLoS One 2010;5(4):e10197.

[8] Swidsinski A, Mendling W, Loening-Baucke V, Ladhoff A, Swidsinski S, Hale LP, Lochs H. Adherent biofilms in bacterial vaginosis. Obstet Gynecol 2005;106:1013–23.

[9] Santiago GL, Tency I, Verstraelen H, Verhelst R, Trog M, Temmerman M, et al. Longitudinal qPCR study of the dynamics of L. crispatus, L. iners, A. vaginae, (sialidase positive) G. vaginalis, and P. bivia in the vagina. PLoS One 2012;7(9):e45281.

[10] Didier SC, Clâudia GD, Vânia L. Bacterial vaginosis: Clinical, epidemiological and microbiological features. HU Revista 2010;36(3): 223-30.

[11] Amsel R, Totten PA, Spiegel CA, Chen KC, Eschenbach D, Holmes KK. Nonspecific vaginitis. Diagnostic criteria and microbial and epidemiologic associations. Am J Med 1983;74:14-22.

[12] Nugent RP, Krohn MA, Hillier SL. Reliability of diagnosing bacterial vaginosis is improved by a standardized method of gram stain interpretation. J Clin Microbiol 1991;29:297–301.

[13] Fethers K, Twin J, Fairley CK, Fowkes FJI, Garland SM, Fehler G, et al. Bacterial vaginosis (BV) Candidate bacteria: Associations with BV and behavioural practices in sexually-experienced and inexperienced women. PLoS One 2012;7(2):e30633.

[14] Vaca M, Guadalupe I, Erazo S, Tinizaray K, Chico M, Cooper P, Hay P. High prevalence of bacterial vaginosis in adolescent girls in a tropical area of Ecuador. BJOG 2010;117:225–8.

[15] Marrazzo JM, Koutsky LA, Eschenbach DA, Agnew K, Stine K, Hillier SL. Characterization of vaginal flora and bacterial vaginosis in women who have sex with women. J Infect Dis 2002;185:1307-13.

[16] Tchamouroff SE, Panja SK. The association between receptive cunnilingus and bacterial vaginosis. Sex Transm Infect 2000;76:144-5.

[17] Sharma AK, Ranjan R, Mehta G. Prevalence and determinants of reproductive tract infections among women. J Commun Dis 2004;36:93-9.

[18] Van de Wijgert J, Morrison C, Cornelisse P, Munjoma M, Moncada J, et al. Bacterial vaginosis and vaginal yeast, but not vaginal cleansing, increase HIV-1 acquisition in African women. J Acquir Immune Defic Syndr 2008;48(2):203–10.

[19] Brotman R, Melendez J, Ghanem K. A case control study of anovaginal distance and bacterial vaginosis. Int J STD AIDS 2011;22(4):231-3.

[20] Koumans E, Sternberg M, Bruce C, McQuillan G, Kendrick J, Sutton M, Markowitz L. The prevalence of bacterial vaginosis in the United States, 2001-2004; associations with symptoms, sexual behaviors, and reproductive health. Sex Transm Dis 2007;34(11):864–9.

[21] Morris MC, Rogers PA, Kinghorn GR. Is bacterial vaginosis a sexually transmitted infection? Sex Transm Infect 2001;77(1):63–8.

[22] Wondemagegn M, Mulat Y, Yohannes Z, Bayeh A. Common causes of vaginal infections and antibiotic susceptibility of aerobic bacterial isolates in women of reproductive age attending at Felegehiwot referral Hospital, Ethiopia: a cross sectional study. BMC Women's Health 2015;15:42.

[23] Jols JA, Smit PW, Kort R, Reid G, Schuren FH, Tempelman H, et al. Microarray-based identification of clinically relevant vaginal bacteria in relation to bacterial vaginosis. Am J Obstet Gynecol 2011;204(4):305.

[24] Gray RH, Kigozi G, Serwadda D, Makumbi F, Nalugoda F, Watya S, et al: The effects of male circumcision on female partners' genital tract symptoms and vaginal infections in a randomized trial in Rakai, Uganda. Am J Obstet Gynecol 2009;200(1):42.

[25] Kenyon C, Colebunders R, Crucitti T. The global epidemiology of bacterial vaginosis: A systematic review. Am J Obset Gynecol 2013;209(6):505-23.

[26] Fabíola AO, Viola P, Katrin L, Jörg H, Iracema M, Francisco F, et al. Sexually transmitted infections, bacterial vaginosis, and candidiasis in women of reproductive age in rural Northeast Brazil: A population-based study. Mem Inst 2007;102(6): 751-6.

[27] Fausto G, Márcia G, Jossimara P, Andréa D, José CP, Steven SW, Marilza VC. Vaginal flora alterations and clinical symptoms in low-risk pregnant women. Gynecol Obstet Invest 2011;71:158–62.

[28] Vaca M, Guadalupe I, Erazo S, Tinizaray K, Chico ME, Cooper PJ, et al. High prevalence of bacterial vaginosis in adolescent girls in a tropical area of Ecuador. BJOG 2010;117(2):225–8.

[29] Edith Á, Andrea R, Lilian M, Luisa FM, Patricia G, Elkin O, et al. The prevalence of and factors associated with C. trachomatis, N. gonorrheae, T. vaginalis, C albicans infection, syphilis, hiv and bacterial vaginosis in females suffering lower genital tract infection symptoms in three healthcare attention sites in Bogotá, Colombia, 2010. Rev Colombiana Obstet Ginecol 2010;63(1):25-35.

[30] Brooks-Smith-Lowe K, Rodrigo S. Prevalence of bacterial vaginosis in Grenadian women of reproductive age. West Indian Med J 2013;62(7):599-603.

[31] Claire CB, Tania D, Lauren C, David C, Karthika D, Oksana O, et al. The etiology of vaginal symptoms in rural Haiti. Int J STD AIDS 2014;25(9): 669–75.

[32] Mathys JR, Marthie ME, Andries WD, Hennie L, Steve AS, Marleen MK. A cross-sectional study on the relationship of age, gestational age and HIV infection to bacterial vaginosis and genital mycoplasma infection. BMJ Open 2015;5:e008530.

[33] Tolosa JE, Chaithongwongwatthana S, Daly S, Maw WW, Gaitán H, Lumbiganon P, et al. The international infections in pregnancy (IIP) study: Variations in the prevalence of bacterial vaginosis and distribution of morphotypes in vaginal smears among pregnant women. Am J Obstet Gynecol 2016;195(5):1198–204.

[34] Bosch FX, Lorincz A, Muñoz N, Meijer CJ, Shah KV. The causal relation between human papillomavirus and cervical cancer. J Clin Pathol 2002;55(4):244-65.

[35] Glass HC, Costarino AT, Stayer SA, Brett C, Cladis F, Davis PJ. Outcomes for extremely premature infants. Anesth Analg 2015;120(6):1337-51.

[36] Moss TJM. The respiratory consequences of preterm birth. Proceed Aust Physiol Soc 2005;36:23-8.

In: Public Health Themes in Grenada … ISBN: 978-1-53618-118-0
Editors: J. Merrick and L. Glasgow © 2020 Nova Science Publishers, Inc.

Chapter 7

RECOMMENDATIONS FOR DEVELOPING PESTICIDE EXPOSURE PREVENTION PROGRAMS IN CARIBBEAN COUNTRIES

Lindonne Glasgow[1,*]*, MSPH, DrPH*
and Alicia C McDonald[2]*, PhD, MPH*
[1]School of Medicine, Department of Public Health and Preventive Medicine, St George's University, Grenada, West Indies and
[2]Department of Public Health Sciences, Pennsylvania State University College of Medicine, Hershey, Pennsylvania, United States of America

ABSTRACT

On a global scale, pesticides are commonly used in agriculture production, despite increasing awareness of the hazardous nature of many of these products. Pesticides have been classified by the World Health Organization (WHO) according to their potential for adverse effects on human health. Community and occupational exposures were found to be associated with

* Correspondence: Dr. Lindonne Glasgow, Assistant Professor, Department of Public Health and Preventive Medicine, St George's University, PO Box 7, True Blue, St George's, Grenada, West Indies. Email: lglasgow@sgu.com.

increased risk for acute and chronic health problems such as reproductive disorders, neurological problems, flu-like symptoms, skin rashes, eye irritation, and nausea. Agricultural workers and members of their households experience high exposure to pesticides through dermal, inhalation, and ingestion routes. Studies have shown that health problems from pesticide exposures are more prominent in low-income countries that also have fewer resources to develop and adopt modern agriculture technologies. In the Caribbean, pesticide use is high in agricultural production, and studies have shown that agricultural workers do not commonly use personal protective equipment. These practices in the Caribbean region increase health risks for agricultural workers and members of their households. Developing effective interventions to improve safety in the use of pesticides among agricultural workers is necessary and should be a public health priority. To our knowledge, there is no published literature that describes approaches to developing and implementing effective interventions to improve pesticide stewardship - that is, the safe use of pesticides, in Caribbean countries. This chapter provides approaches to developing experiential, participatory, and learner-centered interventions aimed at behavior change, to minimize pesticide exposure and health risks among agricultural workers in the Caribbean region.

INTRODUCTION

On the global level, pesticides are commonly used in agriculture production. Increasingly, and more so in recent years, however, studies suggest that some pesticides can have significant negative impacts on human health, increasing risk to various chronic diseases such as Parkinson's disease, end-stage renal disease, and different types of cancers (1–5). Besides, acute and chronic symptoms in humans, such as reproductive disorders, neurological problems, flu-like symptoms, skin rashes, eye irritation, and nausea have been found to be among common health problems that result from exposure to pesticides (6). The World Health Organization (WHO) has classified pesticides based on their toxicological potential for human health and the environment (7).

The WHO expressed concerns about exposure to pesticides, among agricultural workers and other communities, particularly in low-income countries (7). Pesticide exposure can occur through dermal contact, inhalation, and ingestion. Generally, the low-income countries lack innovative practices that are more common in high-income countries to maintain and improve occupational safety (7). Safety precautions in pesticide usage also tend to be limited among agricultural workers in low-income countries as compared to the practice among workers in high-income countries (7). The Caribbean has been described to be on a "pesticide treadmill," indicating the high and increasing usage of pesticides in agriculture production (8). As a result, concerns have been raised about food safety and the health of agricultural workers in the region from pesticide exposure (8).

The agriculture sector remains a significant contributor to the gross domestic product (GDP) in many Caribbean countries (9). As such, it is imperative to take measures to reduce the burden of disease among the workers in the sector. Studies have suggested that unsafe usage of pesticides and poor pesticide protective behaviors, resulting in the increased exposure among workers, are due to the lack of knowledge and misperceptions of the risks associated with the use of the products (6). In the absence of effective preventive interventions, a high percentage of workers in the agriculture sector in the Caribbean continue to be exposed to hazardous pesticides. The Pan American Health Organization (PAHO) has emphasized the need for countries to establish and enforce regulations to address occupational and environmental factors that constitute risks for diseases (10). For the Caribbean, recommendations to minimize pesticide exposures among agricultural workers may also have significant implications for reducing the incidence of diseases.

In order to address the incidence of diseases associated with pesticide exposures in the Caribbean region, public health interventions must target behavioral change among agricultural workers. Studies have found few agricultural workers in the Caribbean region use protective equipment while handling and applying pesticides (11–14). A study conducted in the Dominican Republic found that cytotoxic and genotoxic effects were associated with exposure to pesticides among applicators (15), showing the potential health effects pesticides may have on disease risk. To our knowledge, there is no published literature describing interventions aimed at improving pesticide stewardship- that is, safe use of pesticides, in an effective and participatory manner in the Caribbean. This chapter provides recommendations for experiential, participatory, and learner-centered approaches in developing pesticide exposure prevention programs, focused on behavior change, for agricultural workers in the Caribbean countries. Lastly, this chapter includes a discussion about the benefits of social change for agricultural workers and the regional public health systems.

Application of behavior change theory

Agriculture is the traditional livelihood in many Caribbean countries from colonial times. Although tourism, service, and manufacturing industries variably dominate the highest contributions to GDP across countries, the agriculture sector maintains a prominent role in economies and to ensure food security in the Caribbean. In most of the Caribbean countries, a significant segment of the population engages in commercial or subsistence farming. Small scale farmers dominate the sector (16,) which, in most islands, have only been moderately transformed into using modern technologies. Traditional and labor-intensive methods that resulted in hazardous exposures to pesticides are utilized even in contemporary times (9, 17). Because many traditional practices are the norm, behavior change may be slow or resisted among agricultural workers.

The Transtheoretical model is a suitable framework on which to premise a preventive health program for the Caribbean region. On the belief that people do not change their behavior quickly, the Transtheoretical model postulates that people go through five incremental stages in behavior change: pre-contemplation, contemplation, preparation, action, and maintenance (18). These stages represent a build-up in actions towards compliance and maintaining new behaviors. The model shows a progression from mental processing of information to contemplating action to adopting the action (behavior change) and, finally, to maintain the behavior change. Self-pacing and readiness are core principles that underpin the interventions at every stage. This learner-driven approach to change can easily transform into high acceptance of the interventions by agricultural workers. The progressive approach can also be critical to ensuring agricultural workers have both interest in and absorptive capacity for the behavior change interventions. Apart from applying a model that may be effective for positive behavior change among agricultural workers, the other sections of this paper highlight factors that should also be incorporated across the stages of implementation.

SETTING THE PACE FOR INTERVENTIONS

To develop a health promotion campaign, the first step is to determine the situation in the community. This step is referred to as formative research or situational analysis. This analysis is critical for informing the design of an intervention. Interventions that were developed for other contexts or previously implemented may not offer the best fit in the current environment and time. As for establishing a pesticide protective program, the intention is to investigate the situation pertinent to the handling and application of pesticides by agricultural workers. Community-Based Participatory Research (CBPR) approach is suitable for application in this investigation, requiring the target group, that is, the agricultural workers, to contribute their knowledge and experiences in planning and developing the research. A wide cross-section of the workers should be consulted to create a stakeholder map and tools for the inquiry. Public health practitioners, academicians, and other preventive health experts should participate in this initial research designing consultations to ensure that scientific methods and best practices are considered and appropriately applied at this initial phase. Broad-based participation at this early stage can be advantageous to generate interest and increased participation in subsequent activities.

The formative research should incorporate a variety of themes that address agricultural workers' knowledge, interests, perspectives, attitudes, and practices related to pesticide usage and health. Such information would be valuable to guide in framing messages and activities to address gaps in knowledge about pesticide safety, poor attitudes, and unsafe practices. Data, which describe morbidity and mortality rates related to pesticide use, can be collected from registries and other authoritative sources, such as from government surveillance reports. Analysis of secondary data may serve to provide crucial evidence of the magnitude of the problem in the sector. Representatives for the agricultural workers and institutions, public health practitioners, academicians, policymakers, and other public health experts should review all results and consult in the development of the interventions, ensuring proper alignment of the interventions with the needs and expectations of the agricultural workers.

Goal-Driven Programs

Interventions should be developed with the ultimate goal of reducing the prevalence of health problems among agricultural workers. To achieve this goal, the interventions should focus on addressing gaps in knowledge and practices regarding the safe use of pesticides. Heightening awareness about the possible adverse effects of exposure to pesticides and, at the same time, increasing knowledge about safe practices is paramount to behavior change. Behavior change should aim to increase pesticide stewardship through: 1) use of personal protective equipment such as using masks and gloves, and 2) practicing good agriculture hygiene, such as washing clothes after using pesticides and washing hands before eating and using the toilet. By reducing exposure to pesticides, agricultural workers will also decrease the risk for developing health problems such as cancers and reproductive and neurological disorders (1-5). The support of public health experts and policymakers can be instrumental in affirmative actions to address agricultural workers' health needs.

Interventions should seek to be both systematic and strategic. Purpose-driven interventions can have the most substantial effect on the knowledge, attitudes, and practices of the agricultural workers. Some key components in a campaign to address exposure to hazardous pesticides can include: 1) call for attention to the public health issue and its impact on health, 2) identification of the target group of agricultural workers in which pesticide exposure is present, 3) documentation of current behaviors regarding the use of pesticides, 4) assessment of the potential adverse health effects due to pesticide exposure in the target population, 5) a plan to protect the health of the agricultural workers and their communities, and 6) evaluation of the overall social and economic benefits. Contact information for the program implementers and sources of additional information should be provided to the workers. The interventions should be progressive – reflecting the tenets of the Transtheoretical model, from pre-contemplation to action to maintenance of the new behavior. This approach is highly practical, although the timeframe could vary for individual workers to achieve the goal - safe use of pesticides - and subsequently reduce pesticide-associated health disease and conditions.

COMMUNICATION MEDIA

Three communication tools that are variably but highly accessible to Caribbean agricultural workers are television, radio, and telephone. Within the last decade, telephone access increased significantly in the Caribbean region, in particular, with cellular (or mobile) phone usage. The competition between the increasing numbers of telecommunications service providers and government regulations have been beneficial to keeping the cost of telephone and television services at affordable rates. Messages to be used for mobilization and in the interventions should be prepared in formats for dissemination through these various media to reach the largest cross-section of agricultural workers. Radio is advantageous for use in various locations, including in workplaces such as farms. Using the radio to disseminate information would increase the amount of time for which messages can be aired, even during prime time, at an affordable cost. Radio production is also relatively cheap. Using television is advantageous to disseminate information using interactive formats such as stories, charts, and pictures. These formats may be more suitable for persons with lower literacy.

Television and radio are also suitable for persons with hearing and vision impairment, respectively. Texting, via cellular telephone, allows for disseminating and receiving short instant messages.

ENSURING APPROPRIATENESS IN MESSAGING

Age, literacy, and media appeal must be considered in developing messages to explain pesticide exposure risks and protective measures. While television and radio are more commonly accessed by middle-aged to older people, social media platforms, such as Whatsapp and Facebook, have greater appeal for young people in the Caribbean. Messages should be presented in formats that are suitable for agricultural workers with different literacy levels. The messages may also be crafted for the attention of the other household members and the wider community that interact with and support the agricultural workers. The channels for dissemination of messages will need to be selected based on suitability to accommodate formats such as tables, still charts, interactive charts, pictures, verbal presentations, and short or long text. Local dialects can be useful to express the meaning of some content or to simplify messages (19). Representative groups of agricultural workers' can be consulted to review messages and to provide feedback to improve appropriateness and relevance for the wider group. Segments of the workers' group can also be involved in piloting messages.

MARKETING AND GETTING ATTENTION

Marketing of the pesticide prevention intervention should be conducted through direct and indirect means. Firstly, branding has the benefit of allowing the target group to identify with interventions through the use of distinctive design, content, and images (20). For example, indirect marketing of the programs can include Caribbean- or island-flavored songs, jingles, theatricals, and posters via television and radio. These activities are symbolic of Caribbean traditions and can readily capture the attention of the agricultural workers. Cultural features, such as calypso beat in songs, local theater groups performing plays and displaying national colors on posters, can enhance the marketing strategy to capture the attention of the agriculture workers. Carnival and religious symbols may also be appropriate to grab attention to public health messages in the Caribbean setting.

Secondly, the aim of breakthrough inattention is to attract and engage the target group (20). The messages should be crafted to appeal specifically to the agricultural workers and provide a sense of urgency for behavior change. Some practical and feasible new behaviors should also be presented to attract attention.

Peer-to-peer marketing among agricultural workers may result in increased support for participation in the interventions. Information about time, place, and format for interventions should always be provided in intervention marketing campaigns. Community groups, agriculture organizations, and other influential organizations, such as donor agencies, can be instrumental in marketing programs to the agricultural workers. The influence of gatekeepers and influential local leaders can affect the community's reception to marketing (19). Influential members and leaders can reject intervention or messages, based on how it personally impacts them, and also influence the decisions of the wider group. In such cases, the message or intervention will need to be revised to increase its appeal to both the leaders and workers.

POSSIBLE CHALLENGES AND SOLUTIONS

The choice of the communication channel can determine the reach of messages to agricultural workers. It is beneficial for a wide range of media to be used to disseminate information. This, however, may have cost implications leading to fewer media being used segments of the target population not having access to information. This lack of access to information can have a significant impact on the success of the program. To address this issue, media accessibility and preference for the agricultural workers should be identified in the formative research. In pre-testing messages, the reach through various media should also be investigated. The most widely accessible media should eventually be used in the campaign.

Developing a non-specific message is another challenge. Messages that are not sufficiently tailored for a specific group may not attract interest and participation in the intervention. This challenge can be addressed by doing stakeholder mapping to identify the particular characteristics of the agricultural workers that should be targeted in messaging. Documenting the demographic characteristics of the agricultural workers, such as literacy, age, and preferred communication medium, is also useful for ensuring messages about risk and protection from pesticide exposure, are appropriate and appealing.

An ethical issue may constitute unrealistic and unreasonable promises regarding behavior change and outcomes. Messages can be exaggerated and lead to disappointment when benefits are not perceived as proportionate to the effort for adopting the behavior change. To avoid this challenge, evidenced-based interventions should be adopted, with clearer indications of cause/effect relationships (19). Such an approach may include the application of public health theories and results from scientific studies (20).

The introduction of excessively costly or unaffordable practices to replace current practices can be considered as unethical as it introduces bias by limiting participation of segments of the target group (19). For example, large farmer holders may be able to purchase respirators for use when applying pesticides while small farm holders are deprived of acquiring this protective equipment. If cheaper alternatives are not available, the agriculture workers may be forced to resort to using ineffective methods, such as covering the mouth with a cloth while applying pesticides. The inability of the target group to maintain a behavior will also be counter-productive to achieving intervention goals. Although social marketing can result in ready adoption of alternative behaviors, the capacity, and resources that reside among agricultural workers and in the wider community should be assessed in the formative research and considered in the development of interventions.

METHODS FOR EVALUATING THE EFFECTIVENESS OF PESTICIDE EXPOSURE PREVENTION INTERVENTIONS

Evaluation is an essential component in the intervention cycle and should be planned during the initial development phase. This process should cater to agricultural workers reflecting on their experiences during interventions, identifying changes in behaviors, and evaluating the potential impacts of the changes on their health and well-being. These steps support experiential learning - learning through practice and being able to identify and define the outcomes. Formative, process, and summative evaluations should be conducted. The formative evaluation includes an assessment of the situation – for example, determine which workers use pesticides, how are pesticides applied in work settings, frequency of pesticide use, compliance with good agricultural practices, and pesticide stewardship. Process evaluations should determine whether a behavior is changing during the intervention and what factors contribute to positive or negative responses to the intervention. The summative evaluation should focus on what impact was achieved, unintended effects, and cost-effectiveness of the intervention upon completion. The summative evaluation should indicate the quantity and quality of change from the formative evaluation. Text messaging, surveys, and feedback via radio and television may be used to collect both qualitative and quantitative information for these evaluations. A final report should be prepared and submitted to all stakeholders.

CONCLUSION

Social change is the process of improving the conditions of individuals and communities through the use of interventions (21). The campaign among agricultural workers caters for social change with a focus on the behavior of workers to improve pesticide stewardship in the agriculture sector. Achieving positive behavior change towards minimizing exposure to pesticides has implications for the health and well-being of the Caribbean population. The agriculture industry is one of the oldest establishments in the Caribbean, and many learned traditional behaviors are still dominantly practiced despite increasing evidence of the hazardous nature of some pesticides and their effect on one's health. The recommendations in this paper draw on the Transtheoretical model, which postulates an incremental approach to behavior change. The recommendations, such as applying a self-driven behavior change model in interventions, facilitating community-based participatory learning, and identifying behavior change through reflection support experiential, participatory, and learner-centered approaches in the development and implementation of the interventions to address health risks from pesticide exposures among Caribbean agricultural workers. Social change can also arise from sharing information about innovations and results (20, 22). This intervention may be replicated in local communities with the results from the evaluation of each cycle disseminated to improve subsequent deliveries of the intervention. The results can also be disseminated across the Caribbean countries; however, each country should ensure that the recommendations are adapted to its specific context.

Finally, reducing exposure to pesticides can result in significant improvement in the health outcomes of agricultural workers in Caribbean countries. The spin-off effect is reducing the burden of diseases and the burden on the health care system while allowing resources to be reallocated to development. Generally, an effective campaign on safely using pesticides among agricultural workers in the Caribbean can contribute to protecting their health and improving the overall health status of the region.

REFERENCES

[1] Brouwer M, Schinasi L, Beane Freeman LE, Baldi I, Lebailly P, Ferro G, et al. Assessment of occupational exposure to pesticides in a pooled analysis of agricultural cohorts within the AGRICOH consortium. Occup Environ Med 2016;73(6):359–67.

[2] Tago D, Andersson H, Treich N. Pesticides and health: A review of evidence on health effects, valuation of risks, and benefit-cost analysis. Adv Health Econ Health Serv Res 2014;24:203–95.

[3] Lemarchand C, Tual S, Boulanger M, Levêque-Morlais N, Perrier S, Clin B, et al. Prostate cancer risk among French farmers in the AGRICAN cohort. Scand J Work Environ Health 2016;42(2):144–52.

[4] Goldman SM, Kamel F, Ross GW, Bhudhikanok GS, Hoppin JA, Korell M, et al. Genetic modification of the association of paraquat and Parkinson's disease. Mov Disord 2012;27(13):1652–8.

[5] Lebov JF, Engel LS, Richardson D, Hogan SL, Hoppin JA, Sandler DP. Pesticide use and risk of end-stage renal disease among licensed pesticide applicators in the Agricultural Health Study. Occup Environ Med 2016;73(1):3–12.

[6] Remoundou K, Brennan M, Hart A, Frewer LJ. Pesticide risk perceptions, knowledge, and attitudes of operators, workers, and residents: A review of the literature. Hum Ecol Risk Assess An Int J 2014;20(4):1113–38.

[7] World Health Organization. Preventing disease through healthy environments - Exposure to highly hazardous pesticides: A major public health concern, 2010. URL: http://www.who.int/ipcs/features/hazardous_pesticides.pdf.

[8] University of the West Indies (St. Augustine Campus). Too many chemicals in the crop. 2016. URL: https://sta.uwi.edu/uwitoday/archive/july_2016/article17.asp.

[9] Kinda Campo K-R, Robinson A, Patrice Isaac W-A, Ganpat W. Connecting small farmers in the Caribbean to knowledge, networks, and institutions through ICTs. J Agric Food Inf 2017;18(2):81–95.

[10] Pan American Health Organization. Cancer mortality is declining in some countries of the Americas, 2013. URL: http://www.paho.org/hq/index.php?option=com_content&view=article&id=9135%3A2013-cancer-mortality-declining-some-countries-americas-new-paho-who-report&Itemid=1926&lang=en.

[11] Ragin C, Davis-Reyes B, Tadesse H, Daniels D, Bunker CH, Jackson M, et al. Farming, reported pesticide use, and prostate cancer. Am J Mens Health 2013;7(2):102–9.

[12] Semple H, Johnson K, Arjoonsingh C. Agrochemicals usage and protective clothing among small farmers in Jamaica and Grenada. Caribb Geogr 2005;14(1):15–30.

[13] Forde MS, Robertson L, Laouan Sidi EA, Côté S, Gaudreau E, Drescher O, et al. Evaluation of exposure to organophosphate, carbamate, phenoxy acid, and chlorophenol pesticides in pregnant women from 10 Caribbean countries. Environ Sci Process Impacts 2015;17(9):1661–71.

[14] Henry D, Feola G. Pesticide-handling practices of smallholder coffee farmers in Eastern Jamaica. J Agric Rural Dev Trop Subtrop 2013;114(1):59–67.

[15] Hutter H-P, Khan A, Lemmerer K, Wallner P, Kundi M, Moshammer H. Cytotoxic and genotoxic effects of pesticide exposure in male coffee farmworkers of the Jarabacoa Region, Dominican Republic. Int J Environ Res Public Health 2018;15(8):1641.

[16] Graham B. Profile of the small-scale farming in the Caribbean. Workshop on Small-Scale Farming in the Caribbean, 2012. URL: www.fao.org/3/a-au343e.pdf.

[17] David D, Glenroy E. Characterisation of family farms in the Caribbean: A study of Guyana, Haiti, Jamaica, and Saint Vincent and the Grenadines, 2017. URL: http://repositorio.iica.int/bitstream/11324/6104/1/BVE17109315i.pdf.

[18] Prochaska JO, Di Clemente CC. Transtheoretical therapy: Toward a more integrative model of change. Psychotherapy 1982;19(3):276–88.

[19] Kanj M, Mitic W. Health literacy, 2009. URL: http://www.who.int/healthpromotion/conferences/7gchp/Track1_Inner.pdf.

[20] Glanz K, Rimer BK, Viswanath K, eds. Health behavior: Theory, research, and practice, 5th ed. San Francisco, CA: Jossey-Bass, 2015.

[21] Skendall KC, Ostick DT, Komives SR, Wagner W, eds. The social change model: Facilitating leadership development. San Francisco, CA: 2017.

[22] Parker JC, Thorson E, eds. Health communication in the new media landscape. New York: Springer, 2009.

SECTION TWO:
RESEARCH FROM THE REGION

In: Public Health Themes in Grenada … ISBN: 978-1-53618-118-0
Editors: J. Merrick and L. Glasgow

Chapter 8

Breast Cancer in Grenada, West Indies: A Trend Analysis of Newly Diagnosed Breast Cancer Cases for the Period 2001-2010

Lindsey Moll, MPH,
Moza Hamud, BA,
Victoria Watkins, BS,
Megan Ostlie, BSN,
Zachary Kassirer, MSc,
Kai Wang, MSc,
Vanessa Denny, MD, MSc,
Tolulope Oladimeji, MD, MPH
and Emmanuel Keku, MD, MA, MSPH*
School of Medicine, Department of Public Health and Preventive Medicine, St George's University, Grenada, West Indies

* Correspondence: Dr Emmanuel Keku, Professor, Department of Public Health and Preventive Medicine, St George's University, POBox 7, True Blue, St George's, Grenada, West Indies. Email: ekeku@sgu.edu.

Abstract

Though the burden of breast cancer is on the rise globally, data in the Caribbean region is limited. We examined the trend of breast cancer in the tri-island state of Grenada, Carriacou, and Petit Martinique between 2001 and 2010 in women over 20 years old. A cross-sectional study was conducted. Surveillance and biopsy data from Grenada General Hospital were used to analyze the trend in breast cancer. Data were extracted on biopsies with confirmed breast cancer. The data was collated using an EXCEL spreadsheet and analyzed using EpiInfo to summarize the demographic and pathologic characteristics of each case. Grenada reported 207 breast cancer cases between 2001 and 2010. The incidence rate was 26.4/100,000. St. David's parish had the highest incidence rate (54.5/100,000), and St. Patrick's parish reported the lowest (24.2/100,000). Invasive ductal carcinoma was the most common subtype of breast cancer (76.8%), followed by invasive lobular carcinoma (8.2%), undefined ductal carcinoma (3.4%), mixed carcinoma (2.9%), Ductal in situ carcinoma (2.4%), and invasive adenocarcinoma (1.0%). Other sub-types of breast cancer that were less than 1% include; lobular in situ carcinoma, undefined adenocarcinoma, differentiated carcinoma, undifferentiated carcinoma, invasive squamous cell carcinoma, sarcoma, and others. The majority of the cases occurred in the age range of 40-49 years old. Between 2001 and 2010, Grenada showed a decreasing trend in breast cancer rates, and the incidence rate was lower than those reported by other Caribbean islands. Reasons for elevated incidence rates in St. David deserve further study.

Introduction

Breast cancer is the leading type of cancer frequently diagnosed in women globally, with an estimated 1.4 million incident cases and 459,000 deaths in 2008 (1). Breast cancer account for 25% of all cancer cases and 15% of all cancer deaths among females (2). In the Caribbean region, 24.6% of all cancer diagnoses are breast cancer cases, and 15.8% of all cancer-related deaths are due to breast cancer (3). In 2008, Trinidad and Tobago reported an incidence rate of 36/100 000, and Barbados reported a rate of 74/100 000 (4).

Research has shown that there has been an increase in global incidence rates of breast cancer. There are few studies that have examined the growing incidence rate of breast cancer in the Caribbean region; therefore, further exploration in this region is needed. In the tri-island state of Grenada, Carriacou and Petit Martinique, health service personnel have reported an alarming increase in the number of newly diagnosed breast cancer cases in women under the age of 50 years (5). The purpose of conducting this study was to better understand the incidence of breast cancer amongst the Grenadian population. The objective of the study was to determine the trend (person/place/time) in the newly diagnosed cases of breast cancer in the tri-island state of Grenada, Carriacou, and Petit Martinique during the years of 2001-2010 (6).

OUR STUDY

A descriptive epidemiologic study was performed to analyze the trend(person/place/time) of all the reported diagnosed cases of breast cancer over a defined period of January 1, 2001 through December 31, 2010. The study utilized secondary, passive surveillance data from the Pathology Department at the General Hospital in Grenada, West Indies. The surveillance data provided information on each individual who had undergone breast tissue biopsy at the General Hospital and was confirmed as breast cancer cases. Breast tissue biopsy, followed by histological examination, was used as the primary mode of identifying cancer cases.

Target population

The study area was the Caribbean tri-island state Grenada, Carriacou, and Petit Martinique. Grenada is located northwest of Trinidad and Tobago, northeast of Venezuela and southwest of Saint Vincent and the Grenadines. The target population included all the female citizens and or legal residents of Grenada, Carriacou, and Petite-Martinique.

Study population

The inclusion criterion was outlined as all the confirmed cases of breast cancer in women under the age of 50 years in Grenada for the ten-year period 2001-2010 identified in the Pathology Surgical Entry Book, available at the Grenada General Hospital. For the purpose of the research, the definition of a case was the medically confirmed (breast tissue biopsy followed by histological examination) presence of an invasive/non-invasive ductal or lobular carcinoma of the breast.

The study excluded all breast cancer cases that were not identified in the surveillance data described in the Pathology Surgical Entry Book. All the diagnosed cases of breast cancer in men on the islands of Grenada, Carriacou, and Petit Martinique were excluded from the study. Furthermore, all cases reported out of the demarcated ten-year period that began on January 1, 2001 and ended on December 31, 2010, were excluded from the study.

Ethical Justification

Prior to the start of the research, ethical approval was sought through the Institutional Review Board (IRB) at St. George's University, Grenada-West Indies. Ethical approval was granted. All ethical protocols were observed during the research process.

Data collection

A formal written request of permission to access the surveillance data and perform the research was sent to the Permanent Secretary in the Ministry of Health in Grenada. After permission was granted, the data collection process began.

All the confirmed cases of breast cancer were identified from the Pathology Surgical Entry Book. This book provided data on patient demographics and pathologic characteristics. For this study, the variables under investigation were as follows: date of diagnosis, age at diagnosis, parish of residence, and the specific sub-type of breast cancer. The data collected was inputted into a spreadsheet and exported into EpiInfo for data analysis. One data collector was responsible for the data collection process.

Statistical analysis

Descriptive statistics from EpiInfo were used to summarize the demographic and pathologic characteristics of the identified cases. An analysis of the data was carried out to investigate the frequency of the different breast cancer sub-types amongst the cohort. Annual age-adjusted incidence rates of breast cancer over the specified period were calculated and analyzed on a graph to observe the trend. A time-trend analysis for the reported annual age-adjusted incidence rates was then applied to the data. In addition, the breast cancer incidence rates in the various parishes were assessed and compared.

FINDINGS

There were 207 confirmed cases of breast cancer that were identified from the Pathology Surgical Entry Book (General Hospital) in the tri-Island state Grenada, Carriacou, and Petit Martinique between 2001 and 2010.

Annual age-adjusted incidence rates for the period were calculated and illustrated graphically (see Table 1, Figures 1-2). When a time-trend analysis was applied to the age-adjusted incidence rates, no clear trend was established. Instead, there were relatively unstable and inconsistent changes in the age-adjusted incidence rates across all age categories.

Table 1. Annual age-adjusted incidence rates for breast cancer in Grenada

2001	Number of Cases	Female Population	Crude Rate	WHO World Standard Population	Age-adjusted Rate/100 000
20-29	1	10158	9.8	0.1615	1.6
30-39	4	6203	64.5	0.1471	9.5
40-49	8	5115	156.4	0.1263	19.8
50-59	5	4690	106.6	0.0992	10.6
>60	10	5282	189.3	0.1195	22.6
All Ages	28	31448	526.6	0.6536	64
2002	Number of Cases	Female Population	Crude Rate	WHO World Standard Population	Age-adjusted Rate/100 000
20-29	0	7046	0	0.1615	0
30-39	2	6701	29.8	0.1471	4.4
40-49	4	5526	72.4	0.1263	9.1
50-59	2	3279	61	0.0992	6.1
>60	6	7170	83.7	0.1195	10
All Ages	14	29722	246.9	0.6536	29.6
2003	Number of Cases	Female Population	Crude Rate	WHO World Standard Population	Age-adjusted Rate/100 000
20-29	1	7096	14.1	0.1615	2.3
30-39	3	6747	44.5	0.1471	6.5
40-49	6	5565	107.8	0.1263	13.6
50-59	1	3302	30.3	0.0992	3
>60	6	7220	83.1	0.1195	9.9
All Ages	17	29930	279.8	0.6536	35.4
2004	Number of Cases	Female Population	Crude Rate	WHO World Standard Population	Age-adjusted Rate/100 000
20-29	0	7145	0	0.1615	0
30-39	1	6795	14.7	0.1471	2.2
40-49	7	5604	124.9	0.1263	15.8
50-59	5	3325	150.4	0.0992	14.9
>60	5	7271	68.8	0.1195	8.2
All Ages	18	30140	358.8	0.6536	41.1
2005	Number of Cases	Female Population	Crude Rate	WHO World Standard Population	Age-adjusted Rate/100 000
20-29	0	7195	0	0.1615	0
30-39	1	6842	14.6	0.1471	2.1
40-49	4	5643	70.9	0.1263	9
50-59	3	3348	89.6	0.0992	8.9
>60	2	7322	27.3	0.1195	3.3
All Ages	10	30350	202.4	0.6536	23.3

2006	Number of Cases	Female Population	Crude Rate	WHO World Standard Population	Age-adjusted Rate/100 000
20-29	0	7255	0	0.1615	0
30-39	6	6892	87.1	0.1471	12.8
40-49	13	5683	228.8	0.1263	28.9
50-59	6	3372	177.9	0.0992	17.7
>60	7	7373	94.9	0.1195	11.3
All Ages	32	30575	588.7	0.6536	70.7
2007	Number of Cases	Female Population	Crude Rate	WHO World Standard Population	Age-adjusted Rate/100 000
20-29	0	7277	0	0.1615	0
30-39	10	6939	144.1	0.1471	21.2
40-49	9	5723	157.3	0.1263	19.9
50-59	9	3375	266.7	0.0992	26.5
>60	9	7625	118	0.1195	14.1
All Ages	37	30939	686.1	0.6536	81.6
2008	Number of Cases	Female Population	Crude Rate	WHO World Standard Population	Age-adjusted Rate/100 000
20-29	0	7347	0	0.1615	0
30-39	1	6987	14.3	0.1471	2.1
40-49	8	5763	138.8	0.1263	17.5
50-59	2	3419	58.5	0.0992	5.8
>60	10	7478	133.7	0.1195	16
All Ages	21	30994	345.3	0.6536	41.4
2009	Number of Cases	Female Population	Crude Rate	WHO World Standard Population	Age-adjusted Rate/100 000
20-29	1	7399	13.5	0.1615	2.2
30-39	3	7036	42.6	0.1471	6.3
2009	Number of Cases	Female Population	Crude Rate	WHO World Standard Population	Age-adjusted Rate/100 000
40-49	4	5803	68.9	0.1263	8.7
50-59	4	3443	116.2	0.0992	11.5
>60	1	7528	13.3	0.1195	1.6
All Ages	13	31209	254.5	0.6536	30.3
2010	Number of Cases	Female Population	Crude Rate	WHO World Standard Population	Age-adjusted Rate/100 000
20-29	0	7450	0	0.1615	0
30-39	5	7085	70.6	0.1471	10.4
40-49	3	5783	51.9	0.1263	6.6
50-59	0	3467	0	0.0992	0
>60	9	7583	118.7	0.1195	14.2
All Ages	17	31368	241.2	0.6536	31.1

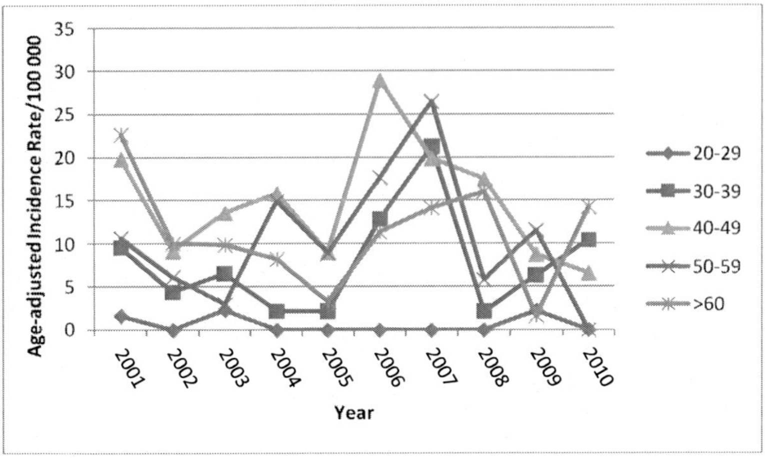

Figure 1. Distribution of newly diagnosed breast cancer using age-adjusted incidence rates (across all age categories).

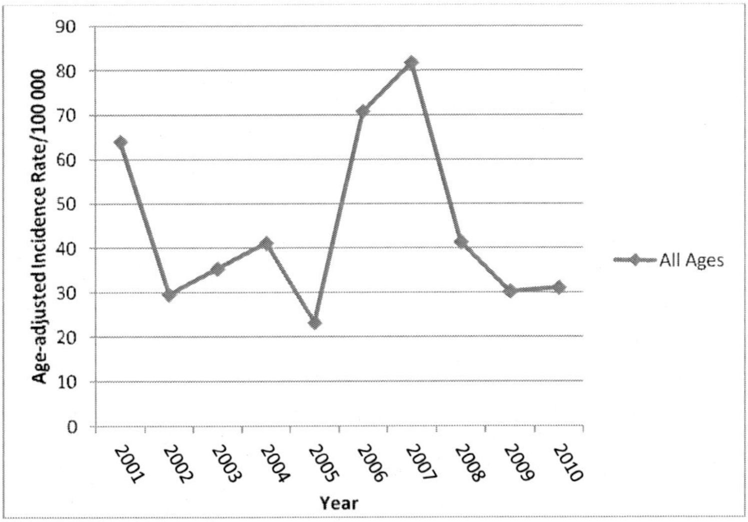

Figure 2. Distribution of newly diagnosed breast cancer of all ages between 2001-2010, using age-adjusted incidence rates.

Distribution of breast cancer by type

The most common type of breast cancer reported in the population was invasive ductal carcinoma (76.8%). This was followed by invasive lobular carcinoma of the breast (8.2%), lobular in situ carcinoma (LCIS) (0.5%), differentiated carcinoma of the breast (0.5%), undifferentiated carcinoma of the breast (0.5%), undefined adenocarcinoma of the breast (0.5%), sarcoma of the breast (0.5%), and invasive squamous cell carcinoma of the breast (0.5%).

Age-distribution

The youngest confirmed case of breast cancer was 26 years old, diagnosed in 2001. The case was reported as residing in the parish of St. John and was diagnosed with invasive ductal carcinoma with no metastasis. The oldest confirmed case of breast cancer in this study was 90 years old and was diagnosed in 2010. The patient was a resident of the parish of St. George and was diagnosed with invasive ductal carcinoma with no metastasis.

Table 2. Summary of breast cancer sub-types in the population, 2001-2010

Sub-type of Breast Cancer	Frequency	% Frequency
Invasive ductal carcinoma	159	76.8
Invasive lobular carcinoma	17	8.2
Ductal in situ carcinoma	5	2.4
Lobular in situ carcinoma	1	0.5
Undefined ductal carcinoma	7	3.4
Invasive adenocarcinoma	2	1.0
Undefined adenocarcinoma	1	0.5
Mixed carcinoma	6	2.9
Differentiated carcinoma	1	0.5
Undifferentiated carcinoma	1	0.5
Invasive squamous cell carcinoma	1	0.5
Sarcoma	1	0.5
Other	5	2.4
Total	207	100

The most commonly occurring age for confirmed breast carcinoma was 46 years. The average age was 53 years, with a standard deviation of 14.53 and a variance of 211.15. The median age was 49 years. Inter-quartile age range distributions were 41 (25%) and 65 (75%) respectively. When an analysis of the incidence rates of breast cancer by age-distribution was applied to the data, the highest rate was noted in the 40-49 age category followed by the >60 and 50-59 age categories (see Table 3).

Table 3. Total incidence rates (un-adjusted) of breast cancer in Grenada 2001-2010

Age Category	Number of Cases	Female Population	Incidence Rate/100 000
20-29	3	10158	29.5
30-39	37	6203	596.5
40-49	65	5115	1270.8
50-59	37	4690	788.9
>60	65	5282	1230.6
All Ages	207	31448	3916.3

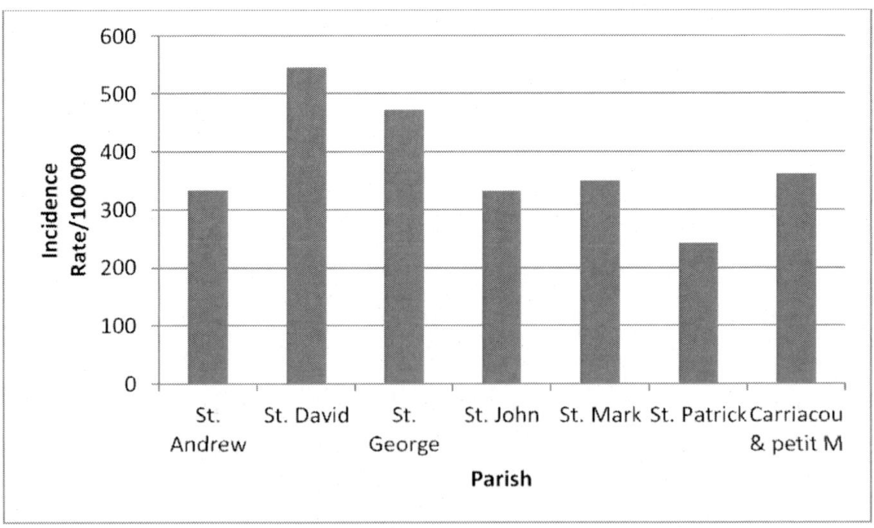

Figure 3. Distribution by parish of newly diagnosed breast cancer in Grenada 2001-2010.

Geographical (parish) distribution

Table 4. Distribution by parish of newly diagnosed breast cancer in Grenada 2001-2010

Parish	Number of Cases	Female Population	Incidence Rate/100 000
St. Andrew	42	12636	332.4
St. David	30	5507	544.8
St. George	90	19033	472.9
St. John	14	4219	331.8
St. Mark	7	2003	349.5
St. Patrick	13	5363	242.4
Carriacou & Petit Martinique	11	3033	362.7
Total	207	46431	2636.5

Table 5. Newly diagnosed breast cancer (%) sub-types by parish between 2001-2010

Type of cancer	St. Andrew	St. David	St. George	St. John	St. Mark	St. Patrick	Carriacou & Petit Martinique
Invasive ductal carcinoma	75	77.8	80	78.6	71.4	69.2	72.7
Invasive lobular carcinoma	5.0	14.8	7.8	7.1	0	7.7	9.1
Ductal in situ carcinoma	5.0	0	3.6	0	0	0	0
Lobular in situ carcinoma	2.5	0	0	0	0	0	0
Undefined ductal carcinoma	5.0	3.7	2.2	7.1	14.3	0	0
Invasive adenocarcinoma	0	0	1.1	0	0	0	0
Undefined adenocarcinoma	0	0	0	7.1	0	0	0
Mixed carcinoma	2.5	0	2.2	0	0	7.7	18.2
Differentiated carcinoma	2.5	0	0	0	0	0	0
Undifferentiated carcinoma	0	0	0	0	0	7.7	0
Invasive squamous cell carcinoma	0	0	0	0	0	7.7	0
Sarcoma	0	0	1.1	0	0	0	0
Other	2.5	3.7	2.2	0	14.3	0	0
Total:	100	100	100	100	100	100	100

The highest incidence rates of breast cancer were reported in St. David (544.8/100 000). The second highest rate was reported in St. George

(472.9/100,000), followed by Carriacou and Petit Martinique (362.7/100,000). The lowest rate was reported in St. Patrick (242.4/100 000) (see Figure 3). Overall, out of all the confirmed cases of breast cancer in each parish, invasive ductal carcinoma was the most common sub-type noted throughout (Tables 4-5).

DISCUSSION

Between January 1, 2001 and December 31, 2010, 207 breast cancer cases were identified. The most recent calculated age-adjusted incidence rate was 31.1/100,000 for the year 2010. Upon regional evaluation, Grenada still has a fairly low incidence rate when compared to Jamaica (56.8/100,000), The Republic of Trinidad and Tobago (36/100,000), and the Dominican Republic (32.7/100,000) (4). From a global perspective, Belgium has the highest incidence rate of breast cancer, with an age-adjusted incidence rate of 109.2/100,000 (4). Compared to other countries around the world, the low incidence rate of breast cancer in Grenada can be due to demographic factors, such as the country having a predominantly black population. The Centers for Disease Control and Prevention (2015) stated that white women had a higher risk of developing breast cancer compared to black women.

Overall, the highest incidence rates across the time period were observed in the 40-49 age category, and the lowest incidence rates overall were observed in the 20-29 age category. Like in many other countries, we can conclude that in Grenada, new breast cancer cases is not a common disease amongst a younger population. Breast cancer is the most common cancer amongst females globally (7); hence, there has been a global rising of attention to the disease. Breast cancer awareness has increased on the island of Grenada in the last decade, and this could explain the periods of increase where more people might have been seeking professional care.

On September 7, 2004 and July 13, 2005, Hurricanes Ivan and Emily hit the island of Grenada. Significant changes were noted in the year 2005, with a downward trend of breast cancer incidence rates observed for all age-categories. The population may have suffered psychological trauma following the environmental disasters and, as a result, may have been oblivious to the statuses of their health, resulting in the decreased identification of cases. More significantly, the disasters caused severe destruction and devastation to the island, both physically (landscape) and economically. The island's water and electrical supplies were interrupted for a long period. With this, health services were only available on a limited scale to the population. This resulted in a major disruption to the health care system and could explain the observed decline in the trend of breast cancer incidence rates.

An unstable economic situation has been reported for Grenada over the last five years. This instability is reflected in the results collected between the years 2007 and 2010 that demonstrate instability and inconsistency (no trend established). Prior to the July 2008 elections, high inflation rates were seen in the price of basic commodities-food and fuel. In 2009, the economic performance was recorded as -5.7% of the GDP. The recession could be an explanation for the downward trend seen in the years 2007 and 2009.

The recession has considerably affected the Grenadian economy and, overall, the functioning of the Grenadian health care system over the years. Grenada's health care system is predominantly universal; however, the system is overburdened and lacks sufficient human and financial resources to offer universal coverage for all. Therefore, this results in long waiting times when patients seek health care services. Reluctantly, many people are forced to pay out-of-pocket for the services they need. To those who cannot afford this service, they are subjected to waiting for long periods of time to have procedures performed, such as breast tissue biopsies. This would result in many cases remaining undiagnosed.

Invasive ductal carcinomas followed by lobular carcinomas have been described as the most common pathologic breast cancer types. Medullary, mucinous and papillary carcinomas of the breast have been described in the literature as rarer histological subtypes of breast cancer (6-8). Medullary cancers have been said to account for 2% of all breast cancers globally (9). It is most commonly found in women who have the mutated BRCA-1 gene. Current research suggests that medullary carcinomas have a more favorable prognosis compared to invasive ductal carcinomas of the breast (6, 8).

Mucinous carcinomas are said to account for approximately 2% of all breast carcinomas globally (10). They are slow growing tumours, with close to none or very slight lymph infiltration, and usually have a more favorable prognosis compared to other types. Tubular carcinomas of the breast account for approximately 1% of all breast cancers, globally (11). This statistic is consistent with the findings of this study. The recurrence rate of this sub-type is very low. Papillary carcinomas of the breast usually does not infiltrate other body parts and normally affect older people (12). This demonstrates a good prognosis. Papillary carcinoma subtypes were noted in very insignificant proportions in the population of this study.

A recent study carried out to assess breast cancer morbidity in peri-menopausal women found that 42.7% of the cases identified from the population were pre-menopausal (13). This study shows that the majority of the population with breast cancer were pre-menopausal women. Fifty one percent of the reported cases in the Grenada population were under the age of 50 years. Furthermore, 34% of the reported cases were between the ages of 30-45 years. With reference to an earlier study, the age of menopause is observed to be 50 years (14). A significantly large proportion of the cases reported were pre-menopausal, and this may suggest the possible existence of a BRCA-1 mutation within the population. BRCA 1 and BRCA 2 mutations are associated with early onset of breast cancer in women (15).

Age is a known risk factor for breast cancer; there is an increased risk with age. However, there is a much poorer prognosis for younger diagnosed cases (16, 17). This is because younger cases have more aggressive forms of breast cancer with poor prognosis (16). With a significantly large percentage of cases in the population identified under the age of 50 years, there is a need for the Grenadian government to design health promotion programs that encourage screening for breast cancer with the goal of early diagnosis.

The survival rate from breast cancer is considerably lower in the younger population. It is believed that this is due to the strong association with BRCA gene mutation (18). In our study population, 19% of all the cases were below the age of 40 years. This is a significant proportion, and preventive measures should be applied to the population to ensure early diagnosis, which increases survival chances and improved quality of life.

Significant spatial distributions (by parish) of breast cancer were described in the findings of the research. Current research is proposing possible associations between geographically distributed environmental toxins and the development of mutations on the BRCA-1 genes (19). The parish of St David reported the highest incidence rate followed by St. George, and St. Patrick having the lowest incident rate. In Grenada, families are normally clustered by geographical region (in this case, parish). With this, further research needs to be conducted to see if an association exists between the distribution (parish) of incidence and familial history of breast cancer and mutation in the BRCA1 gene.

In conclusion, the Ministry of Health in Grenada needs to make a commitment to develop and establish appropriate surveillance systems for breast cancer. A local cancer registry for breast cancer was commissioned in 2008 but, to date, it still requires much work in order to be considered fully functional. A true estimate of the burden of breast cancer on the population can only be analyzed when proper surveillance systems are put into operation.

Furthermore, in the effort of prevention, the Ministry of Health should promote early breast cancer detection through screening by mammography. The American Cancer Society currently has guidelines for age at mammography to begin at 40. Much research has been carried out to assess the benefits of early detection of breast cancer mainly through screening by mammography. Studies have indicated that early detection substantially decreases mortality rates (20, 21). One study claimed that mammography screening had been shown to have the greatest effect on breast cancer mortality reduction in the age group of 50-69 years (19). Another study claimed that early detection through mammography decreases breast cancer mortality by up to 25% (22). It is claimed that the promotion of screening by mammography for women between the ages of 40-49 years results in increased low-grade detections, decreased treatments, and decreased recurrence rates (23). These findings may be applied to the population of this study, which reported an alarming fraction (51%) of the cases as being under the age of 50. In addition to this, continuous awareness campaigns, the promotion of self-breast examinations from age 20, and biennial clinical breast exams should be encouraged.

The limitation of the study was the chosen surveillance medium used to identify the cases of breast cancer in Grenada. The study only reported cases that were identified through breast tissue biopsy and histological examination at the Pathology Department in the General Hospital, Grenada. Consequently, many cases were excluded from participation. Therefore, this would have affected the trend (person/place/time) analysis and resulted in an under-estimation of the true burden of breast cancer in the population.

Acknowledgment

We are grateful to Dr Barrymore Mcbarnette, Chief Oncologist at the Grenada General Hospital for all the assistance given to facilitate the data collection process. We would like to acknowledge Dr Hegamin-Younger for her contribution to the statistical analysis. Finally, we would like to extend our appreciation to Dr Scarlett Stuart, who offered advice on the basis of her medical expertise and passion for the study of Breast cancer.

References

[1] Youlden DR, Cramb SM, Dunn NA, Muller JM, Pyke CM, Baade PD. The descriptive epidemiology of female breast cancer. Cancer Epidemiol June 2012;36(3):237-48.

[2] Torre LA, Bray F, Siegel RL, Ferlay J, Lortet-Tieulent J, Jemal A. Global cancer statistics. CA Cancer J Clin 2015;65(2):87-108.

[3] American Cancer Society. Global cancer facts and figures, 2nd edition. Atlanta, GA: American Cancer Society, 2011.

[4] Global Cancer Control. World cancer report 2008. Lyon: International Agency Reseach Cancer, 2008.

[5] Delpech PA, Haynes-Smith G. Breast self-examination and health beliefs in Grenadian women. Cancer Nurs 2015;38(5):54–9.

[6] Samir S, Fayaz MS, Motawy MM, Abuzallouf S, George T, Abdelhady MM, et al. Medullary carcinoma of the breast: Ten-year clinical experience of the Kuwait Cancer Control centre. J Clin Oncol 2008:26:1-8.

[7] Ferlay J, Shin HR, Bray F, Forman D, Mathers C, Parkin DM. *Estimates of worldwide burden of cancer in 2008.* Int J Cancer 2010;127(12):2893-917.

[8] Albrektsen G, Heuch I, Thoresen S. Histological type and grade of breast cancer tumors by parity, age at birth, and time since birth: a register –based study in Norway. BMC Cancer 2010:10:1-11.

[9] Vincent-Salomon A, Gruel N, Lucchesi C, MacGrogan G, Dendale R, Sigal-Zafrani B, et al. Identification of typical medullary breast carcinoma as a genomic sub-group of basal-like carcinomas, a heterogenous new molecular entity. Breast Cancer Res 2007:9(2):1-15.

[10] Sharma S, Bansal R, Khare A, Agrawal N. Mucinous carcinoma of breast: cytodiagnosis of a case. J Cytol 2011:28(1):42-4.

[11] Sanz MI, Casas FT, Rodriguez GN, Xaurado RF, Gimferrer MC, Perez CA, et al. Clinical features and prognosis of tubular breast cancer. Breast Cancer Res 2011:13(suppl 2):P1.

[12] Benkaddour YA, Hasnaoui SE, Fichtali K, Fakhir B, Jalal H, Kouchani M, et al. Intracystic papillary carcinoma of the breast: report of three cases and literature review. Case Rep Obstet Gynecol 2012;2012:979563.

[13] Butt Z, Haider SF, Arif S, Khan MR, Ashfaq U, Shahbaz U, et al. Breast cancer risk factors: a comparison between pre-menopausal and post-menopausal women. J Pak Med Assoc 2012:62(2):120-4.

[14] Velez MP, Alvarado B, Lord C, Zunzunegui MV. Life course socioeconomic adversity and age at natural menopause in women from Latin America and the Caribbean. Menopause 2010:17(3):552-9.

[15] Peto J, Collins N, Barfoot R, Seal S, Warren W, Rahman N, et al. Prevalence of BRCA1 and BRCA2 gene mutations in patients with early-onset breast cancer. *J Natl Cancer Institute* 1999;91(11):943-9.

[16] Dirier A, Burhanedtin-Zincircioglu S, Karadayi B, Isikdogan, Aksu R. Characteristics and prognosis of breast cancer in younger women. J BUON 2009:14(4):619-23.

[17] Anders CK, Johnson R, Litton J, Phillips M, Bleyer A. Breast cancer before age 40 years. Semin Oncol 2009;36(3):237–49. doi: 10.1053/j.seminoncol.2009.03.001.

[18] Nixon AJ, Neuberg D, Hayes DF, Gelman R, Connoly JL, Schnitt S, et al. Relationship of patient age to pathologic features of the tumor and prognosis for patients with stage I or II breast cancer. J Clin Oncol 1994:2(5):888-94.

[19] Brody JG, Rudel RA. Environmental pollutants and breast cancer. Environ Health Perspect 2003:111(8):1007-19.

[20] Peto R, Boreham J, Clarke M, Davies C, Beral V. UK and USA breast cancer deaths down 25% in year 2000 at ages 20-69 years. Lancet 2000:355(9217):1822.

[21] Mettler FA, Upton AC, Kelsey CA, Ashby RN, Robert NA, Rosenberg RD, et al. Benefits versus risks from mammography: A critical reassessment. Cancer 1996:77(5):903-9.

[22] Snekus E, Kyriakides S, Ohno S, Penault-Llorca F, Poortmans P, Rutgers E, et al. Primary breast cancer: ESMO clinical practice guidelines for diagnosis, treatment and follow-up. Ann Oncol 2015;26(Suppl 5):v8-v30.

[23] Qassem A, Snow V, Sherif K, Aronson M, Weiss KB, Owens DK. Screening mammography for women 40 to 49 years of age: A clinical practice guideline from the American College of Physicians. Ann Intern Med 2007:146:511-5.

In: Public Health Themes in Grenada … ISBN: 978-1-53618-118-0
Editors: J. Merrick and L. Glasgow © 2020 Nova Science Publishers, Inc.

Chapter 9

PROSTATE CANCER IN GRENADA, WEST INDIES: A SEVEN-YEAR TREND ANALYSIS FOR THE PERIOD 2008-2014

Vandyke Jones, MD, MPH, Colby Hansen, BS, Bradley Wainoris, BSN, Caroline Bashour, BS, Sulayman Khan, BS, Charisse Douglas-Jones, MD, Shelly Rodrigo, PhD and Emmanuel Keku*, MD, MA, MSPH

School of Medicine, Department of Public Health and Preventive Medicine, St George's University, Grenada, West Indies

ABSTRACT

Prostate cancer is the second most commonly diagnosed cancer in men worldwide, with countries such as the United States showing a higher

* Correspondence: Dr Emmanuel Keku, Professor, Department of Public Health and Preventive Medicine, St George's University, POBox 7, True Blue, St George's, Grenada, West Indies. Email: ekeku@sgu.edu.

incidence of prostate cancer in African American men. Studies performed in neighboring Caribbean countries show a high incidence of prostate cancer. Grenada is a small island country in the Caribbean with a population that is predominantly of African descent. Currently, there is limited data regarding the burden of prostate cancer in Grenada. This chapter seeks to determine the incidence, distribution, and mortality rate of prostate cancer in Grenada from 2008-2014. A cross-sectional study was performed utilizing secondary surveillance data available from national registries. Analytical software was used to determine the incidence, mortality, and distribution of cases by parish in Grenada during the period of study. Local incidence rate was as high as 91.03/100,000 (average 70.1/100,000). Mortality rate averaged 83.4/100,000. St. John was the parish with the highest recorded rate of 210/100,000 during the study period, with the parishes St. George and St. John having the highest overall 7-year average. Grenada has incidence levels comparable to Caribbean regional figures. There were higher mortality rates than expected. The geographical distribution of cases shows the parish of St. John having the highest individual incidence rate during the period.

INTRODUCTION

Grenada is a tri-island nation consisting of Grenada, Carriacou, and Petite Martinique. It has a population of 105,539 people, 53,008 male, and approximately 89.4% of African ancestry (1). Since the end of the 18th century, the vast majority of the population in the Caribbean region is of African descent (2). The ethnic profile of a geographical region is important to consider when examining disease rates. Prostate cancer has an increased incidence in African American men in the United States, and similar trends are seen in the mortality rate trends during the past 15 years (3). Worldwide, prostate cancer is the second most commonly diagnosed cancer in men in over 12 of the planet's most populated nations (4). In fact, there were 1.1 million men worldwide who were diagnosed with prostate cancer in 2012 alone (5).

Before the advent of screening using prostate-specific antigen (PSA) testing, prostate cancer often went undiagnosed and, therefore, untreated. When PSA testing became more commonly used, the rate of diagnosed prostate cancer began to spike (6). This increase in the number of identified cases was seen in the US during the 1980s; it was also corroborated by similar rises in the incidence of many European countries during the 1990s (4).

According to a study done recently in Barbados, the Caribbean region generally has similarly high rates of prostate cancer in its black populations (7). In fact, Martinique, which is another Caribbean country with similar ethnic profile, had the highest rate of prostate cancer worldwide in 2011 (8). There are also four other Caribbean countries ranked in the top twenty highest prostate cancer incidence rates worldwide, which include Trinidad and Tobago, Barbados, Guadeloupe, and Puerto Rico (9).

According to the National Vital Statistics System, cancer was the number one cause of death among men and women in 2014. In relation to morbidity, prostate cancer has the highest rates; however, prostate cancer was the third most commonly diagnosed after cervical cancer and breast cancer, respectively (10). A study conducted by Asulin et al. revealed that between the years 1990-2000, prostate cancer accounted for 61.4% of the male cancer cases and 53.6% of the cases associated with mortality (11).

Studies have shown that men are less likely to visit their doctor than women (12), and as such, it is quite often that cancer has already progressed to an advanced stage by the time it is diagnosed (13). This would have more of an impact on mortality than an early diagnosis potentially would. The authors of this paper noted a lack of research on prostate cancer in Grenada over the past 15 years. Other cancers, such as cervical and breast cancer, have both been investigated within the past five years (10).

The goal of this chapter is to perform a review of prostate cancer trends in Grenada within the last seven years with the hope of contributing to future interventions to decrease its impact. The specific objectives were to identify the incidence of prostate cancer in Grenada within the last seven years (2008-2014); to identify the mortality of prostate cancer in Grenada during the years (2009-2013) and to determine the distribution, by parish, of prostate cancer incidence and mortality in Grenada (2009-2014).

OUR STUDY

A cross-sectional study was conducted utilizing secondary information derived from the National Cancer Registry, the National Statistics Office, and the Births and Deaths Registry. The analysis of the data was conducted utilizing the software: Microsoft Excel 2016, Epi Info7, and IBM SPSS Statistics 20.

The three existing resources were reviewed for data on prostate cancer during the period extending from 2008-2014. Data from the National Cancer Registry was used to determine the number of prostate cancer cases over that 7-year period among the male population of Grenada. That value was subsequently used to calculate the incidence rate per 100,000 of the male population. A case was defined as a male patient entered into the National Cancer Registry with a diagnosis of prostate cancer with corresponding histopathological confirmation. The age standardization rate was also calculated (ASR).

The National Cancer Registry also provided geographical information permitting the categorization of the cases by parish in Grenada. Grenada has seven parishes: Carriacou, St. Andrew, St. David, St. George, St. John, St. Mark, and St. Patrick. The Grenada Births and Deaths Registry was consulted in order to determine the deaths between the years 2009-2013 due to prostate cancer. The cases in which prostate cancer was the primary cause of death were included in this study.

FINDINGS

The data for prostate cancer incidence was collected from the period between January 2008 and December 2014. During this time period, 263 men were diagnosed with prostate cancer with a histopathological confirmation. The collection period for the data on the mortality rate of prostate cancer was January 2009 to December 2013. During this time period, there were 200 recorded deaths in which prostate cancer was the primary cause. Table 1 reports the distribution of new diagnoses of prostate cancer each year from 2008-2014. The distribution showed that 2014 had the highest frequency, with 50 new cases (19.1%) that year, closely followed by 2008, which had 39 new cases (14.8%). 2013 had the lowest frequency with 23 new cases (8.7%). Table 1 and Figure 1 also show the distribution of prostate cancer cases according to parish in Grenada. The parish of St. George had the greatest proportion of cases with 117 cases (44.5%). It was followed by the parish of St. Andrew with 19.8% of the cases (52). St. Mark and Carriacou had the lowest proportion of cases over the collection period with 4.2% and 4.9%, respectively.

Table 1. The frequency of new prostate cancer cases by year 2008-2014 and by parish

Variables		Frequency	Percentage (%)	Cumulative Total
Years	2008	39	14.8	14.8
	2009	48	18.3	33.1
	2010	40	15.2	48.3
	2011	33	12.5	60.8
	2012	30	11.4	72.4
	2013	23	8.7	80.9
	2014	50	19.1	100
Total		263	100%	100%
Parishs	Carriacou	13	4.9	4.9
	St. Andrew's	52	19.8	24.7
	St. David's	22	8.4	33.1
	St. George's	117	44.5	77.6
	St. John's	27	10.3	87.9
	St. Mark's	11	4.1	92.
	St. Patrick's	21	8.0	100
Total		263	100	100%

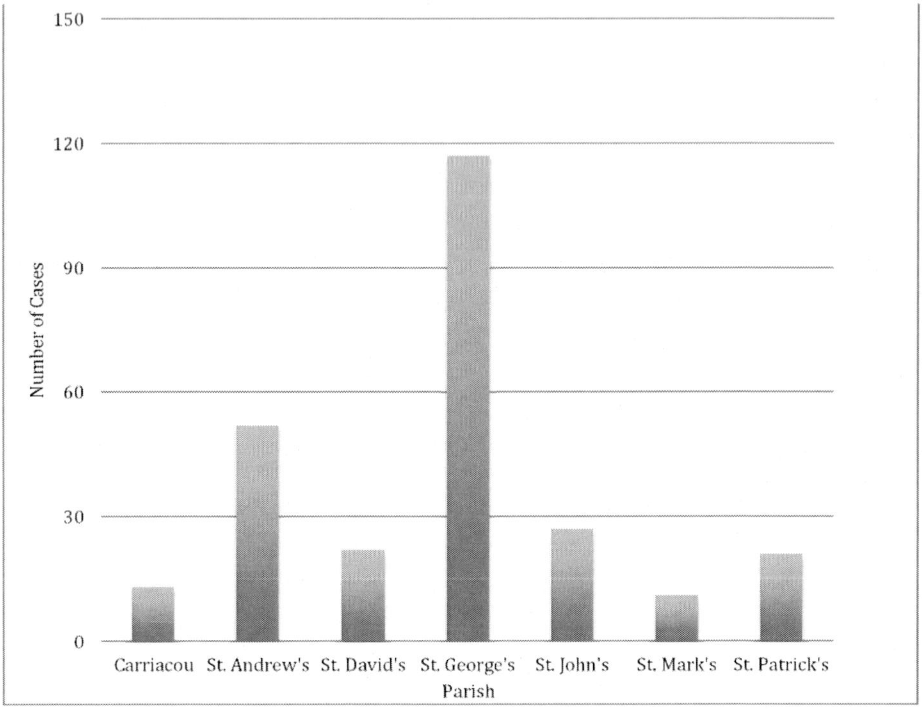

Figure 1. Frequency of new prostate cancer cases by Parish in Grenada 2008-2014.

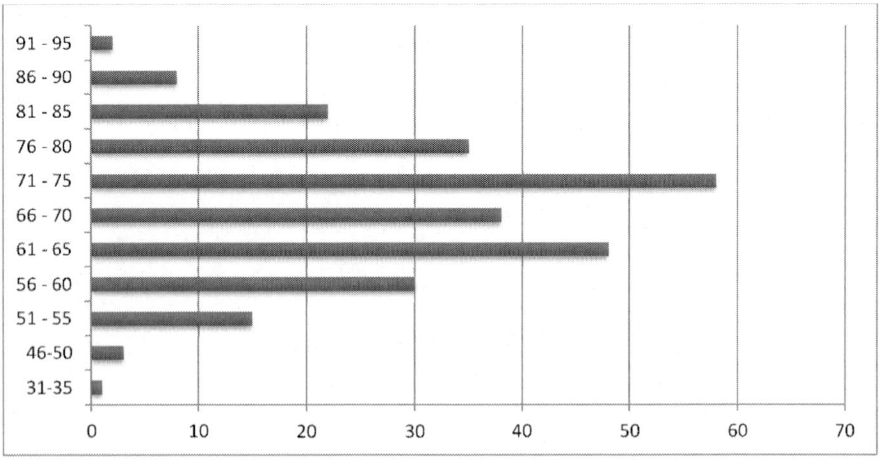

Figure 2. Prostate cancer distribution by age group in Grenada, 2008-2014.

Figure 2 shows the distribution of new prostate cancer cases by age group. The 71-75 year age group has the highest occurrence of new cases over the collection period, with the 61-65 age group having the second highest number of new cases of prostate cancer. The age group with the lowest number of cases was 31-35 years, with just one case in 2014, which was the year with the highest incidence overall. This patient was diagnosed at age 32 years. The average age for diagnosis of prostate cancer in Grenada during this period was 68–72 years, which was also the most commonly occurring age in the data set. Figure 3 and Table 2 present the deaths attributed to prostate cancer in the study period 2009-2013. The number of deaths from prostate cancer showed a progressive increase with age until it peaked and then declined. The age group, which had the most prostate-related deaths, was 71-75, which is also where we saw most of the new cases. The mean age of death primarily due to prostate cancer is around 76.7 years, with 78 years being the most common age of death; similar trends for prostate cancer mortality appear in the UK (7) as well as in the United States (8).

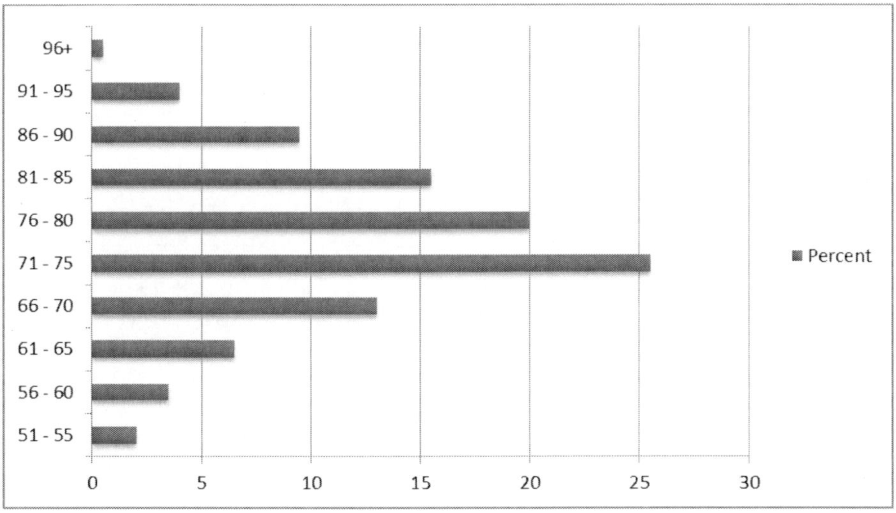

Figure 3. Prostate cancer mortality in Grenada, 2009-2013.

Table 2. Prostate cancer mortality by age group, Grenada, 2009-2013

		Frequency	Percent
Valid	51 - 55	4	2.0
	56 - 60	7	3.5
	61 - 65	13	6.5
	66 - 70	26	13.0
	71 - 75	51	25.5
	76 - 80	40	20.0
	81 - 85	31	15.5
	86 - 90	19	9.5
	91 - 95	8	4.0
	96+	1	0.5
	Total	200	100.0

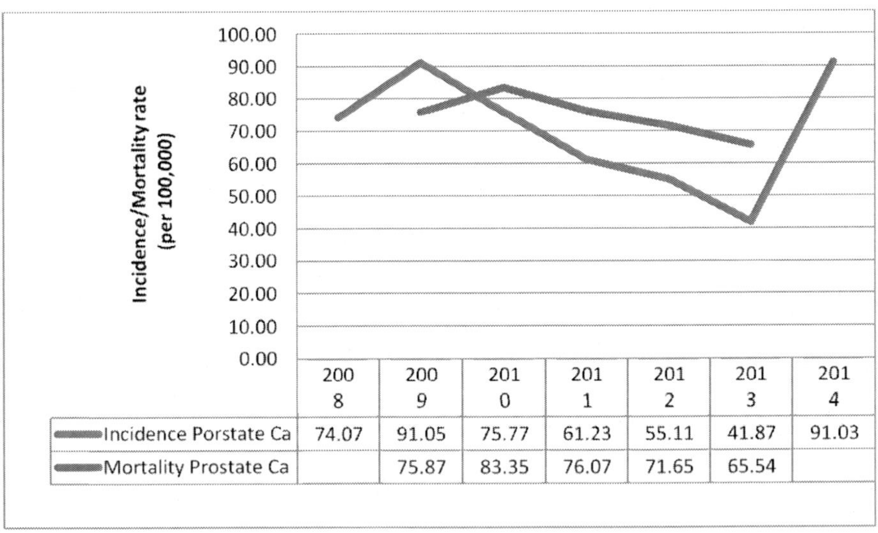

Figure 4. Prostate cancer in Grenada, incidence (2008-2014) vs. mortality (2009-2013).

Figure 4 presents the incidence of prostate cancer per 100,000 as it compares to the mortality rate. Unlike what is seen in the US (8), but similar to the trend in Barbados (9), the mortality rate appears to be relatively high and has surpassed the incidence rate from 2010-2013. The highest incidence seen was in 2014 (91.03), with the lowest rate noted in 2013(41.87). The highest mortality rate was in 2010 (83.35), which then declined to the lowest rate in 2013 (65.54). Figure 5 shows the age-specific incidence of prostate cancer for the Grenadian male population as it compares to the US population of African American men and the overall incidence in the US. In all cases, the age group of 65-74 years had the highest incidence. The incidence in the US nearly doubled the incidence in Grenada. Of all the cases, the 20-49 year age group has the fewest cases among all the countries whose populations were compared. The population standardized incidence rate of Grenadian men when calculated according to the Surveillance, Epidemiology and End Results (SEER) US 2000 population was 60.47, though, among Grenadian men, it averaged 70.89 and was as high as 91.03 in 2014. The incidence in Grenada is lower than the Barbadian incidence rate over the 2002-2008 study period (158.80) (9).

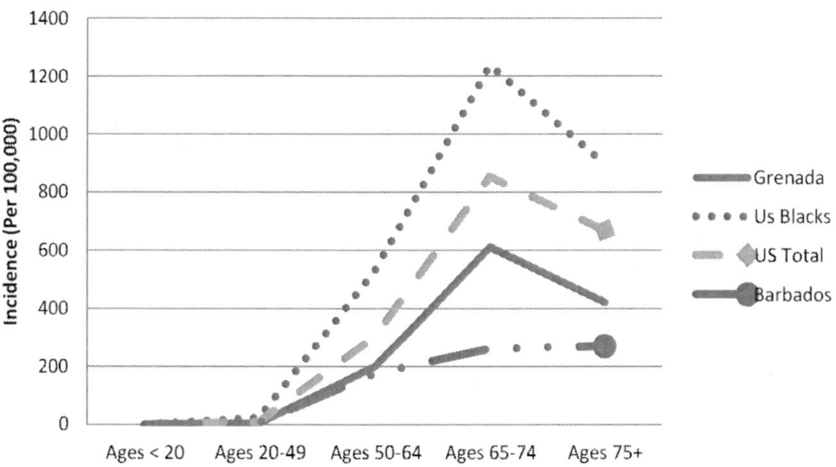

*Population standardization was not done to US 2000 population as the other regional and US Black population were seen as sufficiently similar not to warrant it.

Figure 5. Age specific incidence of prostate cancer in Grenada (2008-2014) * Barbados (2002-2008) and US (2006-2012).

Figure 6 shows the incidence rate throughout the 7-year study period with respect to the seven parishes in Grenada (per 100,000). The highest recorded incidence during this period was in the parish of St. John in 2010, which was as high as 208.48; this is about three times higher than the national rate during that year. St. John retained the highest incidence rate for three consecutive years (2009-2011) and again in 2014. St. George had the highest rate in 2008 (112.42), Carriacou in 2011 (105.67), and St. Mark in 2013 (132.5) despite having two years without any cases (2010, 2011). Figure 7 shows a graphical representation of the distribution of the cases by parishes over the 7-year period. St. George had the highest number of cases of prostate cancer (117), and St. Andrew had the second highest (52 days). St. Mark had the lowest number of cases (11).

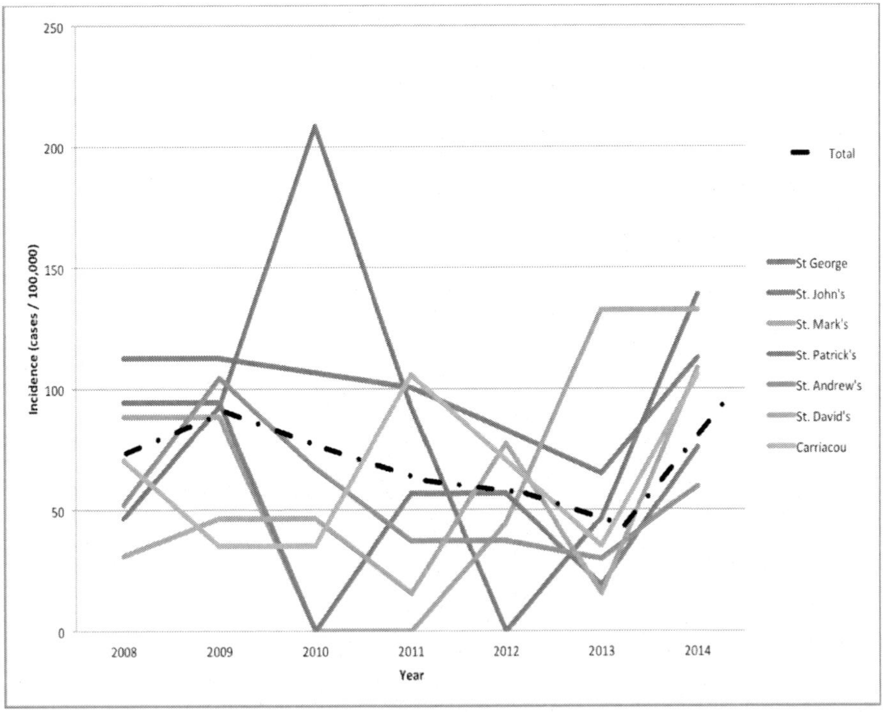

Figure 6. Distribution of incidence rates by parish between 2008-2014.

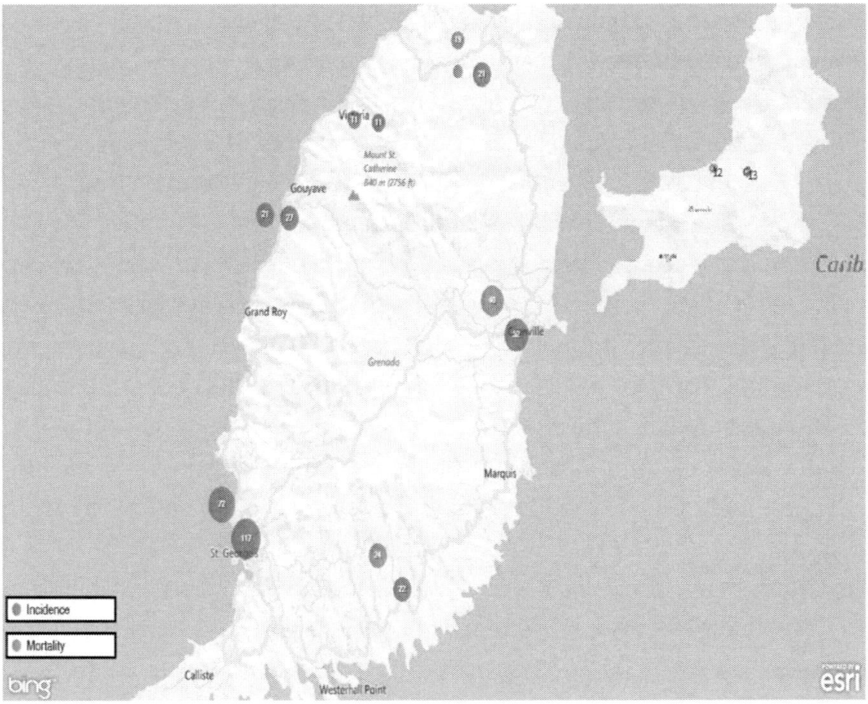

Figure 7. Distribution of prostate cancer incidence rates (2008-2014) and mortality rates (2009-2013) by parish in Grenada.

DISCUSSION

A prostate cancer registry was first established in Grenada by Dr. Robert Yearwood, and from 1996-2007 reportedly, it had recorded 300 cases of prostate cancer (8). Grenadian males, during the seven-year study period from 2008-2014, had a total of 263 incident cases. Grenada's incidence per 100,000 for prostate cancer in its male population had an incidence rate in 2014 was 91.03/100,000. During the 7-year study period, the average incidence was 70.1. According to the World Cancer Research Fund (WCRF), the incidence rate recorded in Grenada in both 2009 and 2014 (91.05 and 91.03 /100,000 respectively), would place Grenada as having the 18th highest incidence of prostate cancer globally (5).

The 2004 study conducted in Grenada by Asulin et al., which was done between 1990-2000, recorded an incidence rate of 61.4 /100,000, which was lower than our currently recorded national 7-year incidence rate. This implies that there has been an increase in the number of new cases over the past 14 years in Grenada. According to the study by Gibson et al. from 1998-2002, the average incidence in Jamaica was 65.6/100,000, which was still lower than the 7-year average in our study in Grenada (11).

The Grenadian incidence rate over the collection period was still lower than that recorded in Barbados by Hennis et al. (7) in 2011, which was 160.4/100,000 for their 7-year study between 2002-2008. This rate ranked Barbados as number 4 by the WCRF (5). The trend between 2009-2013 showed a decrease in the prostate cancer incidence rates in Grenada from 91.05/100,000 to 41.87/100,000, which was similar to the pattern shown in the US rates according to SEER for that time period (2009-2012). During that period, black Americans showed an incidence rate that was higher at 223.7/100,000 (8). However, Grenada showed a rise in its incidence rates once again up to 91.03/100,000 in 2014. The mortality rate for prostate cancer between 2009-2013 was 83.4/100,000. This rate was higher than the incidence rate between 2010-2013, a trend that was not seen in the other compared populations in the region or amongst African Americans in the US (11).

The rate in the previous study done in Grenada was lower at 53.6/100,000. This mortality rate was also higher than the 7-year average incidence in Barbados of 63.7/100,000 and in African Americans in the US of 82.7/100,000. It is suspected that this difference may be attributed to the limited screening and treatment options currently available in the country. Additionally, it was observed in a previous study that male patients tend to visit their doctors less frequently than females resulting in diagnoses occurring at a more advanced stage of cancer (4).

The parishes with the highest individual 7-year average incidence rates were St. George, St. John, St. Mark, and Carriacou, respectively (98.90, 89.35, 69.41 and 69.42 per-100,000). These parishes all share the western coast of the Caribbean Sea. As far as the author of this study is currently aware, there is no comparative study done in the Caribbean, which considers the distribution of prostate cancer incidence rates by location with which this finding can be compared. Strengths in the study are:

- Histopathological confirmation is the most accurate form of definitive prostate cancer diagnosis.
- Use of a functional cancer registry.
- Use of updated census data (2011)
- Regional comparisons to recently conducted studies.

Weaknesses in the study are:

- Loss of data: There is a private urology practice on the island, which occasionally sends patients to external diagnosis labs outside of Grenada. These patients were not included in the data from the hospital pathology laboratory, making the true incidence rates slightly higher than those reported.
- Co-morbidities are not always considered in the cause of death. For our study, the morbidity figures were compiled from prostate cancer being either a definitive or a probable cause of death.
- Undocumented cases may contribute to reduced prostate cancer diagnoses. As discussed in the paper, men tend to neglect visiting their physicians, which may contribute to unreported cases. Along with this, a lack of screening in specific age groups could contribute to the undocumented cases.

In conclusion, prostate cancer incidence rates in Grenada are overall trending high compared to other regional rates. Prostate cancer mortality was higher than expected; in some years, it was higher than the incidence rate. The distribution of prostate cancer by parish shows higher incidences in the parish of St. John and all of the other west coast (Caribbean Sea) parishes. Further studies are needed to formulate and investigate hypotheses to explain and corroborate some of these findings. In addition, major public health concerns have been raised in terms of the high local incidence rates as well as the geographical distribution of the cases. These also need to be addressed.

ACKNOWLEDGMENTS

The author of this paper will like to recognize the assistance and contributions of the following persons: The Department of Public Health and Preventative Medicine, School of Medicine, St. George's University Grenada; Dr Allister Antoine, Dr Francis Martin and Mrs Angela Joseph at the Ministry of Health of Grenada; and Dr Barrymore McBarnett and Ms Leandra Charles at the oncology department (national cancer registry) of the Grenada General Hospital.

REFERENCES

[1] Central Intelligence Agency. The world factbook: Grenada, 2018. URL: https://www.cia.gov/library/publications/the-world-factbook/geos/gj.html.

[2] Appiah A, Gates HL. Africana the encyclopedia of the African and African American experience. New York: Basic Civitas Books, 1999.

[3] Centers for Disease Control and Prevention. USCS data visualizations. URL: https://gis.cdc.gov/cancer/USCS/DataViz.html.

[4] Cancer patterns, Trends and burden. URL: http://www.iarc.fr/en/publications/books/iarc50/IARC_Ch4.2.1_web.pdf.

[5] Cancer today. Global cancer observatory. URL: http://gco.iarc.fr/today/fact-sheets-cancers.

[6] Yossepowitch O. Prostate cancer in men with serum PSA of <4ng/ml: Under-diagnosed or over-treated? Eur Urology 2008;53(4):686–8.

[7] Hennis AJM, Hambleton IR, Wu S-Y, Skeete DH-A, Nemesure B, Leske MC. Prostate cancer incidence and mortality in Barbados, West Indies. Prostate Cancer 2011;2011:1–10.

[8] Belpomme D, Irigaray P. Environment as a potential key determinant of the continued increase of prostate cancer incidence in Martinique. Prostate Cancer 2011;2011:1–8.

[9] Prostate leading newly diagnosed cancer among men; breast cancer leads for women. Bethesda, ND: NIH-National Cancer Institute, 2004.

[10] Avi A T Bahadoor - Yetman, Riley L, Gibbons A, Fields PJ, Mapp-Alexander V, Hage R, et al. Prevalence of cervical cancer and associated mortality in Grenada: A ten-year analysis (2000 - 2010). Rev Panamericana Salud Publica 2016;39(4):194-9.

[11] Asulin Y, McCann TJ, McCarty CW, Hage RW, Rooney PJ, Macpherson CNL. Cancer incidence and mortality in Grenada 1990-2000. West Indian Med J 2005;53(6):368-73.

[12] Thomas K. Common men's health conditions (urology). URL: https://www.loyolamedicine.org/urology/mens-health-conditions.

[13] Bailey L. Study: African American men say doctor visits are often a bad experience. URL: https://news.umich.edu/study-african-american-men-say-doctor-visits-are-often-a-bad-experience/.

[14] Data on prostate cancer in Grenada. Prostate cancer Caribbean 2008. URL: https://pccaribbean.wordpress.com/site-map/grenada/data/.

[15] Ancient Egyptian medicine. URL: http://medlibrary.org/medwiki/Ancient_Egyptian_medicine.

[16] Haas GP, Delongchamps N, Brawley OW, Wang CY, de la Roza G. The worldwide epidemiology of prostate cancer: perspectives from autopsy studies. Can J Urol 2008;15(1):3866-71.

[17] Cancer incidence statistics. Cancer research UK 2020. URL: https://www.cancerresearchuk.org/health-professional/cancer-statistics/incidence#heading-One.

[18] SEER Prostate Cancer by age group 1975-2012. URL http://seer.cancer.gov/faststats/selections.php#Output

[19] Hennis AJM, Hambleton IR, Wu S-Y, Skeete DH, Nemesure B, Leske MC. Prostate cancer incidence and mortality in Barbados, west indies. Prostate Cancer 2011;2011:565230. doi:10.1155/2011/565230.

[20] Haas GP, Delongchamps N, Brawley OW, Wang CY, de la Roza G. The worldwide epidemiology of prostate cancer: perspectives from autopsy studies. Can J Urol 2008;15(1):3866-71.

[21] Gibson T, Hanchard B, Waugh N, Mcnaughton D. Thirty-year trends in incidence and age-distribution of prostate cancer in Kingston and St Andrew, Jamaica, 1978–2007. West Indian Med J 2014;60(1):9-12.

In: Public Health Themes in Grenada … ISBN: 978-1-53618-118-0
Editors: J. Merrick and L. Glasgow © 2020 Nova Science Publishers, Inc.

Chapter 10

EPIDEMIOLOGIC SURVEILLANCE OF AMPUTATION IN GRENADA, 2010-2017

Shawn Charles[1], MD, MPH and Lindonne Glasgow[2,*], MSPH, DrPH
[1]Ministry of Health, Social Security and International Business, St George's, Grenada
[2]Department of Public Health and Preventive Medicine, St George's University, St George's, Grenada, West Indies

ABSTRACT

The prevalence of limb amputation related to peripheral arterial disease (PAD) and diabetes has attracted global attention as a major health problem. Recently published studies, however, are virtually absent on diabetes foot and lower limb complications in the Caribbean region. A

* Correspondence: Dr Lindonne Glasgow, Assistant Professor, Department of Public Health and Preventive Medicine, St George's University, POBox 7, True Blue, St George's, Grenada, West Indies. Email: lglasgow@sgu.com.

retrospective descriptive study was conducted in Grenada, a small Caribbean island, with secondary data from January 2010 to December 2017 of patients having amputations at the Grenada General Hospital. Data on demographics, reason for amputation, type of amputation, and comorbidities were also collected in the study. A total of 654 persons were recorded that had an amputation at the General Hospital; 370 (56.6%) males, 284 (43.4%) females, and median age 64 years (<1 to 105 years). The overall annual incidence of amputations ranged from 50.5 to 102.4 per 100,000 per year. Lower limb amputations ranged from 39.0 to 87.8 per 100,000 per year. Diabetes was comorbidity in 51.1% of amputations. Amputations can have negative effects on the quality of life of individuals. With indications of a potential global increase in the number of persons with diabetes, effective and timely diabetes prevention and management programs are of utmost importance in Grenada to address risk factors for amputations. Other Caribbean countries may benefit from this study, which creates awareness of the significance of the issue and the relevance for interventions to improve health outcomes in the region.

INTRODUCTION

The prevalence of limb amputation related to peripheral arterial disease (PAD) and diabetes has attracted global attention as a major health problem (1). An amputation is the removal of part of, or an entire, limb by surgery or trauma. Diabetes can cause microvascular and macrovascular complications that compromise immune response and blood circulation in the limbs resulting in the need for amputation to preserve life and health (2). Worldwide, between 40-60 million people are affected by diabetic foot and lower limb complications (3). Data from 12 countries in Europe and Australasia participating in the VASCUNET collaboration show the prevalence of diabetes among people who had amputations ranged from 25.7% in Finland to 74.3% in Slovakia, while the mean annual incidence of major amputations varied between 7.2/100,000 in New Zealand and 41.4/100 in Hungary (1). In a study in Canada, 81% of persons who had a lower limb amputated also had diabetic complications (4). In the United States, the Centers for Disease Control and Prevention (CDC) reported a decline in leg and foot amputations among people with diabetes from 1996-

2008 (5); however, a recent study reported a reverse in the trend between 2009-2015 (6). The CDC reported that 108,000 diabetes-related amputations were done in 2014 (7). The likelihood of having an amputation related to diabetes increased 4.9 times among people ≥65 years (1).

Overall, the risk for lower limb amputation is 10-fold higher among people with diabetes as compared to non-diabetic people (8), rendering diabetes as a significant cause of amputation and needing interventions for preventing the surgery. Lower limb amputation is the most common type of amputation among people with diabetes, while upper limb amputation related to diabetes is significantly fewer and usually associated with traumatic injury (8). Limb amputation is associated with emotional disturbances and trauma as well significant decline in the quality of life of the individual, particularly when there is minimal support to provide for basic needs and to access appropriate health care (9). High mortality rate, comorbidities, and high health care cost are major issues that contribute to poor health outcomes among people who had amputations (8).

This study describes the trends in amputations at the General Hospital in Grenada over eight years, 2010–2017. Grenada is a small island located in the southern part of the Caribbean archipelago, with a population of approximately 111,500 people. Few studies have been published recently on the prevalence and incidence of diabetic foot and limb complications and amputations in Caribbean countries. Older studies show an increasing rate of diabetes and related health problems, including amputations, in some Caribbean countries (10). In a study published in 2004, Barbados had among the highest rate of lower extremity amputations in the world (10). This study is, therefore, of value in determining the prevalence and potential impact of amputation in the Grenadian population. Other Caribbean countries may benefit from this study, which creates awareness of the significance of the issue and the relevance for interventions to improve health outcomes in the region.

Our study

A descriptive retrospective study was conducted using secondary data collected for the surveillance of amputations performed at Grenada General Hospital from the period 1st January 2010 to 31st December 2017. Grenada General Hospital is the main general medical and public surgical hospital in the state. It is the final referral hospital for both the public and private health sectors. It is a 198-bed facility, and the services offered include; accident and emergency, internal medicine, pediatrics, general surgery, obstetrics and gynecology, intensive care, ophthalmology, orthopedics, oncology, radiology, and laboratory services.

The Epidemiology and Information Department of the Ministry of Health routinely collects data on amputation as part of its surveillance of all health events in the country. Data on amputations were gathered from the paper-based operating theatre and surgical ward registers. A descriptive analysis of these data was undertaken to characterize the occurrence of amputations in Grenada.

The data elements selected for analysis included age, sex, parish of residence, dates of admission and discharge, reason for amputation, type of amputation, and comorbidities. The data were entered into a Microsoft Excel spreadsheet and analyzed to identify trends in the occurrence of amputations and the frequency of accompanying comorbidities.

Our findings

A total of 654 patients underwent one or more amputations at the General Hospital during the study period. Of that total, 370 (56.6%) were male, and 284 (43.4%) were female. The average age of the patients who had amputations varied by year, ranging from 63.2-65.9 years in 2011-2017. In 2010, the average age was 56.3 years. Table 1 shows the distribution of patients by sex.

Table 1. Distribution of patients that had amputations by sex

Sex	2010		2011		2012		2013		2014		2015		2016		2017		Total	
	No.	%	No.	%	No.	%	No.	%	No.	%	No.	%	No.	%	No.	%	No.	%
Female	19	35.8	28	42.4	43	44.8	34	45.3	59	52.2	38	39.2	41	41.4	22	40.0	284	43.4
Male	34	64.2	38	57.6	53	55.2	41	54.7	54	47.8	59	60.8	58	58.6	33	60.0	370	56.6
Grand Total	53	100.0	66	100.0	96	100.0	75	100.0	113	100.0	97	100.0	99	100.0	55	100.0	654	100.0

Table 2. Number and proportion of persons having amputations distributed by parish

Parish	2010		2011		2012		2013		2014		2015		2016		2017		Total	
	No.	%	No.	%	No.	%	No.	%	No.	%	No.	%	No.	%	No.	%	No.	%
St. Andrew	17	32.1	15	22.7	14	14.6	12	16.0	18	15.9	16	16.5	18	18.2	7	12.7	117	17.9
St. David	7	13.2	13	19.7	12	12.5	8	10.7	14	12.4	20	20.6	11	11.1	11	20.0	96	14.7
St. George	22	41.5	19	28.8	37	38.5	20	26.7	45	39.8	22	22.7	31	31.3	14	25.5	210	32.1
St. John	1	1.9	4	6.1	10	10.4	15	20.0	10	8.8	12	12.4	12	12.1	9	16.4	73	11.2
St. Mark	1	1.9	4	6.1	6	6.3	6	8.0	8	7.1	4	4.1	3	3.0	3	5.5	35	5.4
St. Patrick	3	5.7	9	13.6	13	13.5	8	10.7	12	10.6	8	8.2	9	9.1	6	10.9	68	10.4
Carriacou	2	3.8	2	3.0	3	3.1	6	8.0	6	5.3	5	5.2	2	2.0	4	7.3	30	4.6
Cruise ship	-	0.0	-	0.0	1	1.0	-	0.0	-	0.0	-	0.0	-	0.0	-	0.0	1	0.2
NA	-	0.0	-	0.0	-	0.0	-	0.0	-	0.0	10	10.3	13	13.1	1	1.8	24	3.7
Grand Total	53	100.0	66	100.0	96	100.0	75	100.0	113	100.0	97	100.0	99	100.0	55	100.0	654	100.0

Table 3. Incidence of amputations in Grenada by year

Year	Overall per 100,000	Upper limb amputations per 100,000	Lower limb amputations per 100,000	Finger/hand amputations per 100,000	Forearm/arm amputations per 100,000	Toe amputations per 100,000	Partial foot amputations per 100,000	BKA per 100,000	AKA per 100,000
2010	50.5	11.4	39.0	11.4	0.0	12.4	1.0	21.9	3.8
2011	61.9	8.4	53.4	8.4	0.0	15.0	2.8	30.0	5.6
2012	91.1	15.8	75.3	14.9	0.9	18.6	2.8	36.2	17.7
2013	69.1	12.9	56.2	12.0	0.9	20.3	1.8	25.8	8.3
2014	102.4	14.6	87.8	13.7	0.9	11.0	6.4	44.8	25.6
2015	89.0	10.9	78.1	9.1	1.8	20.9	6.4	32.7	18.2
2016	90.2	2.7	87.5	0.9	1.8	22.5	0.9	42.4	21.6
2017	48.4	2.7	45.8	2.7	0.0	18.8	0.0	24.2	2.7

BKA: Below knee amputations, AKA: Above knee amputations.

The parish with the largest proportion of cases over the eight-year period was St. George (32.1%), followed by St Andrew (17.9%). The years with the highest incidence of amputations were 2012 (91.1/100,00), 2014 (102.4/100,000), and 2016 (90.2/100,000). Tables 2-3 show the parish/residence of the patients having amputations and incidence per year.

Type of amputation and diagnosis

Overall, lower limb amputation was the most common type of amputation at the Grenada General Hospital. Below-knee amputation (BKA) was the most frequent procedure (281, 42.8%) followed by removal of toes and above-knee amputation (AKA). Upper limb amputation was more common in males and individuals in younger age groups. Loss of finger(s)/hand was more common than amputation at the forearm or arm. The most common reason for amputations in the upper limbs was injury. Tables 4-6 show the total number of amputations and the type and cause of upper limb amputations.

Table 4. Number and percentage of amputations, 2010-2017

Location of amputation	No.	%
Finger(s)/Hand	79	12.0
Forearm/Arm	7	1.1
Toe(s)	152	23.2
Partial foot (Trans metatarsal)	24	3.7
Below knee	281	42.8
Above knee	113	17.2
Total	656	100.0

*At least one patient had multiple amputations.

A total of 152 toe amputations were recorded, which represented 23.2% of the total. The highest number of toe amputations was in 2015 (23) and 2016 (25).

Table 5. Distribution of amputations of finger(s)/hand by gender and year

	2010		2011		2012		2013		2014		2015		2016		2017		Total	
	No.	%	No.	%	No.	%	No.	%	No.	%	No.	%	No.	%	No.	%	No.	%
Finger/hand amputation																		
Males	11	91.7	8	88.9	13	81.3	11	84.6	11	73.3	6	60.0	1	100.0	2	66.7	63	79.7
Females	1	8.3	1	11.1	3	18.8	2	15.4	4	26.7	4	40.0	-	-	1	33.3	16	20.3
Total	12	100.0	9	100.0	16	100.0	13	100.0	15	100.0	10	100.0	1	100.0	3	100.0	79	100.0
Forearm/arm amputation																		
Males	-	-	-	-	1	100.0	-	-	1	100.0	2	100.0	2	100.0	-	-	6	85.7
Females	-	-	-	-	-	-	1	100.0	-	-	-	-	-	-	-	-	1	14.3
Total	-	-	-	-	1	100.0	1	100.0	-	-	2	100.0	2	100.0	-	-	7	100.0

Table 6. Diagnosis or reason for upper limb amputation

Diagnosis/reason for amputation	Amputations of fingers/hand		Amputations of forearm/arm	
	No.	%	No.	%
Infection (including osteomyelitis, abscesses, etc.)	22	27.8	2	28.6
Gangrene	11	13.9	-	-
Injury	42	53.2	4	57.1
Congenital (polydactyly)	3	3.8	-	-
Cancer	1	1.3	-	-
Other	-	-	1	14.3
Total	79	100.0	7	100.0

The number of partial foot (trans metatarsal) amputations was 24 (3.7%) in total. The highest number of these procedures was in 2014 and 2015 with seven (7) and eight (8) cases, respectively. Below-knee amputations were the most common type of lower limb amputation with a total of 281 (42.8%) procedures during the eight-year period. The largest number of below-knee amputations were recorded in 2014 (49) and 2016 (47). A total of 113 (17.2%) above-knee amputations were recorded during the eight-year period, with the highest number in 2014 (28) and 2016 (24). Gangrene was listed as the most common reason for toe, below-knee, and above-knee amputations, while infections were the most common reason for partial foot amputations. Tables 7-8 show the number, type, and cause of lower limb amputations.

Comorbidities

Of the 656 amputations, 335 (51.1%) patients had diabetes, 107 (16.3%) had hypertension, and 33 (5.0%) had peripheral vascular disease recorded as comorbidity. The highest proportion of amputations was of the lower extremities among patients with diabetes as a comorbidity. Table 9 shows comorbidities in patients that had amputations by gender. Table 10 shows the number of amputations in patients with diabetes.

Table 7. Lower limb amputation by year

	2010		2011		2012		2013		2014		2015		2016		2017		Total	
	No.	%	No.	%	No.	%	No.	%	No.	%	No.	%	No.	%	No.	%	No.	%
Toe amputation																		
Males	9	69.2	8	50.0	12	60.0	9	40.9	2	16.7	20	87.0	15	60.0	11	52.4	86	56.6
Females	4	30.8	8	50.0	8	40.0	13	59.1	10	83.3	3	13.0	10	40.0	10	47.6	66	43.4
Total	13	100.0	16	100.0	20	100.0	22	100.0	12	100.0	23	100.0	25	100.0	21	100.0	152	100.0
Partial foot amputation (trans metatarsal)																		
Males	1	100.0	2	66.7	1	33.3	1	50.0	5	71.4	5	62.5	1	100.0	-	-	15	62.5
Females	-	-	1	33.3	2	66.7	1	50.0	2	28.6	3	37.5	-	-	-	-	9	37.5
Total	1	100.0	3	100.0	3	100.0	2	100.0	7	100.0	8	100.0	1	100.0	-	-	24	100.0
Below knee amputation																		
Males	11	47.8	17	53.1	19	48.7	15	53.6	26	53.1	17	47.2	27	57.4	19	70.4	151	53.7
Females	12	52.2	15	46.9	20	51.3	13	46.4	23	46.9	19	52.8	20	42.6	8	29.6	130	46.3
Total	23	100.0	32	100.0	39	100.0	28	100.0	49	100.0	36	100.0	47	100.0	27	100.0	281	100.0
Above knee amputation																		
Males	2	50.0	3	50.0	9	47.4	5	55.6	9	32.1	11	52.4	13	54.2	-	-	52	46.0
Females	2	50.0	3	50.0	10	52.6	4	44.4	19	67.9	10	47.6	11	45.8	3	100.0	61	54.0
Total	4	100.0	6	100.0	19	100.0	9	100.0	28	100.0	21	100.0	24	100.0	3	100.0	113	100.0

Table 8. Diagnosis or reason for lower limb amputations

Diagnosis or reason for amputation	Toe amputations		Partial foot amputations		Below knee amputations		Above knee amputations	
	No.	%	No.	%	No.	%	No.	%
Infection	64	42.1	15	62.5	81	28.8	30	26.5
Gangrene	68	44.7	8	33.3	175	62.3	71	62.8
Injury	12	7.9	-	-	1	0.4	-	-
Congenital (polydactyly)	6	3.9	-	-	-	-	-	-
Cancer	-	-	-	-	1	0.4	1	0.9
Ischemia	1	0.7	-	-	21	7.5	8	7.1
Ulcer	1	0.7	-	-	-	-	-	-
Other (e.g., necrosis unspecified)	-	-	1	4.2	2	0.7	3	2.7
Total	152	100.0	24	100.0	281	100.0	113	100.0

Table 9. Distribution of comorbidities among patients who had amputations

Comorbidity	Diabetes Mellitus		Hypertension		Renal Failure		Congestive heart failure		Peripheral Vascular Disease		Cerebrovascular accident		Unknown/none	
	No.	%	No.	%	No.	%	No.	%	No.	%	No.	%	No.	%
Female	177	52.8	73	68.2	5	55.6	5	62.5	16	48.5	4	80.0	-	-
Male	156	46.6	34	31.8	4	44.4	3	37.5	17	51.5	1	20.0	-	-
Total	335	100.0	107	100.0	9	100.0	8	100.0	33	100.0	5	100.0	159	100.0

Table 10. Number and proportion of types of amputations in patients with diabetes

Location of amputation	Total No. of amputations	Amputations with diabetes recorded as a comorbidity	
		No.	%
Finger(s)/Hand	79	9	11.4
Forearm/Arm	7	1	14.3
Toe(s)	152	79	52.0
Partial foot (Trans metatarsal)	24	18	75.0
Below knee	281	163	58.0
Above knee	113	65	57.5
Total	656	335	51.1

DISCUSSION

The rising prevalence of noncommunicable diseases is a global problem that has negative implications for small island states, such as Grenada and the other Caribbean islands, with limited and stretched resources for health care systems. Few recent studies have been published, estimating the prevalence and incidence of diabetes foot and limb complications and amputations in Caribbean countries. In the absence of collecting and analyzing data, a dearth may remain in recognizing and understanding the "true" burden of amputation on the population and the health care system. This study is among the first in Grenada to provide information showing trends in the incidence of all types of amputations in the recent period. Given the scantiness of recently published information, this study may also create awareness of the significance of the issue in the Caribbean region and spur heightened action to address the risk factors, primarily diabetes, and peripheral arterial disease.

The findings in this study were consistent with that of other countries. Among 12 countries in Europe and Australasia, between 25-75% of persons who had amputations also had diabetes (1). It was found that 50% of the persons in Grenada who had an amputation during the reporting period also had diabetes. This pattern affirms the value of strengthening diabetes prevention and management programs as important interventions towards curbing the number of amputations. The data in Grenada is suggestive of the possibility of having prevented about half of the amputations. Additionally, as in other international countries, the incidence of lower limb amputation in Grenada was significantly higher than upper limb amputations. Owing to the high incidence, preventive interventions should also be streamlined to address the specific risk factors for lower limb amputation.

Behrendt et al. (5) reported that people above 65 years in the United States were at higher risk for amputation. In Grenada, the average age of the persons who had amputations ranged from 63.2-65.9 years in the latter seven years of reporting. In the first reporting year, the average age was 56.3 years. While older people are more likely to experience poor health, having an amputation can significantly decrease the quality of life for the individual. Given that average life expectancy in Grenada is approximately 71 years, having an amputation translates into prolonged years of disability. The health, economic, and emotional consequences may be more dire after retirement when the individual has less access to financial resources for care and likely to become dependent on others. In 2004, a study was published citing diabetes foot care was a problem in Barbados and that the country had among the highest rate of lower extremity amputations in the world (10). Limited access to prosthetic devices and rehabilitation services in the region were also deemed to increase hardship for persons who had amputations (10). These conditions may not have improved much in the Caribbean region, particularly, as data is also lacking to highlight the extent of this problem and the need for redress.

Currently, there is no national or community-based program in Grenada to provide psychosocial and other support for people who had amputations. Additionally, until the National Health Insurance (NHI) is commissioned in Grenada, older people, in particular, may be confronted with a high cost for health services, particularly for services provided at private facilities. Behrendt et al. (2018) found that countries with fee-for-service reimbursement had a lower incidence of major amputations compared to a higher incidence in countries with population-based reimbursement system. This finding shows a potentially important function of the NHI in the management of major amputations. Driven by financial reward, a fee-for-service- system may serve to motivate health care workers to provide high quality care for patients to prevent or to reduce the risk for amputation. Serious consideration should, therefore, be given to ensure the NHI facilitates adequate preventive care for Grenadians.

The results show a higher incidence of upper limb amputation among men in Grenada with injury as the major cause. There was less variability between the number of men and women who had lower limb amputations, highlighting the need for prevention and care equally for both genders. Geiss et al. (5) found the number of persons, particularly aged 18-64 years (young and middle-aged adults), who had amputations in the United States increased between 2009-2015 compared to the CDC's findings for 1996-2008 (5). The trends in the United States and in Grenada suggest the need for all age groups and genders to be targeted by interventions, rather than selected groups. In Brazil, Santos (11) found that men lived longer following amputation, losing more years of healthy life. Healthy life expectancy must be considered in planning with the aim of improving the quality of life for men who had amputations and ensuring that adequate services and are provided, including health education (11).

Global data and projections do not give reassurance for a decrease in amputations. The World Health Organization (WHO) estimates show that about 422 million people were affected by diabetes in 2014, rising from 108 million in 1980 (12). The number of people with diabetes worldwide has increased steadily, and the number is expected to continue to rise (8). PAD, the other main cause of amputation, has affected an increasing number of people, estimated at 202 million (1). Considering the high and increasing prevalence of noncommunicable diseases in Grenada and other Caribbean countries (13, 14), not only are appropriate measures needed to prevent and manage diabetes, but these measures need to be implemented in a timely manner. While the number of amputations may appear insignificant, the overall social and economic burden is huge, extending to family and community members. Retrofitting physical infrastructure and social adjustments may also incur a significant burden on society.

Based on human rights, deliberate efforts should be made to relieve the trauma and discomfort associated with illness. Traumatic experiences may persist for several months after an amputation. Quite often, persons having amputations, especially those of the lower limbs, are pitied and/or stigmatized and, as such, the individual may withdraw from the society and normal functions. In the absence of adequate rehabilitation services, the level of the disability created by the amputation is magnified. Support groups and networks may serve an important role in rehabilitation and reintegration in the society of people who had amputations. The physical and social infrastructure must also be adequate for use by people with disabilities.

Recent publications on diabetes complications and amputation in the Caribbean are virtually non-existent. In the absence of data, there may not be sufficient understanding of the significance of amputation on the population health outcomes. The need for strengthening current interventions may not be sufficiently highlighted. As such, this study is useful to address the information gap to inform policy and interventions in Grenada. Other Caribbean countries may benefit from this study, which creates awareness of the significance of the issue and the relevance for Caribbean population health outcomes. Amputation can have serious effects on quality of life and may also put a strain on resources to make adjustments to accommodate persons with severe disabilities. These burdens, however, can be managed through the timely implementation of appropriate measures to address risk factors. Finally, Behrendt et al. (1) suggest that countries should also focus on improving data collection and analysis of amputation procedures and results, ensuring standardization of procedural and diagnosis codes with international protocols.

ACKNOWLEDGMENTS

The authors thank the Ministry of Health, Social Security, and International Business for providing access to the data; particularly the staff at the

Epidemiology and Information Department. The staff at the General Hospital is also specially thanked for collecting and inputting the data in the registers. Funding was not provided by any institution for this study. The authors declare that they have no conflict of interest. Informed consent was obtained from each individual participant involved in this study. This study was conducted in accordance with the 1964 Declaration of Helsinki and its subsequent amendments.

REFERENCES

[1] Behrendt C-A, Sigvant B, Szeberin Z, Beiles B, Eldrup N, Thomson IA, et al. International variations in amputation practice: A VASCUNET report. Eur J Vasc Endovasc Surg 2018;56(3):391–9.

[2] Weledji EP, Fokam P. Treatment of the diabetic foot - to amputate or not? BMC Surg 2014;14:83.

[3] International Diabetes Federation. Diabetes atlas: Individual, social and economic impact, 9th ed. Belgium: IDF, 2019.

[4] Kayssi A, de Mestral C, Forbes TL, Roche-Nagle G. A Canadian population-based description of the indications for lower-extremity amputations and outcomes. Can J Surg 2016;59(2):99–106.

[5] Centers for Disease Control and Prevention. CDC report finds large decline in lower-limb amputations among US adults with diagnosed diabetes. CDC Online News Release 2012. URL: https://www.cdc.gov/media/releases/2012/p0124_lower_limb.html.

[6] Geiss LS, Li Y, Hora I, Albright A, Rolka D, Gregg EW. Resurgence of diabetes-related nontraumatic lower-extremity amputation in the young and middle-aged adult U.S. population. Diabetes Care 2019;42(1):50–4.

[7] Centers for Disease Control and Prevention. National diabetes statistics report: Estimates of diabetes and its burden in the United States. Atlanta, GA: US Department Health Human Services, 2014.

[8] Al-Thani H, Sathian B, El-Menyar A. Assessment of healthcare costs of amputation and prosthesis for upper and lower extremities in a Qatari healthcare institution: a retrospective cohort study. BMJ Open 2019;9(1):e024963.

[9] Davie-Smith F, Coulter E, Kennon B, Wyke S, Paul L. Factors influencing quality of life following lower limb amputation for peripheral arterial occlusive disease: A systematic review of the literature. Prosthet Orthot Int 2017;41(6):537–47.

[10] Hennis A, Fraser HS. Diabetes in the English-speaking Caribbean. Rev Panam Salud Pública 2004;15(2):90–3.

[11] Santos KPB dos, Luz SCT da, Mochizuki L, d'Orsi E, Santos KPB dos, Luz SCT da, et al. Burden of disease from lower limb amputations attributable to diabetes mellitus in Santa Catarina State, Brazil, 2008-2013. Cad Saude Publica 2018;34(1). URL: http://www.scielo.br/scielo.php?script=sci_arttext&pid=S0102-311X2018000105006&lng = pt&tlng = pt.

[12] World Health Organization. Diabetes 2019. URL: https://www.who.int/news-room/fact-sheets/detail/diabetes.

[13] Pan American Health Organization. PAHO/WHO Data - Visualization. PLISA Health Information Platform for the Americas. URL: https://www.paho.org/data/index.php/en/indicators/visualization.html.

[14] Barreto SM, Miranda JJ, Figueroa JP, Schmidt MI, Munoz S, Kuri-Morales PP, et al. Epidemiology in Latin America and the Caribbean: Current situation and challenges. Int J Epidemiol 2012;41(2):557–71.

In: Public Health Themes in Grenada … ISBN: 978-1-53618-118-0
Editors: J. Merrick and L. Glasgow

Chapter 11

HAZARD AND RISK ASSESSMENT OF RAINWATER HARVESTING SYSTEMS IN CARRIACOU, GRENADA

Lindonne Glasgow**, MSPH, DrPH and Jeremy Mendes, BSc
Department of Public Health and Preventive Medicine,
St George's University, St George's, Grenada, West Indies

ABSTRACT

The structure and operation of 20 rainwater harvesting systems in households in Carriacou were observed to identify hazards and estimate the risk associated with the systems. A semi-qualitative assessment methodology was adopted from the World Health Organization and International Water Association Water Safety Plan Manual. A matrix was used to calculate risk scores based on the frequency and severity of

---

* Correspondence: Dr Lindonne Glasgow, Assistant Professor, Department of Public Health and Preventive Medicine, St George's University, POBox 7, True Blue, St George's, Grenada, West Indies. Email: lglasgow@sgu.com.

hazardous events. This study focused on three types of hazards: physical (esthetics), chemical and microbial. The observations were conducted in June, 2019. Of the nine parameters assessed, more than 50% of the 15 concrete tanks received high to very high scores in six areas. More than 50% of the five plastic tanks also received high to very high scores in six areas. When the overall risk score was calculated, three systems received low scores, ten systems received medium scores, and seven systems received high scores. Overall, the findings are indicative of moderate risk associated with rainwater harvesting systems in households in Carriacou. Public health safety can be improved through educating householders, regular monitoring of the systems, and enforcement of safety measures, such as first flush devices and filters. These findings can be applied to develop guidelines for the replication of rainwater harvesting technology on the mainland in Grenada.

INTRODUCTION

Rainwater harvesting is well recognized for obtaining potable water in many countries (1). The technology is commonly used in dry areas and where surface water is virtually non-existent. Harvested rainwater is also used to supplement municipal supplies with the additional benefits of risk substitution, low service and maintenance cost, and quality service (1, 2). The technology is considered environmentally friendly, reducing runoff that can cause flooding and soil erosion (3).

Rainwater harvesting is significant for public health (4). Harvested rainwater can become contaminated at several points along the system – catchment, conveyance, storage - up to levels that exceed recommended guidelines. Microbial contamination of the water can result in significant health problems; usually, severe diarrhea and vomiting, leading to other secondary problems and death, particularly in young children (5). Poor sanitation in the environment is a major factor that contributes to high bacterial concentration in rainwater systems (6, 7). Failing to treat harvested rainwater, such as by application of chlorine tablets, and improper installation of safety devices, such as for first flush diversion and filtering debris from the water, also make the systems prone to contamination (7). Contaminants, such as chemicals and microorganisms, can enter stored rainwater from soils through cracks in underground tanks. The materials used to construct the system can also be hazardous, and leached into the water, posting a threat to human health from consumption of the water (8).

Although only a few major outbreaks of gastrointestinal illnesses were reported in Caribbean countries from the consumption of harvested rainwater, there were health challenges in some countries. Salmonella outbreaks were found to be associated with the consumption of rainwater in Trinidad and Jamaica (9). In some situations, technical issues presented challenges in ensuring the systems were designed for safety and efficiency (10). Another significant issue was the discovery of elevated levels of pollutants from African origin, including arsenic and pesticides, deposited in cisterns in the Caribbean region (11–13).

This research was conducted as a pilot study to identify hazards and estimate the risk associated with rainwater harvesting systems in Carriacou, a small dependency in the State of Grenada. The structure and operation of the systems were analyzed using a semi-qualitative matrix approach published by the World Health Organization (WHO) and the International Water Association (14). Risk scores were calculated based on the frequency and severity of hazardous events associated with the location and operation of the systems. To our knowledge, this semi-qualitative matrix methodology has not been applied to conduct risk assessment in previous studies in Carriacou. The results from this study should allow for better streamlining of interventions to improve water safety in Carriacou and on the mainland in Grenada. The information can also be used to inform the designing of future research, with a wide range of variables, to get in-depth knowledge of the significance of rainwater harvesting for public health in Grenada and other Caribbean islands. Financial support for this study was provided by the Windward Island Research Foundation (WINDREF) at St. George's University in Grenada.

OUR STUDY

This research involved observations and assessment of rainwater harvesting systems in Carriacou in the State of Grenada to identify potential hazardous events and evaluate the risk related to those events. Two systems were randomly selected from among households in the larger communities and one system from among households in the smaller communities for observation and evaluation. A total of 20 systems were included in this study. Four systems were in the communities in the southern part of the island, three systems in communities in the northern part, and 13 systems in communities in the central part of the island. Table 1 shows the community and number of systems included in the study.

Table 1. Selected communities and the number of systems included in the study

Community	Number of Systems Assessed
Laurenston	2
L'Esterre	2
Dunfries	1
Hillsborough	1
Harvey Vale	1
Brunswick	2
Grand Bay	1
Mt. Royal	1
Windward	2
Bogles	1
Prospect	1
Beausejour	1
Six Roads	1
Hermitage	2
Mt. Dor	1
Total	20

Observation and evaluation

The approach for this study was adopted from the WHO and the International Water Association *Water Safety Plan Manual* (14). Specific parameters were considered in the assessment and a matrix provided for calculating risk scores from potentially hazardous events based on the frequency of events and severity. This study focused on three types of hazards: physical (esthetics), chemical and microbial. The observations were conducted on June 29-30, 2019. Information on frequency and type of maintenance was deduced from a survey conducted in Carriacou in collaboration with the Caribbean Regional Pilot Program for Climate Resilience (PPCR). All other information for the assessment was deduced from the observations of the systems.

Table 2. Semi-quantitative risk matrix approach for calculation and interpretation of risk score

		Severity or consequence				
		Insignificant or no impact - Rating: 1	Minor compliance impact - Rating: 2	Moderate aesthetic impact - Rating: 3	Major regulatory impact - Rating: 4	Catastrophic public health impact - Rating: 5
Likelihood or frequency	Almost certain / Once a day - Rating: 5	5	10	15	20	25
	Likely / Once a week - Rating: 4	4	8	12	16	20
	Moderate / Once a month - Rating: 3	3	6	9	12	15
	Unlikely / Once a year - Rating: 2	2	4	6	8	10
	Rare / Once every 5 years - Rating: 1	1	2	3	4	5

Risk score	<6	6-9	10-15	>15
Risk rating	Low	Medium	High	Very high

Source: *WHO Water Safety Plan Manual* (2009). Available at http://apps.who.int/iris/bitstream/handle/10665/75141/9789241562638_eng.pdf?sequence=1&isAllowed=y.

Table 3. Hazardous event, likelihood and severity scores used for calculating risk scores

Hazard	Severity Score	Events Frequency Score									
		1	2	3	4	5	6	7	8	9	10
		Windy	No filtering device	No first flush device	Crack in underground cistern	Concrete roof	No yearly maintenance of tank/ filter/gutter	Mosquito larvae/ algae	Animals on compound with cistern	Agriculture/ agrochemical use in vicinity	Catchment/ system close to road
		Daily (5)	Daily - dirt, leaves, debris, dead animals in catchment area (5)	Weekly - accumulated matter on catchment area (5)	Daily - particulates, chemicals, microorganisms (5)	Weekly - accumulated matter (4)	Daily - accumulated matter (5)	Daily - uncovered storage tank (5)	Daily - excreta, urine, (5)	Monthly - agrochemicals (3)	5 Daily - fine particles (5)
Esthetics											
Mosquito larvae/algae	Major impact: Physical contamination (4)							X			
Leaves, debris	Major impact: Physical contamination (4)	X	X	X			X				
Fine particles	Moderate Impact: color and taste change (3)	X	X	X	X	X	X				X

Hazard	Severity Score	Events Frequency Score									
		1	2	3	4	5	6	7	8	9	10
Chemical											
Light industrial activities	Major impact: Chemical contamination (4)			X			X				
Traffic exhaust and dirt	Minor impact: color change (2)			X			X				X
Agrochemicals	Catastrophic public health impact (5)			X	X		X			X	
Microbial											
Excreta from rats, bats, etc. dead animals, etc.	Catastrophic public health impact (5)			X							
Excreta, urine from dogs, sheep, chickens, etc.	Catastrophic public health impact (5)				X				X		
Sewage from septic tank/pit latrine	Catastrophic public health impact (5)				X						

Evaluation and calculation of risk scores

Table 2 shows the semi-quantitative matrix from the *WHO Water Safety Plan Manual* (2009). The likelihood/frequency of a hazardous event and the severity were both measured on a scale of 1-5. The likelihood of an event was ranked as rare (1 point), unlikely (2 points), moderate (3 points), likely – once a week (4 points) and almost certain – once a day (5 points). The severity was ranked as insignificant or no impact (1 point), minor compliance impact (2 points), moderate esthetic impact (3 points), major regulatory impact (4 points), catastrophic public health impact (5 points). The risk scores were derived from multiplying the number corresponding to the likely frequency of the event (3 monthly, 4 weekly, and 5 daily) by the hazard severity score for specific likely events (4 mosquito larvae/algae, 4 leaves and debris, 3 fine particulates, 4 light industrial activities, 2 traffic exhaust and dirt, 5 agrochemicals, 5 excreta from rats, bats, etc. dead animals, etc. in the catchment area, 5 excreta, urine from dogs, sheep, chickens, etc. on the compound, 5 sewage from septic tank/pit latrine).

A maximum of 25 points was achievable, indicating that the highest level of risk was associated with the specific hazard. In cases where several hazardous events were present, the most regular frequency score was used in the calculation. A risk score <6 reflects low risk, 6-9 reflect medium risk, 10-15 reflect high risk, and >15 reflect very high risk. Table 3 shows the hazardous events and likelihood and severity scores used in calculating the overall risk scores for the systems in Carriacou.

FINDINGS

Of the 20 systems observed, five had plastic storage tanks, and 15 had concrete cisterns for storage, located fully or partially below ground level. Of the nine parameters, more than 50% of the 15 concrete tanks received high to very high risk score, attributable to six events (leaves and debris; fine particulates; chemicals from light industrial activities; chemicals from traffic exhaust; microbes in excreta and dead vectors (catchment area); and microbes from animal excreta and urine (tank area)). Of the nine parameters, more than 50% of the five tanks received high to very high risk score, attributable to seven events (mosquito/algae; leaves and debris; fine particulates; chemicals from light industrial activities; chemicals from traffic; chemical from agricultural activities; and microbes from excreta and dead animals (catchment area)). When the overall risk score was calculated, three systems received low risk scores, ten systems received medium risk scores, and seven systems received high risk scores. Table 4 shows the number of systems deriving specific risk scores for each event.

Table 4. Number of systems attracting specific risk scores by event and type of system

Hazard	Number of Systems with Concrete Tanks	Systems with Plastic Tanks
Esthetics		
Mosquito larvae/algae	VH – 2 L- 13	VH – 3 L - 2
Leaves, debris	VH - 14 L-1	VH – 4 L-1
Fine particulates	0	L – 1 H- 2 VH - 2
Chemical		
Chemicals from catchment area (industrial activities, compounds, adhesives, etc)	VH - 11 H-1 L-3	VH - 3 H-1 L-1
Chemicals from traffic exhaust and dirt	VH-10 H-3 L-2	VH - 3 H -1 L-1
Agrochemicals		
Microbial		
Microorganisms from animal excreta, dead animals, etc. in catchment area	VH – 12 L-3	VH - 1 L-4
Contamination from animals on compound	VH-2 L - 13	0
Microorganisms from septic tank/pit latrine	VH-3 L-12	0

VH – Very High, H – High, L- Low, M- Medium.

Discussion

For many years, the Caribbean Public Health Agency (CARPHA) and other public health agencies have encouraged the use of rainwater harvesting technology in Caribbean countries to augment municipal supplies and as a measure to mitigate climate change impacts in areas that are prone to water-stress (15–18). Rainwater harvesting systems are, however, also highly susceptible to pollution from various sources and have implications for public health when the contaminated water is consumed. In the study in Carriacou, there was moderate public health risk associated with consuming water from the systems, which received a mixture of high, very high a low scores attributable to specific hazard and likely frequency of the events. Half of the systems received overall scores in the category of medium risk. A medium-level risk score indicates a moderate presence of environmental factors that have the potential to compromise the quality of harvested rainwater, and that could affect human health. The presence and effect of those factors may vary by season. For example, during the dry season, due to windier conditions and low volume of water in tanks, there may be an elevation in the concentration of pollutants. According to the WHO, weather, chemicals, microorganisms, and organic matter can have mild to significant impacts on the quality of harvested rainwater (1).

A few systems did not have filters to prevent the entry of pollutants into storage tanks. Diversion of the first set of water was also not commonly practiced. In the absence of filters/mesh and first flush devices, debris can be easily transported into tanks and compromise the physical, chemical, and microbial quality of the water. Organic matter facilitates the growth of microorganisms, protect organisms from the effects of disinfection, and increase the demand for chlorine in water (8). Concrete roof, which was present in some households in Carriacou, is usually flatter than galvanize roof and favors lodgment and buildup of particulates on the uneven surface. Dissolved solids can increase the turbidity of the water and affect the taste and appearance. Systems that do not contain filters or first flush devices are more prone to changes in the quality of water from weather events. The WHO encouraged the use of effective devices to minimize the entry of organic matter into harvested rainwater, as well as the practice of regular maintenance of systems and disinfection of the water (8).

Fishing is the dominant livelihood in Carriacou. The island is also well known for its boat building trade. Many chemicals that are toxic to humans are used in the construction of boats. Carriacou is windy, and chemicals can be easily transported to water collection surfaces and later washed into the storage tanks. On the small island, applying pesticides in residential areas by spraying also increases the potential for chemical pollution of the water. The concentration of pollutants may be lower in the wet season due to the regular exchange of stored water. In the dry season, however, the concentration of pollutants may be elevated due to the low volume of water present in the tanks. The deposition of chemical pollutants from African origin, carried in dust blows that typically occur in the dry season, and detected in water tanks in the Caribbean (11–13) is proof that large quantities of particulates can be transported in the wind and accumulate to levels that may pose a risk to human health. Health problems such as cancer, neurological and developmental disorders, and irritation may result from exposure to toxic chemicals (19). Residents should be encouraged to improve safety practices, including the installation of flush diversion valves. Flush systems can be manually operated and require human intervention for effective use in each rainy period. A more practical approach is to install an automated system that also requires low maintenance. An effective flush system can significantly reduce pollutants in stored rainwater. This can eventually reduce the incidence of waterborne disease on the island, although the incidence is generally low in the wet season with an increase in the dry season.

Rearing livestock, poultry, and other domesticated animals such as cats and dogs in close vicinity to cisterns can constitute a biohazard for ingress of polluted groundwater into cracked tanks. Cats and rats can also climb onto catchment areas, such as on roofs, and deposit excreta which can introduce pathogens to rainwater systems. Animal fences were not commonly seen in Carriacou although animals were left untethered. This situation may increase the risk for transmission of disease-causing organisms from animal sources to humans. Salmonella outbreaks were found to be associated with the consumption of rainwater in Trinidad and Jamaica (9). Zoonotic diseases can cause serious illnesses in humans and even death (20). Precautions should be taken to prevent animals and animal waste in the immediate vicinity of rainwater harvesting systems.

This pilot study was conducted, including 20 systems in Carriacou. The small sample size is not representative of households in Carriacou, and the results of this study only provide an indication of some environmental factors that may have an impact on public health in Carriacou through the water sector. Further research is needed to understand better the magnitude and extent to which the events, identified in this study, affect the quality of the harvested rainwater. It is important to identify public health risks in the water sector in Caribbean countries for several reasons: water is becoming scarce as a direct consequence of climate change (15); rainwater harvesting systems are increasingly used as a source for potable water, globally and in the Caribbean (1, 10); waterborne diseases account for a significant burden on the health care systems in the region (21, 22); and the region, comprising mostly of small island states, has limited resources to combat waterborne infectious diseases.

Other countries, such as Antigua, Barbuda, St. Lucia, and Barbados, in which rainwater harvesting is a common practice, may benefit from this pilot study to guide water quality studies. This study can be used as a reference to inform steps to improve water safety in the most precarious situations. Irrespective of the countries in which studies are conducted, it is beneficial to share data and technical resources to strengthen the capacities for monitoring rainwater harvesting systems in the Caribbean region. Finally, agencies such as CARPHA, the Pan American Health Organization (PAHO) and the Caribbean Development Bank (CDB) should collaborate with regional governments and local organizations to mobilize and provide resources for the introduction of new technologies in the region and to improve water safety for the Caribbean people.

ACKNOWLEDGMENTS

The authors are grateful to St George's University, the Windward Island Research Foundation (WINDREF), and the Produce Chemical Laboratory in Grenada for their various support for this study. Funding for this study was provided by the Windward Island Research Foundation (WINDREF), Small Research Grant Initiative (#SRGI 19004). The authors declare that they have no conflict of interest. Informed consent was obtained from each individual participant involved in this study. This study was conducted in accordance with the 1964 Declaration of Helsinki and its subsequent amendments.

REFERENCES

[1] World Health Organization. Rainwater harvesting [Internet]. SEARO. South-East Asia Regional Office: WHO, 2017. URL: http://www.searo.who.int/entity/water_sanitation/topics/rainwater/en/.

[2] Peters EJ. Rainwater potential for domestic water supply in Grenada. Water Manag 2006;159(3):147–53.

[3] Rahman S, Khan MTR, Akib S, Din NBC, Biswas SK, Shirazi SM. Sustainability of rainwater harvesting system in terms of water quality. ScientificWorldJournal 2014;2014:721357.

[4] Nijhof S, Jantowski B, Meerman R, Schoemaker A. Rainwater harvesting in challenging environments: Towards institutional frameworks for sustainable domestic water supply. Waterlines 2010;29(3):209–19.

[5] Karim MR. Microbial contamination and associated health burden of rainwater harvesting in Bangladesh. Water Sci Technol 2010;61(8):2129–35.

[6] Hamilton K, Reyneke B, Waso M, Clements T, Ndlovu T, Khan W, et al. A global review of the microbiological quality and potential health risks associated with roof-harvested rainwater tanks. Clean Water 2019;2(1). URL: http://dx.doi.org/10.1038/s41545-019-0030-5.

[7] Clasen TF, Alexander KT, Sinclair D, Boisson S, Peletz R, Chang HH, et al. Interventions to improve water quality for preventing diarrhoea. Cochrane Database Syst Rev 2015;10:CD004794.

[8] World Health Organization. Guidelines for drinking-water quality. WHO Press, 2011. URL: http://apps.who.int/iris/bitstream/10665/44584/1/9789241548151_eng.pdf.

[9] Guidance on use of rainwater tanks. Commonwealth of Australia, 2010. URL: https://www1.health.gov.au/internet/main/publishing.nsf/Content/0D71DB86E9DA7CF1CA257BF0001CBF2F/$File/enhealth-raintank.pdf.

[10] Peters EJ. Success and success factors of domestic rainwater harvesting projects in the Caribbean. J Sustain Dev 2016;9(5). URL: http://dx.doi.org/10.5539/jsd.v9n5p55.

[11] Griffin DW, Garrison VH, Herman JR, Shinn EA. African desert dust in the Caribbean atmosphere? Microbiology and public health. Aerobiologia (Bologna) 2001;17:203–13.

[12] Griffin DW. Atmospheric movement of microorganisms in clouds of dust and implications for human health. DOI Clin Microbiol Rev Clin Microbiol Rev 2007;20(3):459.

[13] Schmidt LJ. When the dust settles, 2001. URL: https://earthobservatory.nasa.gov/Features/Dust/.

[14] Bartram J, Corrales L, Davison D, Gordon B, Howard G, Rinehold A, et al. Water safety plan manual [Internet]. Geneva: World Health Organization, 2009. URL: http://www.who.int/water_sanitation_health/publication_9789241562638/en/.

[15] Dempewolf L, Boodram N, Corbin C, Cox C, Clauzel S, Vogel H, et al. Rainwater harvesting in the Caribbean-State of play 2015. URL: http://www.aidis.org.br/PDF/cwwa2015/CWWA 2015 Paper_GWP-C Dempewolf.pdf.

[16] Global Water Partnership-Caribbean. Mainstreaming rainwater harvesting (RWH) to build climate resilience in the Caribbean water sector 2016. URL: http://www.gwp.org/globalassets/global/toolbox/case-studies/americas-and-caribbean/cs_caribbean_final_final_final.pdf.

[17] Caribbean Environmental Health Institute. Findings of a knowledge, attitude, practice and behavior study on rainwater harvesting and investigation of microbial water quality of stored rainwater. Castries, St. Lucia: Caribbean Environmental Health Institute, 2011.

[18] Caribbean Environmental Health Insitute. Rainwater - Catch it while you can: A handbook on rainwater harvesting in the Caribbean 2009. URL: https://www.caribank.org/uploads/2013/08/em-rainwater-handbook-caribbean.pdf.

[19] Bergmann Å, Heindel JJ, Jobling S, Kidd KA, Zoeller RT, eds. State of the science of endocrine disrupting chemicals - 2012. Geneva: WHO, 2013. URL: http://www.who.int/ceh/publications/endocrine/en/.

[20] King L. Neglected zoonotic diseases. In: The causes and impacts of neglected tropical and zoonotic diseases: Opportunities for integrated intervention strategies. Washington, DC: National Academies Press, 2011:A13. URL: https://www.ncbi.nlm.nih.gov/books/NBK62511/.

[21] Glasgow LM, Forde MS, Antoine SC, Pérez E, Indar L. Estimating the burden of acute gastrointestinal Illness in Grenada. J Health Popul Nutr 2013;31(4 Suppl1):17-29.

[22] Gabriel OO, Jaime A, Mckensie M, Auguste A, Pérez E, Indar L. Estimating the burden of acute gastrointestinal illness: A pilot study of the prevalence and

underreporting in Saint Lucia, Eastern Caribbean. J Health Popul Nutr 2013;31(4 Suppl 1):S3:17-29.

In: Public Health Themes in Grenada … ISBN: 978-1-53618-118-0
Editors: J. Merrick and L. Glasgow © 2020 Nova Science Publishers, Inc.

Chapter 12

KNOWLEDGE, ATTITUDES AND PRACTICES REGARDING RAINWATER HARVESTING IN CARRIACOU, GRENADA

Lindonne Glasgow**, MSPH, DrPH and Jeremy Mendes, BSc
Department of Public Health and Preventive Medicine,
St George's University, St George's, Grenada, West Indies

ABSTRACT

Rainwater harvesting is well established in Carriacou, a small dependency island in the State of Grenada in the Caribbean. Owing to a high dependence on rainwater for domestic purposes, it is essential to regularly monitor practices and the quality of water on the island. This pilot study was conducted to assess the knowledge, attitudes, and practices of residents in 20 households in Carriacou. A survey was administered face to face to

* Correspondence: Dr Lindonne Glasgow, Assistant Professor, Department of Public Health and Preventive Medicine, St. George's University, POBox 7, True Blue, St George's, Grenada, West Indies. Email: lglasgow@sgu.com.

the residents in June, 2019. The survey questions led to the collection of information on household water supply, knowledge about and attitudes to rainwater harvesting, rainwater harvesting practices, and the use and treatment of rainwater for domestic purposes. Fifteen respondents stored water in concrete tanks, while five used plastic tanks for storage. The overwhelming majority of respondents stated they used the water for one or more of the following purposes: drinking, bathing, cooking, cleaning, flushing toilet, and washing vehicles. More than half of the respondents stated that water was always available from their household system. Eighteen respondents reported they did maintenance at least once per year. Four respondents did not have a mesh to filter the water entering the tank, and 16 respondents did not practice first flush diversion. Water safety education programs can be beneficial to improve rainwater harvesting practices in Carriacou. Monitoring practices and providing support for improvements may greatly benefit the water sector on the island and minimize the risk of waterborne illnesses.

INTRODUCTION

Rainwater harvesting is becoming more commonplace to augment municipal supplies. The technology is regarded as reliable to mitigate the impacts of climate change and with significant potential to reduce the risk of contracting pathogenic waterborne illnesses, particularly in areas where wastewater recycling is practiced (1, 2). Rainwater harvesting is a common practice in the Caribbean countries, especially in Trinidad, Antigua and Barbuda, Tortola, Barbados, and the Bahamas. Increasingly, the need to collect and store water to maintain adequate supplies is recognized as the region experiences harsher and extended dry seasons (3–5). About 500,000 Caribbean residents depend entirely or mostly on harvested rainwater to meet domestic, recreational, and agricultural water needs (6). Although governments have taken steps to extend the supply of pipe-borne water in some countries, rainwater harvesting is also promoted as an environmentally friendly approach to supplement municipal supplies (7–9).

The points of collection, conveyance, and storage are susceptible to pollution. Wind and water can be vehicles to transport dust, chemicals, and bio-waste from the vicinity into the system. Studies have shown microbial and chemical pollution resulting from poor environmental sanitation and usage of hazardous construction materials for the systems (2, 10–12). Additionally, discharges from industrial activities are significant sources of pollution from deposition on catchment areas and directly into storage tanks. In addition, studies have shown elevated levels of pollutants in cisterns in the Caribbean from trans-national sources, such as arsenic from dust blows originating from as far as the Sahara desert region in North Africa (13, 14).

Rainwater harvesting is the primary source of water in Carriacou, a small dependency island in the State of Grenada. Grenada is located in the southern part of the Caribbean. Approximately 5,000 persons reside in Carriacou. Surface water is virtually non-existent on the island, and it is not uncommon for most residents to experience a shortage of water during the dry season. The dry season typically lasts from January-June. During the dry season, there is an elevated risk of pollution from wind transportation. At the same time, the concentration of pollutants can build up faster in the small volume of water in storage tanks. Syndromic data from the Ministry of Health in Grenada show a consistent peak in the number of cases of diarrheal illness during the dry season each year (15), which may be indicative of the higher concentration of pollutants in water. The findings from the Burden of Illness (BOI) study in Grenada in 2008-2009 highlighted the need for closer monitoring of water safety practices, both on the mainland and in Carriacou and Petite Martinique.

This pilot study was conducted in partnership with the Caribbean Regional Pilot Program for Climate Resilience (PPCR) with a small sample of residents to investigate knowledge, attitude and practice (KAP) regarding rainwater harvesting in Carriacou. The regional project was designed to provide information on the feasibility and need for replicating rainwater harvesting technologies on the mainland in Grenada. In this study, we collected information on household water supply, knowledge about and attitudes to rainwater harvesting, rainwater harvesting practices, and the use and treatment of rainwater for domestic purposes. The study was conducted in the first month of the rainy season. The results of this study should inform future research with larger samples to obtain a more comprehensive understanding of the quality of water for potable uses. The findings also provide insights on some appropriate interventions for water safety in Carriacou. Lastly, the findings will complement the PPCR to propose recommendations for safety in adopting rainwater harvesting technologies on the mainland, where communities also experience water shortage from pipe-borne sources during the dry season.

OUR STUDY

This pilot study was conducted with residents in 20 households across 15 communities in Carriacou. Two households were randomly selected in larger communities and one household in smaller communities. A total of four households were selected in the communities in the southern part of the island, three households in the communities in the northern part, and 13 households in communities in the central part of the island. The geographic spread in the sampling was representative of the number of communities and residents in the respective parts of the island. Table 1 shows the communities and number of households included in this pilot study.

Through the PPCR, a 3-day consultation was held in St. Lucia in March, 2019 to develop and test a questionnaire for use in the regional study in three Caribbean islands - Grenada, Jamaica, and St. Lucia. This questionnaire was modified slightly for use in the study in Carriacou. The modified questionnaire was further piloted with a small group, and the recommendations were incorporated to improve comprehension and answer choices suitable for the context on the island.

At the household level, one adult above 18 years, preferably the head of the household, was selected to participate. The survey was administered face to face by trained surveyors on June 29-30, 2019 in the first month of the rain season. Questions were included to collect information about household water supply, knowledge about and attitudes to rainwater harvesting, rainwater harvesting practices, and use and treatment of rainwater for domestic purposes. Participants were required to provide written consent before being interviewed. Responses were recorded on the questionnaire and later entered into a database for analysis.

Table 1. Number of households selected in each community in Carriacou for inclusion in the study

Community	Number of systems assessed
Laurenston	2
L'Esterre	2
Dunfries	1
Hillsborough	1
Harvey Vale	1
Brunswick	2
Grand Bay	1
Mt. Royal	1
Windward	2
Bogles	1
Prospect	1
Beausejour	1
Six Roads	1
Hermitage	2
Mt. Dor	1
Total	20

FINDINGS

Of the 20 respondents in the pilot study, 14 (70.0%) were males, and 6 (30.0%) were females. The majority of respondents (15, 75.0%) also identified themselves as the head of the households. Half (10, 50.0%) of the respondents were between 41-65 years, and more than half (12, 60.0%) had lived in the community for more than 26 years. The majority (14, 70.0%) of respondents lived in concrete houses, and 14 (70.0%) also had toilet facilities with a flush to septic tank system. Table 2 shows the demographic characteristics of the respondents.

Table 2. Demographic characteristics of the respondents

	Number	Percentage		Number	Percentage
Gender			Floor material		
Male	6	30.0	Dirt/Sand	0	0
Female	14	70.0	Wood	6	30.0
			Plywood	0	0
Position in household			Concrete	14	70.0
Head	15	75.0			
Other member	5	25.0	Roof material		
			Thatch	0	0
Age (years)			Wood	0	0
18-24	1	5.0	Galvanize/metal	17	85.0
25-40	4	20.0	Clay/shingles	0	0
41-65	10	50.0	Concrete	3	15.0
65+	5	25.0			
			External wall material		
Household Size			Dirt	0	0
1-3	7	35.0	Plywood	1	5.0
4-7	12	60.0	Galvanize	2	10.0
8+	1	5.0	Concrete	14	70.0
			Wood	3	15.0
Residence in community (years)					
<1 year	0	0	Toilet facility		
1-5	2	10.0	Flush to septic	15	75.0
6-10	1	5.0	Pit latrine	5	25.0
11-25	5	25.0	Bucket	0	0
26+	12	60.0	Bush/field	0	0

Household water supply

Residents were asked about the main source of water for their households, disruptions, and alternative sources. Fifteen (75.0%) respondents reported a private concrete cistern was the main source of water for the household, while 5 (25.0%) reported a private plastic tank was used. More than half of the respondents (12, 60.0%) reported water was always available from the private supply, 6 (30.0%) stated water was available for most of the year, and 2 (10.0%) reported water was available for about half of the year or less. Nine (45.0%) respondents stated they had the most disruptions during the period of December to May. Of the respondents who experienced shortages during the year, 5 (55.5%) stated they sourced water from friends and neighbors as an alternative. About one-third of the respondents (6, 30.0%) stated their supply was more than adequate throughout the year, 10 (50.0%) stated adequate and 4 (20.0%) stated they experienced scarcity for the household.

Rainwater harvesting practice

In reporting on the location of the storage facility, 19 respondents stated the facility was underground. Almost half of the respondents (9, 45.0%) reported they did not make preparations to secure their systems during the passage of a hurricane, storm or an earthquake; half (10, 50.0%) did not have a water line indicator in their system, and 4 (20.0%) did not have a mesh to filter the water entering the tank. The majority, 16 (80.0%), did not use a first flush system. A little more than half (12, 60.0%) of the respondents reported they treated the water before consumption; six added bleach, two added chlorine tablets, and three had small fishes to consume mosquitoes and larvae.

Only two (10.0%) respondents reported they used additional filtration or treatment methods after the water left the tank. Half of the respondents also stated they did not have a mesh to stop mosquitoes from going up into the pipes. Eighteen (90.0%) respondents reported they did maintenance or cleaning of the system. Table 3 shows the type and frequency of maintenance by respondents. Six (30.0%) respondents stated they felt they should do more maintenance while 13 (65.0%) felt they did not need to do additional maintenance.

Table 3. Frequency and type of maintenance performed by respondents

	Number	Percentage		Number	Percentage
Maintenance/cleaning			Clean Storage tank		
Yes	18	90.0	Every 5 years	1	5.0
No	2	10.0	Every 2 years	3	15.0
			Yearly	4	20.0
Maintenance			Dry season	6	35.0
Every 4-5 years	1	5.0	Twice yearly	1	5.0
Every 3 years	3	15.0	3-4 months	1	5.0
Every 2 years	2	10.0			
Dry season	6	30.0	Clean roof/gutters		
Twice yearly	2	10.0	Yes	16	80.0
Occasionally	1	5.0	No	4	20.0
No response	2	10.0			
			Clean roof/gutters		
Clean storage tank			Every 2 years	8	40.0
Yes	18	90.0	Yearly	4	20.0
No	1	5.0	Dry season	1	5.0
			Twice yearly	1	5.0
			Every 3 months	1	5.0

Use and appearance of drinking rainwater

The overwhelming majority of the respondents (19-20, 95.0-100%) reported they used the harvested rainwater for one or more of the following purposes: drinking, bathing, cooking as well as for cleaning, flushing toilet, and washing vehicles. Nine (45.0%) also used the water for lawns/gardens. Eighteen (90.0%) respondents stated the water tasted good, and a similar proportion felt it was safe for drinking. Sixteen (80.0%) respondents stated the water was clear during most of the year.

Knowledge and attitude to rainwater harvesting

Respondents were asked to state their level of agreement with statements that demonstrate their knowledge and attitude to rainwater harvesting. The most variance in the responses was to the question of whether the government was responsible for providing residents in Carriacou with safe water. While six (30.0%) of respondents agree, only two (10.0%) strongly agreed, five (25.0%) neither agreed nor disagreed, and seven (35.0%) disagreed. The responses differed more significantly on the question of the safety of using chlorine to treat drinking water. Five (25.0%) respondents strongly agreed that chlorine was safe to treat the water, seven (35.0%) agreed, three (15.0%) were neutral, and five (25.0%) disagreed. There was also variance in the responses regarding the safety of water after diverting the first set from the tank. Almost half (9, 45.0%) of the respondents neither agreed nor disagreed that the water was safer from using a first flush system, seven (35.0%) disagreed and four (20.0%) respondents, in total, strongly agreed and agreed. Table 4 shows the respondents' agreement with the statements.

Table 4. Respondents level of agreement with statements regarding rainwater harvesting

	Number	Percentage		Number	Percentage
Untreated rainwater is safe to drink			Rainwater treated with bleach is safe to drink		
Strongly agree	3	15.0	Strongly agree	5	25.0
Agree	10	50.0	Agree	7	35.0
Neutral	3	15.0	Neutral	3	15.0
Disagree	4	20.0	Disagree	5	25.0
Strongly disagree	0	0	Strongly disagree	0	0
Diverting the first set or rainwater makes the water safe to drink			Untreated rainwater is safe for bathing		
Strongly agree	2	10.0	Strongly agree	10	50.0
Agree	2	10.0	Agree	7	35.0
Neutral	9	45.0	Neutral	3	15.0

Table 4. (Continued)

	Number	Percentage		Number	Percentage
Disagree	7	35.0	Disagree	0	0
Strongly disagree	0	0	Strongly disagree	0	0
Filtered rainwater is safe to drink			Untreated rainwater is safe for cooking		
Strongly agree	9	45.0	Strongly agree	8	40.0
Agree	8	40.0	Agree	12	60.0
Neutral	3	15.0	Neutral	0	0
Disagree	0	0	Disagree	0	0
Strongly disagree	0	0	Strongly disagree	0	0
Boiled rainwater is safe to drink			It is the responsibility of government to supply us with safe water		
Strongly agree	15	75.0	Strongly agree	2	10.0
Agree	4	20.0	Agree	6	30.0
Neutral	1	5.0	Neutral	5	25.0
Disagree	0	0	Disagree	7	35.0
Strongly disagree	0	0	Strongly disagree	0	0

DISCUSSION

Rainwater harvesting is considered a safe alternative to municipal water supplies having a lower risk of contamination from sources such as lead pipes and chemicals and microorganisms in recycled water (1). Rainwater systems, however, are susceptible to microbial and chemical pollution, in particular (11, 16, 17). Constant monitoring is necessary to ensure that a consistent and safe supply of water is available in communities that are prone to experience water stress. KAP studies can be beneficial to understand risk and inform appropriate interventions to improve water safety. The findings from the BOI study in 2008-2009 and other studies in Carriacou suggest there is a need for close monitoring of the rainwater harvesting systems.

The results of this study indicate there is some level of efficient management of water supply by residents in Carriacou, with about half of the respondents stating they had a consistent supply of water throughout the year. This study did not focus on the extent and practices related to the management of supply. In the context of climate change mitigation, the issue is important, relating to the efficiency of the technologies that are currently used versus alternative technologies. The results show extremely high dependency on rainwater for drinking, cooking, bathing, laundry, and cleaning. This high dependence on harvested rainwater shows, not only the social impact of the practices but also the public health implications relating to water quality in Carriacou.

While there was a general positive indication about the management of water supplies in households, about half of the respondents also stated their supply was only "adequate" with an additional 20.0% stating they experienced scarcity. Together, these statistics indicate a potentially high risk for water shortage by a significant segment of the Carriacouan population. Climate change exacerbates this challenge, calling to attention the need to monitor and manage the balance between water demand and supply. The size of households, rainfall patterns, and other factors should be given consideration in determining what systems are adequate for households. Currently, pipe-borne water is the main supply on the mainland in Grenada. In promoting the replication of rainwater harvesting on the mainland, it may be best to develop policies that support diligence in water supply and address the gaps found in this pilot study in Carriacou. This approach can ensure that the measure becomes an effective climate change mitigation strategy and attract long term use by a significant segment of the population.

There were notable differences in the responses regarding the government's responsibility for providing safe water for residents in Carriacou. Several factors may account for the differences, including individual perception about the need and influence of laws and policies to direct the management of individual and communal water supplies. In the absence of a structured program by the government that actively directs and monitors rainwater harvesting in Carriacou, residents are left to make choices regarding how they manage household supplies. This autonomy may translate into little understanding and appreciation of the government's responsibility for oversight of public health, which also extends into the water sector. The government's failure to construct a modern water system on the island at the time of the interview may be another reason for the mixed responses.

Governments have ultimate responsibility for public health (18), and their agencies should ensure water safety measures are implemented and maintained within their jurisdictions. In the BOI study in 2008-2009, the third highest prevalence of acute gastrointestinal illness (AGI) was found in Carriacou and Petite Martinique (15). Despite a few reports of major issues related to water consumption in the dependency islands, a monitoring system is still prudent to maintain a potable quality of water in all households on the island and to reduce the seasonal increases in AGI cases. Inconsistency in the responses regarding the use of chlorine for sterilization also shows a possible need for education and health promotion to demonstrate best practices in rainwater harvesting including the WHO recommended usage of chlorine tablets for sterilization (10), first flush system and filters or mesh to reduce the potential for pollution of water in storage tanks.

More than half of the residents reported they did not make preparations to prevent disruption of their water supply in the event of a disaster, such as a hurricane or an earthquake. Given the island's close proximity to Kick 'em Jenny, an active submarine volcano, attention should be given to ensure there is a safe and consistent supply of water in the event of an emergency situation. Grenada and its dependencies are also located within the Atlantic Ocean's hurricane track, which could increase vulnerability to catastrophic climatic events. Ensuring a safe supply of water during an emergency reduces the chances of water- and/or food-related mortality and morbidity.

The results indicate most of the respondents performed maintenance of their rainwater system. The extent of maintenance parts of the system (collection surfaces, conveyance, and storage facility) was not investigated in this study. While most of the respondents stated they did yearly maintenance, some also felt they should do more. This may be an indication of the need for training to maintain the systems. Financial constraints may also limit maintenance, especially in households headed by women. The replicating the technology in Grenada, residents should be made aware of associated costs and educated on plans to provide for the maintenance of the system. All parts of a rainwater harvesting system should be systematically maintained as a measure to ensure the water is safe for consumption. The following recommendations may also be appropriate to address gaps and improve rainwater harvesting management in Carriacou as well as for application in replicating the technology on the mainland in Grenada:

- Conduct a follow-up risk assessment study in Carriacou with a representative sample to identify hazards and estimate the risk associated with the conditions. The information from this study should be used in the development or modification of interventions to improve water safety in Carriacou.
- Conduct community-based national education programs on best practices in rainwater harvesting technology. The messages should be communicated through various channels to ensure reach to the widest cross-section of the population.
- Establish a team/unit with responsibility for all activities related to rainwater harvesting at the national level.
- Monitor the condition of rainwater harvesting systems and operations on a regular basis. Ensure systems contain all appropriate safety devices such as first flush devices, rodent-proof, and drain taps in plastic tanks.
- Create policies that promote safety in rainwater harvesting. Address non-compliance with public health policies.
- Conduct a national survey to collect baseline data from residents on the mainland prior to the construction of systems. Post-training and post-adaptation surveys should also be conducted to evaluate differences in knowledge, attitudes, and practices.

Although a small sample was included in this study, useful information was provided on household water supply, knowledge about and attitudes to rainwater harvesting, rainwater harvesting practices, and the use and treatment of rainwater for domestic purposes in Carriacou. Recommendations are made to address gaps and to improve the management of rainwater harvesting systems in Carriacou. The recommendations can be referenced in the regional PPCR initiative to highlight an evidence-based approach in its work. Further studies are needed, however, to validate the situation in Carriacou. Meanwhile, the Government of Grenada, through the Environmental Health Department, can begin to take steps towards replication with improved practices on the mainland while ensuring an appropriate supportive environment for rainwater harvesting practice to thrive. Climate change has significant impacts on water supply and quality. Water security, however, is crucial for public health and to ensure a high quality of life for all the citizens.

Acknowledgments

The authors are grateful to St. George's University, the Windward Island Research Foundation (WINDREF), and the Produce Chemical Laboratory in Grenada for their various support for this study. Funding for this study was provided by the Windward Island Research Foundation (WINDREF), Small Research Grant Initiative (#SRGI 19004). The authors declare that they have no conflict of interest. Informed consent was obtained from each individual participant involved in this study. This study was conducted in accordance with the 1964 Declaration of Helsinki and its subsequent amendments.

References

[1] World Health Organization. Rainwater harvesting. South-East Asia Regional Office: WHO, 2017. URL: http://www.searo.who.int/entity/water_sanitation/topics/rainwater/en/.

[2] Rahman S, Khan MTR, Akib S, Din NBC, Biswas SK, Shirazi SM. Sustainability of rainwater harvesting system in terms of water quality. ScientificWorldJournal 2014;2014:721357.

[3] Caribbean Rainwater Harvesting Handbook. Rainwater: A handbook on rainwater harvesting in the Caribbean. The Caribbean Environmental Health Institute. 2009. URL: https://www.caribank.org/uploads/2013/08/em-rainwater-handbook-caribbean.pdf.

[4] Caribbean Environmental Health Institute. A programme for promoting rainwater harvesting in the Caribbean region, 2006. URL: http://www.caribbeanrainwater harvestingtoolbox.com/Media/Print/Programme to Promote RWH in the Cabbean Region.pdf.

[5] United Nations Environmental Programme. Climate change in the Caribbean and the challenge of adaptation. Panama City: United Nations Environmental Programme, 2008. URL: http://www.pnuma.org/deat1/pdf/Climate_Change_in_the_Caribbean_Final_LOW20oct.pdf.

[6] Global Water Partnership-Caribbean. Mainstreaming rainwater harvesting (RWH) to build climate resilience in the Caribbean water sector, 2016. URL: http://www.gwp.org/globalassets/global/toolbox/case-studies/americas-and-caribbean/cs_caribbean_final_final_final.pdf.

[7] Peters EJ. Success and success factors of domestic rainwater harvesting projects in the Caribbean. J Sustain Dev 2016;9(5). URL: http://dx.doi.org/10.5539/jsd.v9n5p55.

[8] Dempewolf L, Boodram N, Corbin C, Cox C, Clauzel S, Vogel H, et al. Rainwater harvesting in the Caribbean-State of play, 2015. URL: http://www.aidis.org.br/PDF/cwwa2015/CWWA 2015 Paper_GWP-C Dempewolf.pdf.

[9] Caribbean Environmental Health Insitute. Rainwater - Catch it while you can: A handbook on rainwater harvesting in the Caribbean, 2009. URL: https://www.caribank.org/uploads/2013/08/em-rainwater-handbook-caribbean.pdf.

[10] World Health Organization. Guidelines for drinking-water quality. WHO Press, 2011. URL: http://apps.who.int/iris/bitstream/10665/44584/1/9789241548151_eng.pdf.

[11] Chubaka CE, Whiley H, Edwards JW, Ross KE. A review of roof harvested rainwater in Australia. J Environ Public Health 2018;2018:6471324.

[12] Gwenzi W, Nyamadzawo G. Hydrological impacts of urbanization and urban roof water harvesting in water-limited catchments: A review. Environ Process 2014;1(4):573–93.

[13] Griffin DW, Garrison VH, Herman JR, Shinn EA. African desert dust in the Caribbean atmosphere?: Microbiology and public health. Aerobiologia (Bologna) 2001;17:203–13.

[14] Holmes CW, Shinn EA, Rodrigues F. The atmospheric transport and deposition of arsenic and other metals in southeastern United States. URL: https://wwwbrr.cr.usgs.gov/projects/GWC_chemtherm/FinalAbsPDF/holmes.pdf.

[15] Glasgow LM, Forde MS, Antoine SC, Pérez E, Indar L. Estimating the burden of acute gastrointestinal Illness in Grenada. J Health Popul Nutr 2013;31(4 Suppl1):17-29.

[16] Kirs M, Moravcik P, Gyawali P, Hamilton K, Kisand V, Gurr I, et al. Rainwater harvesting in American Samoa: Current practices and indicative health risks. Environ Sci Pollut Res 2017;24(13):12384–92.

[17] Stewart C, Kim ND, Johnston DM, Nayyerloo M. Health hazards associated with consumption of roof-collected rainwater in urban areas in emergency situations. Int J Environ Res Public Health 2016;13(10). URL: http://www.ncbi.nlm.nih.gov/pubmed/27754454.

[18] Bhattacharya D. Public health policy: Issues, theories, and advocacy. San Francisco, CA: Jossey-Bass, 2013.

In: Public Health Themes in Grenada … ISBN: 978-1-53618-118-0
Editors: J. Merrick and L. Glasgow

Chapter 13

ASSESSMENT OF RECREATIONAL WATER QUALITY IN THE SOUTHERN COASTAL AREAS OF GRENADA

Sabrina Compton**, BSc, MPH
and Martin Forde, ScD, REng
Department of Public Health and Preventive Medicine,
St George's University, St George's, Grenada

ABSTRACT

The microbial quality of recreational coastal waters along the southwestern coast of Grenada was assessed. A total of 120 samples taken from 12 sites were analyzed for enterococcus faecalis, fecal coliform, pH, temperature. Two samples per day from six sites were collected bi-weekly between 8 a.m. and 12 p.m. during the period of November-December 2008. Rainfall data for the sampling period was obtained from the Grenada Meteorological Office. The highest percentage of sampling days exceeding

* Correspondence: Ms. Sabrina Compton, , Instructor, St George's University, Department of Public Health and Preventive Medicine, PO Box 7, St George's, Grenada, WI. Email: scompton@sgu.edu.

the World Health Organization's (WHO) recommended limits for enterococcus faecalis was recorded at two sites—Beausejour-Bay (70%) and Carenage-Bay ((60)%). The Carenage-Bay sampling site had the highest percentage of sampling days exceeding recommended limits for total fecal coliform ((60)%). Overall, 30% of the samples analyzed showed enterococcus faecalis and total coliform levels above the recommended limits. Other measured variables were inconsistent with increased microbial content. No correlation was observed between rainfall and enterococcus faecalis. This study found that the majority of beaches along the Southwestern coast of Grenada exceeded the recommended limits by WHO for fecal coliform and enterococcus faecalis period.

INTRODUCTION

In 2017, the United Nation World Water Development Report stated that over 80% of all wastewater worldwide, released into the environment, was untreated (1). On a global level, countries are working towards ensuring good water quality for sustainable growth and productivity in accordance with the Sustainable Development Goal 6 (SDG 6) (2). In order to measure the achievement of this sustainable development goal, water quality measures have been established for recreational waters, both freshwater and coastal water bodies. Poor recreational water quality measurements are usually associated with health problems and environmental concerns (3). On the other hand, high quality recreation water indicators have a concomitantly reduced level of adverse health problems (3). Many European countries have reported excellent recreational bathing waters in the last 40 years, which they have attributed to robust water quality monitoring systems (4).

In the Caribbean, recreational waters are almost exclusively located on the coasts of small island states. These coastal recreational waters can be contaminated through point and non-point sources such as agricultural and industrial runoffs, sewage discharges, and industrial effluents (5). Contamination of the coastal environment has been found to be associated with an increase in the incidence of infectious diseases (6). Some diseases and infections acquired through bathing in contaminated waters include acute febrile respiratory illness, infections of the eye, ear, nose and throat, and serious infections such as meningitis, hepatitis A, typhoid fever and poliomyelitis (7). Other diseases caused by bathing in contaminated recreational waters or consumption of contaminated seafood include swimmer's itch, gastroenteritis, dermatitis, viral hepatitis, and dysentery (8).

Environmental problems arise when sewage is discharged inappropriately into coastal areas. This can lead to very high nutrient loads from phosphates and nitrates, which cause localized eutrophication, which in turn is associated with toxic algal blooms (7). The temperature and pH levels can also play a significant role in coastal water quality since both affect the growth and multiplication of aquatic organisms and fecal indicator organisms (5). Caribbean countries, which depend on coral reefs as a natural defense for coastal areas and for the survival of fish populations, already face social and economic threats as a result of the degradation and loss of reefs (9).

Coastal waters are used for several activities, including transportation, food production, hydroelectricity generation, and for the deposition of sewage and industrial waste (7). In the Caribbean, many islands market themselves through the promotion of clean, white sandy beaches; safe for swimming, snorkeling, diving, and bathing. Beach recreational activities are largely hosted around holiday activities and festivals. Not many Caribbean countries, however, have given sufficient attention to the importance of monitoring their recreational water quality. Regulations for sewage treatment and other sources of contamination, such as agricultural runoff, are either non-existent or not adequately implemented in the Caribbean countries. In 2012, the Caribbean Regional Fund for Wastewater Management (CREW) estimated that approximately 85% of the wastewater entering the Caribbean Sea was not treated (10). As a result, many Caribbean coastal water areas are vulnerable to contamination, and those who use these areas are exposed to pathogenic microorganisms that can cause severe infections.

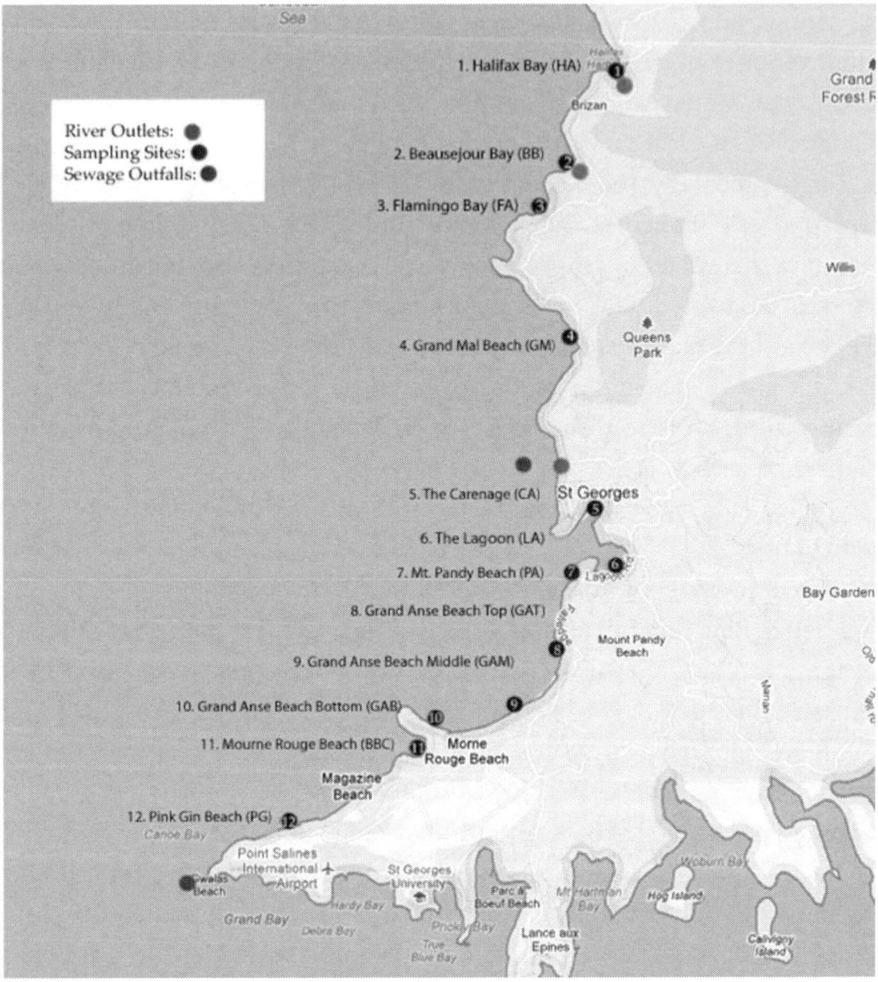

Figure 1. Sampling sites, river outlets, and sewage outfalls along the West coast of Grenada.

Grenada, approximately 133 square miles, is located 12.07° North and 61.0° West and is home to approximately 110,000 people. The island is divided into seven parishes with the parish of St. George, located in the South West, being the most populated with approximately 37,057 residents (11) (see Figure 1). The capital city, St. George's, is also located in this parish, which is the most developed on the island. One of the areas most visited by tourists is Grand Anse, located in the south of St. George parish and popular for shopping and the Grand Anse Beach. Wastewater, mainly greywater from residential, commercial, and industrial establishments, from the Grand Anse area is channeled through a 15-mile conveyor and discharged to a marine outfall. There is currently no secondary treatment of sewage in Grenada. During the rainy season, because of the island's mountainous topography, there is also severe soil erosion and land degradation (12) which affects the quality of the coastal recreational waters. Due to recent changes in the climate, however, rainfall has become less predictable and there has been a 61% increase in rainfall during the dry season (January to May) over the period 1990-2009 (13). Coastal dynamics also play an intrinsic role in determining the status of water quality (14). Closed bays are subjected to higher concentrations of contaminants since they have a low renewal frequency compared to open bays (15).

A study investigating the prevalence of *escherichia coli* and *enterococcus faecalis* in coastal environments located in the Southern parts of Grenada was limited to four coastal sites located on the furthest end of the parish of S. George (16). In another study conducted in 2006 on the West coast of Grenada near the St John's Bay river, measurements of *enterococcus faecalis* levels were taken and found to be low (17). A report from the Government of Grenada's Epidemiological Department stated that gastroenteritis was one of the major acute illnesses affecting infants on the island. Approximately 1067 cases were reported in March 2012 as compared to 319 reported in March 2011(18).

In recognition of the importance of having adequate monitoring systems in place, the Caribbean Environmental Health Institute (CEHI), subsumed into the Caribbean Public Health Agency (CARPHA) as at January 2012, produced and published guidelines for the region's coastal water quality (7). The recommended limits for marine waters for *escherichia coli* is 126 CFU/100 ml, for fecal coliform 200 CFU/100 ml, and for *enterococcus faecalis* 35 CFU/100 ml (7). In assessing water quality, multiple microbial indicators are used to make correlations between the number of microbes and possible contamination. According to the WHO, *enterococcus faecalis* meets all regulatory parameters standards as opposed to total coliform, which is not specific to fecal material (19). The United States Environmental

Protection Agency ((EPA)) also recommended the use of *enterococcus faecalis* as the best indicator for assessing recreational water health risk (20). It is expected that by assessing Grenada's coastal waters using WHO and EPA recommended indicators, data can be obtained to provide a better understanding of the quality of the coastal waters of the Southern part of Grenada.

In this study, the quality of recreational waters of Grenada's most populated coastal regions was assessed and compared with WHO and EPA recommended standards. Sources of possible contamination were examined along with possible health-related outcomes to determine whether water quality monitoring is necessary to ensure safe water-related recreational activities in Grenada.

OUR STUDY

A cross-sectional sampling for *enterococcus faecalis* and fecal coliforms in the coastal waters located in the Southwestern regions of Grenada was taken from November 4th to December 3rd, 2008.

Sample sites

Of the 45 beaches in Grenada, 12 beaches located in the South Western region of the island were selected for this study. The 12 sampled sites were Halifax-Bay ((HA)), Beausejour-Bay ((BA)), Flamingo-Bay ((FB), Grand-Mal (GM), Carenage-Bay (CA), the Lagoon (LA), Mt-Pandy-Beach (PA), Morne-Rouge-Beach (BBC), Pink-Gin-Beach (PG), and Grand-Anse-Beach (GA) (see Figure 1). The GA site, which is approximately three miles long, was divided into three zones: Grand-Anse-Top (GAT), Grand-Anse-Middle (GAM), and Grand-Anse-Bottom (GAB). Each of these sampling areas is subjected to major exposures to contaminants from various water sources such as rivers, stormwater runoff, and sewage discharge. All of the Grand

Anse (GA) sampling sites were heavily patronized by the local residents and tourists. The Grand Mal (GM) area is also a heavily populated zone and subject to runoffs from construction sites. GM site also has a sewer outfall that empties directly into its waters from the Queens Park area. Two of the other sampling sites, the Lagoon (LA) and the Carenage (CA) sites, are major docking areas for ships, cargo boats, yachts, and barges.

Physical parameters

To better assess the quality of the recreational waters, physical parameters such as surface temperature, pH, amount of rainfall, and general weather conditions were recorded. Temperature was measured directly after sampling and noted in degrees Celsius.

Rainfall

Rainfall data for the sampling period was obtained from five meteorological stations operated by the Grenada Meteorological Office. These meteorological stations were chosen based on their location and the direction of the runoff water caused by the rainfall. The chosen stations were located in Vendomme, Mardigras, Annandale, Botanical Gardens, and the Maurice Bishop International Airport. Rainfall data, measured in millimeters (mm), was collected to allow for investigation of possible relationships between water quality and land runoff associated with rainfall. For this study, a low level of rainfall was defined as levels < 10 mm, a moderate level of rainfall as $10 > 100$ mm, and a high level of rainfall as >100 mm.

Sample collection

Water samples were collected during the rainy season, between November 4 to December 3, 2008. Samples were collected bi-weekly for five weeks. Six sites were visited each day, and two samples were taken at each site, amounting to 24 samples per week. Samples were collected between 8 a.m. and 12 p.m. so that any variation in the levels of contamination due to downpours, wind direction, and tidal levels could be evaluated. Serial dilution techniques were used to reduce the density of the organisms present in the samples and to improve measurement accuracy.

The equipment and reagents used for collecting water samples were prepared according to protocols specified by the EPA (20). All equipment was sterilized using detergent and hot water, followed by distilled water. Sampling bottles were autoclaved for 15 minutes up to 121°Celsius and kept closed after sterilization. All samples were taken 5 ft offshore and at a depth of 40 cm below the surface every Monday and Thursday of the week. This sampling protocol was recommended, given the majority of beach users occupy up to this area and where subsurface currents move much slower compared to surface currents (22). For each sample, 100 ml of water was collected leaving space for the sample to be shaken. Testing was done within one hour of sampling. Samples that were not analyzed within this timeframe were refrigerated at or below 4°Celsius.

FINDINGS

Fecal coliform counts for HA, PB, GAM, BB, and FB were above recommended acceptable limits for 10% of the sampling days. This was the lowest observed percentage compared to all other sampled sites. Both BBC and PG sampling sites exceeded recommended fecal coliform limits 20% and 30% of collected samples, respectively, followed by GM, LA, GAT, and GAB in which 40% of samples at these sites exceeded the recommended acceptable limits. At CA, 60% of sampling days were above the recommended limits and was the highest in comparison to all other sites sampled (see Figure 2).

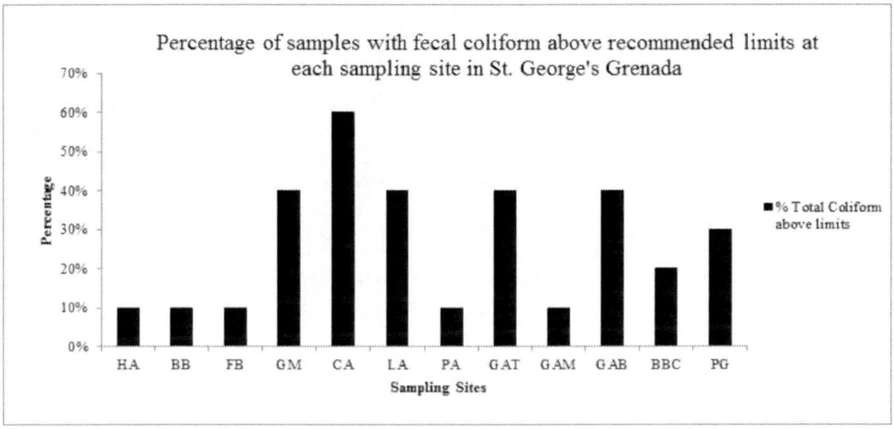

Figure 2. Fecal coliform levels above recommended limits by sampling sites for November 4 to December 3, 2008.

Enterococci faecalis

The recommended acceptable *enterococcus faecalis* limits were exceeded at all sampled sites except FB. PA exceeded recommended limits in 20% of sampling days, and GM, LA, GAT, GAM, GAB, and BBC exceeded recommended limits for 40% of the sampling days. Sample sites LA and GAB had counts over 200 CFU/100 ml on 50% of those sampling days and GAT on all of those days. HA and CA showed similar results exceeding recommended limits on 60% of the sampling days, however, CA level reached counts > 200 CFU/100ml on all sampling days, whilst HA remained below 200 CFU/100ml in all samples. BB exceeded recommended limits on 70% of the sampling days, with 57% of those samples reaching counts above > 200CFU/100 ml (see Figure 3).

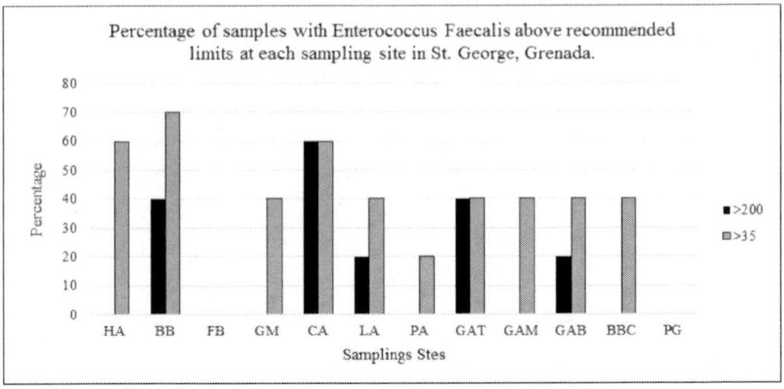

*Black bars indicate percentage of *Enterococcus faecalis* counts > 200 CFU/100 ml samples out of the total that exceeded recommended limits. Example: BB shows percentage of samples exceeding recommended limits (35 CFU/100 ml) in grey (70%) and percentage of samples exceeding 200 CFU/100 ml (40%) of the total in black. NB: This is to emphasize the severity of contamination.

Figure 3. Percentage of *Enterococci faecalis* above recommended limits by sampling site in St. George's Grenada for November 4 to December 3 2008.

Temperature

The temperature for all bays ranged 20.4-31.6°C (see Figure 4). The greatest temperature range was recorded for CA, 20.4°C to 30.1°C.

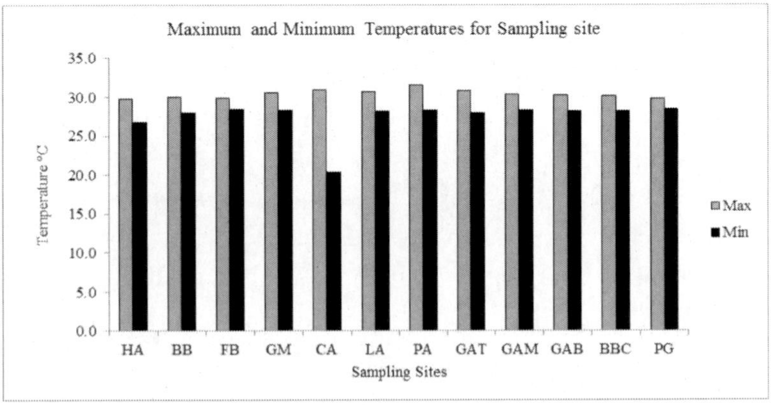

Figure 4. Maximum and minimum temperatures by sampling site for the period November 4 to December 3, 2008.

pH

Recorded pH readings remained within the acceptable range for all sampling sites throughout November, 2008.

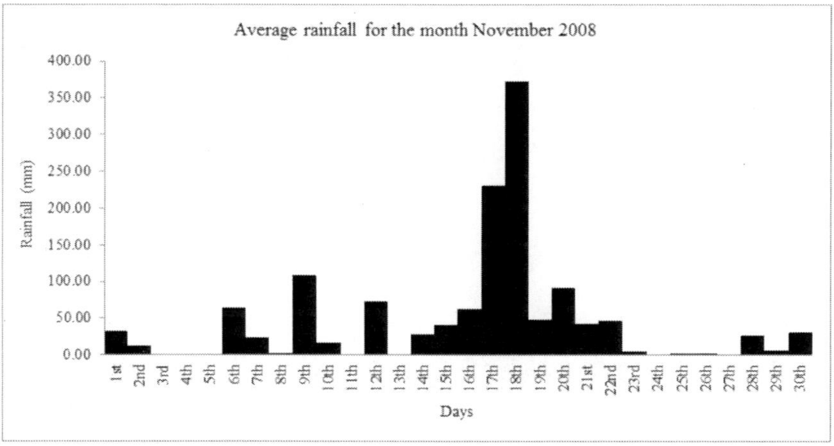

Figure 5. Average rainfall for the month of November in St. Georges, Grenada.

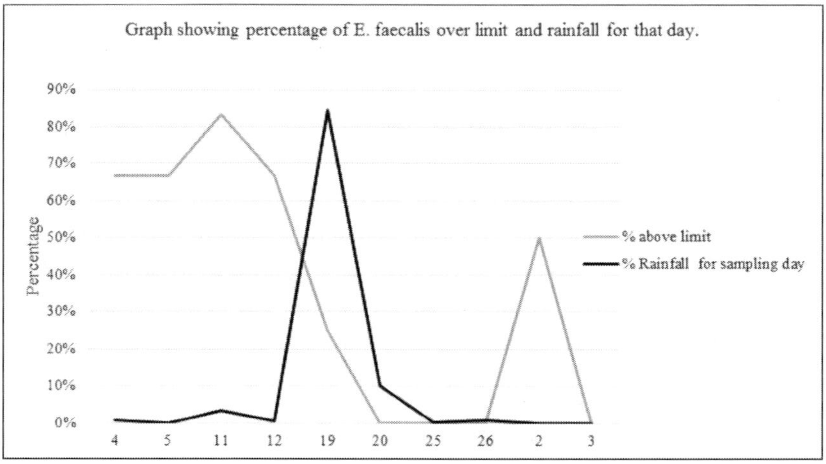

Figure 6. Percentage of enterococcus faecalis above limit and rainfall for the same sampling day.

Rainfall

High levels of rainfall were reported on the following sampling days: November 12, 19, and 20 (see Figure 5). It was observed that the rainfall pattern varied greatly with the corresponding high microbial counts (see Figure 6). Chi square analysis revealed that rainfall and *enterococcus faecalis* were independent as observed throughout the sampling period (χ: 0.63, p: 0.42).

DISCUSSION

Several studies have shown the presence of fecal indicator organisms in coastal waters of Grenada (16, 23, 24). In 2008, an assessment of samples collected from the HA revealed readings that exceeded recommended fecal coliform levels for 10% of the sampling days when the amount of rainfall was low on the same day and moderate the previous day. This study found that *enterococcus faecalis* counts exceeded recommended acceptable levels for 60% of the samples when rainfall levels were low on the same day and moderate 24-hours before testing. Temperatures in the HA bay ranged from 26.8- 29.8°C.

This level was observed with the lowest temperature and exceeding levels of *enterococcus faecalis* and moderate levels of rainfall on the same day and high on the previous day. Halifax Bay is an enclosed bay and subjected to low water renewal and high accumulation of sediment. The area is in the vicinity of the island's main landfill. Runoff from the landfill most likely also accounted for the increased microbial levels recorded at this location by Garrido-Perez in 2008 (15).

BA samples exceeded recommended fecal coliform levels at a similar rate as HA (10%) when rainfall levels were low on the same day and on the previous day. *Enterococcus faecalis* levels exceeded recommended levels in 70% of the sampling sites which, correlated with low, moderate levels of rainfall on the same day, and low-high levels of rainfall 24 hours before testing. This was the highest recorded percentage amongst all tested sites.

Of these samples, 57% were >200.5 CFU/100ml and showed a low correlation with high levels of rainfall. Studies have shown that high rainfall has been associated with increased microbial counts (24). The temperatures measured in BA ranged from 28-30.0°C. Further, no strong correlations were noted with temperature, exceeding levels of *Enterococcus faecalis,* and high levels of rainfall, either on the same day and 24 hours before testing. A reason why rainfall correlations may have been weak is that the BA is more open and, therefore, more amenable to the flushing of any contaminants (15). The *enterococcus faecalis* levels may be high for this location due to continuous contamination by untreated septic tanks that enters the river, as indicated by previous studies (25). The marine estuary located at the mouth of this bay can also present major problems when contaminated from upland sources (26).

The FB samples exceeded the recommended fecal coliform levels at rates similar to HA and BA (10%) when rainfall levels fell at low levels on the same day and moderate on the previous day. The temperatures measured in this bay ranged from 28.4-29.9°C. Recorded *enterococcus faecalis* levels did not exceed recommended levels at any sampling site. Highest rainfall levels 24 hours before and on the same day resulted in the lowest level of *enterococcus faecalis,* which pattern was also observed in previous studies (27). This may have been as a result of protective factors such as increased dilution, the absence of potential sources of pollution, such as runoff from drains, and the bay's long distance from residential areas. No observed correlations could be made between either temperature and high levels of *enterococcus faecalis* or high levels of rainfall on the same day and 24-hours before testing.

The GM samples exceeded recommended acceptable fecal coliform limits for 40% of the sampling days when rainfall levels were low on the same day and low to moderate on the previous day. The temperature at this bay ranged from 28.3-30.6°C. *Enterococcus faecalis* levels exceeded recommended limits for 40% of the samples, however, none exceeding 200 CFU/100 ml. This correlated with low levels of rainfall on the same day and low to moderate levels 24-hours before testing. There was no correlation with the lowest temperature and exceeding levels of *enterococcus faecalis* and high levels of rainfall both on the same day and 24-hours before testing. The BM beach is an open area, therefore, frequent flushing of contaminants with high levels of rainfall may be the reason for the low microbial counts occurring with rainfall. Other parameters such as tidal flow and height could have been important factors that help explain the increase in microbial indicators at this sample site (28). The observed occurrence of a high level of fecal coliform and *enterococcus faecalis* with high temperatures may also be the cause of conflicting results. Temperature is known to affect the rate at which bacteria grow and multiply (5). Other factors, such as contamination from rivers, may have played a role in the increased microbial counts (7).

The CA samples exceeded recommended fecal coliform levels on 60% of the sampling days when rainfall levels fell to low to moderate levels on the same day and low, moderate, and high levels on the previous day. Temperature at this bay ranged from 20.4-31.0°C. This was the highest range noted for the month at all sites and may have been due to the area being completely surrounded by concrete infrastructure which contributes to a higher rate of runoff and flushing when rainfall occurs. *Enterococcus faecalis* levels exceeded recommended levels in 60% of the sampling sites, exceeding >200.5 CFU/100 ml on all days, and was not observed to occur in conjunction with high levels of rainfall. The high level of *enterococcus faecalis* could be attributed to the densely populated Carenage area which is a docking station for barges, cargo boats, and ships. Runoff from these facilities drains directly into the site. Studies have suggested *enterococcus faecalis* level increase in such areas (7, 19). Low levels of *enterococcus faecalis* were observed with high levels of rainfall, which may have been due to dilution of contaminated water. The LA samples exceeded recommended fecal coliform levels 60% of the sampling days when rainfall levels fell to low l on the same day and low to moderate on the previous day. Temperature on that bay ranged from 28.2-30.7°C. *Enterococcus faecalis* levels exceeded recommended levels in 40% of the sampling sites, exceeding >200.5 CFU/100 ml on 50% of those days and was not observed to occur in conjunction with high levels of rainfall. High level of *enterococcus faecalis* could be attributed to the highly developed commercial activities in the area as well as a docking station for barges, cargo boats, and ships. Runoff from facilities also drains directly into the site. Construction activities were noted to have occurred during that period (30). Low levels of *enterococcus faecalis* were observed with high levels of rainfall, which may be due to the dilution of contaminated water, similar to the situation at CA. PA samples exceeded recommended fecal coliform levels 40% of the sampling days when rainfall levels fell at mostly low levels on the same day and low levels the previous day although one day was noted to produce heavy rainfall. Temperature at this bay ranged from 28.2-30.7°C. *Enterococcus faecalis* levels exceeded recommended levels in 20% of the sampling sites and were observed when rainfall levels fell at mostly low to moderate levels on the same day and low levels the previous day. A number of protective factors were present on this beach, including the high amount of flora and absence of drains emptying directly unto to beach.

GA samples (top, middle, and bottom) exceeded recommended fecal coliform levels in 40%, 10%, and 40% samples, respectively, when rainfall levels were at mostly low to high levels on the same day and low the previous day. Temperature at these sites ranged from 28.0-30.8°C (GAT), 28.3-30.4°C (GAM) and 28.2-30.2°C (GAB). *Enterococcus faecalis* counts exceeded recommended levels in 40% of the sampling sites GAB, GAM, and GAT. GAT and GAB, however, reported samples exceeding level >200.5 CFU/100ml in 40% and 20% of all samples, respectively. This was thought to be associated with drains which were observed to empty runoff directly into the swimming area of both sites (GAT and GAB) but were not present at GAM. There are several factors affecting this beach, including being frequently populated with tourists and local residents engaging in recreational activities.

BBC exceeded recommended fecal coliform levels on 20% of the sampling days when rainfall levels fell at mostly low levels on the same day and low levels the previous day, although one day was noted to produce heavy rainfall. The temperatures measured at this bay ranged from 28.2 - 30.1°C. *Enterococcus faecalis* levels exceeded recommended levels in 20% of the sampling sites and did not occur in conjunction with high levels of rainfall.

PG exceeded recommended fecal coliform levels 30% of the sampling days, which was in conjunction with low to moderate rainfall the same day and low the previous day. Temperatures measured at this bay ranged from 28.5°-29.7 C. *Enterococcus faecalis* levels did not exceed recommended levels. This may be mostly due to the open bay and high flushing which may have carried contaminants away from the sample site.

Limitations of this study include possible errors in sample collection and preparation. These samples were collected over 12 years ago in 2008 and, therefore, it might be questioned whether the same results would be achieved today if a new batch of samples were collected. It should be noted that most of the factors that likely contributed to the observed high microbial levels, such as high levels of development and anthropogenic activity, have further increased over the years (31). Additionally, the St. George's sewage outfall still releases untreated sewage and no major improvements in the quality of the water have been found (31, 32).

In conclusion, measurements of two recreational water quality indicators, fecal coliform and *enterococcus faecalis*, at 12 coastal sites located along the southwestern end of Grenada found results that exceed acceptable WHO recommended limits. The sampling site with the highest percentage of samples exceeding recommended levels was BB (70%), which is most likely due to sewage leakages from points along the river leading into this bay. Following BB were HA and CA (60%), LA GAT, GM, GAM, BBC, LA, and GAB (40%). FB (0%) had the best compliance with WHO's recommendations and had no samples that exceeded the recommended limits. The sampling site with the highest levels of fecal coliform was CA (60%), followed by GAT, GAB, GM and LA (40%), PG (30%), BBC (20%), and PB, BB, HA, PB (10%), respectively. The amount of rainfall and *enterococcus faecalis* was shown to have a negative association, possibly due to several factors affecting site flushing and protective mechanisms. Due to inconsistencies in the correlations between rainfall and microbial contamination, it is recommended that water quality monitoring systems be put in place to ensure that persons frequenting the beaches located along the southwestern coast are made aware of the safe days for swimming in these areas. Given that this study was done within an approximate one-month time period, this assessment should be replicated, extending over other months of the year, which can allow for a better assessment of the relationship between rainfall and microbial indicators. Additionally, an extended period of monitoring is necessary so that a comparative analysis can be done between the dry and wet seasons in Grenada. It is also anticipated that the data from this study will provide key information for the Government of Grenada on where best to install proper drainage systems to ameliorate the risk of contaminating coastal sites.

REFERENCES

[1] Koncagül E, Tran M, Connor R, Uhlenbrook S. The United Nation World Water Development Report 2019. Italy: UNESCO; 2019 p. 2. Sustainable Development Goals. Geneva: United Nations, 2019.

[2] Schets FM, De Roda Husman AM, Havelaar AH. Disease outbreaks associated with untreated recreational water use. Epidemiol Infect 2011;139(7):1114–25.

[3] Palaniappan M, Gleick PH, Allen L. Clearing the waters: The focus of water quality solutions. Nairobi: UNEP, 2010.

[4] European Environment Agency. European bathing water quality in 2018. EEA Report No.3. Copenhagen, DK: European Environment Agency, 2019.

[5] IMO/FAO/UNESCO-IOC/WMO/WHO/IAEA/UN/UNEP. Protecting the oceans from land based activities. Hague: GESAMP; 2001.

[6] Bartram J, Rees G. Monitoring bathing waters: A practical guide to the design and implementation of assessment and monitoring programmes. New York: WHO, 2000.

[7] Why treat wastewater: environmental, health and legal considerations. New York: USAID, UNEP, 1997.

[8] Burke L, Maidens J. Reefs at risk in the Caribbean. Washington, DC: World Resources Institute, 2004.

[9] Caribbean Regional Fund for Wastewater Management (CReW). Testing a prototype. New ork: UNEP, 2012.

[10] Fast facts. Mgovernance.net, 2020. URL: https://www.mgovernance.net/.

[11] Forde M, Neff B. Impact of development on water supply and treatment in Grenada: New York: IANAS, UNESCO, 2015.

[12] Infante R. Climate change indicators for the Caribbean region: general trends in temperature and precipitation (1900–2009). Curr J Appl Sci Technol 2018;26(4):1-8.

[13] Caitlin O. Scopel JH, Sandra L. McLellan. Influence of nearshore water dynamics and pollution sources on beach monitoring outcomes at two adjacent Lake Michigan beaches. J Great Lakes Res 2006;32(3):543–52.

[14] Garrido-Perez MC. Microbial indicators of feacal contamination in waters and sediment of beach in waters and sediments of beach bathing zones. Int J Hyg Envir Health 2008; 211(5-6):510-7.

[15] Amadi VA, Kotelnikova S. The prevalence of antibiotic resistant fecal indicator organisms escherichia coli and enterococcus faecalis in the coastal environments, Grenada: WINDREF, 2008.

[16] Patel R, Pedersen K, Kotelnikova S. The bacteriological analysis and health risks in the urban estuary of St. George's Bay, Grenada, West Indies. J Environ Health 2010;73(2):22-6.

[17] Gonzalez M. Comminicable disease report, Grenada: Epidemiology Unit, Ministry of Health, Grenada, 2012.

[18] WHO. Guidelines for safe recreational water envornmental, coastal and fresh waters. Geneva: World Health Organisaton, 2003.

[19] United States Environmental Protection Agency. Fecal bacteria. URL: https://archive.epa.gov/water/archive/web/html/vms511.html.

[20] Environmental Propection Agency. National recommended water quality criteria: Aquatic life criteria table. Wasington, DC: EPA, 1986.

[21] Pidwirny M. Surface and subsurface ocean currents: Ocean current map. URL: http://www.physicalgeography.net/fundamentals/8q_1.html.

[22] Grenada Bureau of Standards. Specifications for effulent from industrial processes dischargeed into the environment. No GDS 79). St George's: Grenada Bureau of Standards, 2006.

[23] Ahn HJ, Grant BS. Coastal water quality impact of storm water runoff from urban watershed in soutern California. Environ Sci Techno. 2005;39(16):5940-53.

[24] Patel R. The ecological distribution of viable indicator organisms and associated health risks form St George's Bay in Grenada. Unpublished, 2007.

[25] Vasconcelos GJ, Swartz RG. Survival of bacteria in seawater using a diffusion chamber apparatus in situ. Appl Environ Microbiol 1976;31(6):913–20.

[26] Albritton H. Fecal coliform and Entercocci relationahip to rainfall and runoff in rural water shed reveal intrinsic diffenrces between fecal pollution indicators. American Geophysical Union Fall Meeting Abstracts, 2009.

[27] Adelzaher AM, Wright EM. Presence of pathogens and indicator microbes at non point source subtropical recreational marine beach. Appl Environ Microbiol 2009;76(3):724-32.

[28] Davies MC, Long AJ. Survival of fecal microorganisms in marine and fresh water sediments. Appl Environ Microbiol 1995;61(5):1888-96.

[29] Socio-economic monitoring in adjacent communities of the Grand Anse Marine Protected Area. St George's: Grenada, 2017:53-4.

[30] Homer F. Grand Anse Marine Protected Area Management Plan 2016-2020. Grenada: Fisheries Division, 2016.

In: Public Health Themes in Grenada … ISBN: 978-1-53618-118-0
Editors: J. Merrick and L. Glasgow © 2020 Nova Science Publishers, Inc.

Chapter 14

METABOLIC SYNDROME, ANXIETY, AND DEPRESSION IN ARUBAN ADULTS

Sibel Dikmen, BS, Marquesa Moore, BS, Ezinma Schwiers, BA and Prakash VAK Ramdass*, MD, MPH

Department of Public Health and Preventive Medicine,
St. George's University School of Medicine, St George's, Grenada

ABSTRACT

Metabolic syndrome is a collection of risk factors that include insulin resistance, dyslipidemia, visceral adiposity, and hypertension. Studies have shown contrasting results regarding its association with anxiety and depressive symptoms. The primary aim of this study was to evaluate the association of metabolic syndrome and the severity of anxiety or depression. Our objectives were to estimate the prevalence of anxiety and depression in Aruba. We conducted a cross-sectional study in Aruba in November 2016. Participants were assessed for metabolic syndrome using

* Correspondence: Dr. Prakash VAK Ramdass, Associate Professor of Clinical Epidemiology, St George's University School of Medicine, Department of Public Health and Preventive Medicine, St George's, Grenada, West Indies. Email: prakash.ramdass@gmail.com.

the harmonized criteria and were screened for depression and anxiety using the Patient Health Questionnaire-9 and the General Anxiety Disorder-7 questionnaires, respectively. We used the $\chi 2$ test/ Fisher's Exact test to compare proportions, and the unpaired t-test to compare continuous variables between groups. Statistical significance was reported at the 0.05 significance level. Our sample included a total of 181 participants, 103 (56.9%) of whom were women. A total of 67 (37.0%) people reported signs of anxiety, while 72 (39.8%) people reported signs of depression. In comparing metabolic syndrome status, there was a statistically significant difference for severity of anxiety ($p = 0.013$) but not for severity of depression ($p = 0.228$). The mean PHQ9 ($p = 0.027$) and the mean GAD7 ($p < 0.001$) scores were both significantly higher in people without metabolic syndrome. Participants with metabolic syndrome had decreased levels of anxiety and depression. There is a high prevalence of anxiety and depression in Aruba.

INTRODUCTION

Metabolic syndrome (MetS) is a collection of risk factors that include insulin resistance, dyslipidemia, visceral adiposity, and hypertension (1). Studies have shown there is a direct relationship with metabolic syndrome and the development of cardiovascular diseases (2) and type 2 diabetes mellitus (3). Moreover, the risk of myocardial infarction and cerebrovascular disease triples in those with metabolic syndrome (3). However, in addition to having an increased risk of cardiovascular diseases, metabolic syndrome has been shown to have an increased association of mood disorders, notably anxiety (4) and depressive symptoms (5). Those with metabolic syndrome components manifest a low-moderate, chronic inflammatory state (6). Concurrently, inflammation has been related to the development of some depressive disorders (7). Other studies suggest that chronic systemic inflammation might explain the link between metabolic syndrome and anxious-depressive syndromes (6).

The relationship between mood disorders and metabolic syndrome has been considerably investigated. However, there are contrasting findings which are likely due to variation in sample demographics. Nonetheless, these investigations have shown to be commonly rooted in the correlation between mood and anxiety disorders with an increased risk of cardiovascular morbidity and mortality (8). In addition, a study by Ellouze et al. showed that patients with type 2 diabetes and depression displayed poorer glycemic control and less medication compliance as compared to those without concurrent depression (9). Thus, there may be other clinical implications relating to pharmacological treatment of patients with metabolic syndrome components and mood disorders. Therefore, a better understanding of the relationship between metabolic syndrome and anxiety or depression can potentially target their etiologies and consequently, provide a foundation for the development of novel therapies.

The primary aim of this study was to evaluate the association of metabolic syndrome and the different levels of severity of anxiety or depression in a sample of Aruban adults. Our objectives were to screen participants with the General Anxiety Disorder-7 (10) questionnaire and the Patient Health Questionnaire-9 (11) to estimate the prevalence of anxiety and depression, respectively. We hypothesized that there would be a positive association between metabolic syndrome and increasing levels of severity of anxiety and depression.

Our study

This study was approved by the institutional review board of Xavier University School of Medicine, Aruba. Written informed consent was obtained from all study participants. A cross-sectional study was conducted at Xavier University School of Medicine, in November 2016, during its Annual Health Fair.

The health fair was held at the campus of Xavier University School of Medicine, from 7 AM to 11 AM. Participants were recruited by announcements on local radio and television, and by flyers posted at popular supermarkets four weeks before the event.

We collected data on sociodemographic variables, health behaviors, depression, anxiety, and metabolic syndrome by using a structured questionnaire. The interviews were conducted in English, Papiamento, and Spanish. Occupation was based on the International Standard for Classification of Occupations (ISCO-08) (12) and was grouped as professionals, skilled workers, unemployed, and retired.

Assessment of depression and anxiety

We screened participants for depression and anxiety with the Patient Health Questionnaire-9 (PHQ9) (11) and the General Anxiety Disorder-7 (GAD7) (10) questionnaires, respectively. Participants were asked whether they had experienced symptoms of depression or anxiety within the past two weeks. Depression and anxiety were categorized as mild, moderate, or severe, using the cut-off points of 5, 10, and 15, respectively.

Assessment of metabolic syndrome

Metabolic syndrome was defined according to the harmonized clinical criteria (1) which require that at least three of the following five criteria have to be met: fasting plasma glucose (≥100 mg/dL and or diabetes medication), triglycerides (≥150 mg/dL and or drug treatment for elevated triglycerides), HDL cholesterol (<40 mg/dL in males and <50 mg/dL in females and or drug treatment for reducing HDL cholesterol), blood pressure (systolic ≥130 mm Hg and or diastolic ≥85 mm Hg and or use of antihypertensive medication), and waist circumference (ethnicity and country-specific cut-off; we used the International Diabetes Federation (13) cut-offs for Europid: 94 cm for men and 80 cm for women). If patients had met the criteria for metabolic syndrome, they were contacted by the laboratory with the results and were recommended to visit their health care provider.

Measurements and biochemical analyses

Waist circumference was measured with a soft tape, on standing subjects, at the level of the umbilicus. Blood pressure was measured on the right arm using a manual mercury sphygmomanometer after the subject had rested for 10 minutes. Systolic and diastolic blood pressures were recorded as the first and last Korotkoff sounds, respectively.

Venous blood samples were taken from the antecubital vein after an overnight fast (participants were advised to fast overnight) and serum total cholesterol was measured by standard enzymatic assays within 4 hours of collection. Blood glucose level was measured using a glucometer (ACCU-CHEK® Active strips in Accu-Chek® Active test meter, Roche Diagnostics, Germany).

Statistical analyses

Data were analyzed using SPSS version 24 (IBM Corp., Armonk, NY, USA). Descriptive statistics (mean ± standard deviation [SD] or percentages) were computed for socio-demographic factors and the prevalence of metabolic syndrome according to the severity of depression and anxiety. We used the unpaired *t*-test to compare continuous variables and the $\chi 2$ test/ Fisher's Exact test to compare proportions between groups. Statistical significance was reported at the 0.05 significance level.

FINDINGS

Our sample included a total of 181 participants, 103 (56.9%) of whom were women. Most of the participants (38.1%) were between the ages of 51-70 years. Hispanics comprised 51.4% of the sample. Metabolic syndrome was present in 21.5% of the participants. A total of 67 (37.0%) people showed signs of anxiety, of which 13 (7.2%) of them had severe anxiety. Similarly,

72 (39.8%) people showed signs of depression, 11 (6.1%) of whom met the criteria for severe depression. Detailed characteristics of the sample are shown in Table 1.

Table 1. Sociodemographic characteristics of the study participants (n=181)

Variables	
Sex, n (%)	
Men	78 (43.1)
Women	103 (56.9)
Age, n (%)	
18 – 30	32 (17.7)
31 – 50	42 (23.2)
51 – 70	69 (38.1)
≥ 71	38 (21.0)
Race, n (%)	
Hispanic	93 (51.4)
Caucasian	8 (4.4)
Mixed	21 (11.6)
Other	59 (32.6)
Occupation, n (%)	
Professional	50 (27.6)
Skilled	49 (27.1)
Unemployed	41 (22.7)
Retired	41 (22.7)
Education, n (%)	
High school	95 (52.5)
Undergraduate	38 (21.0)
Graduate	23 (12.7)
Other	25 (13.8)
Exercise, n (%)	
No regular exercise	60 (33.1)
1-2 hours/ week	55 (30.4)
>2 hours/ week	66 (36.5)
Alcohol consumption, n (%)	
Never	101 (55.8)
Current	80 (44.2)
Smoking, n (%)	
Never	164 (90.6)
Current	17 (9.4)

Variables	
Metabolic syndrome, n (%)	
Yes	142 (78.5)
No	39 (21.5)
Anxiety, n (%)	
None	114 (63.0)
Mild	35 (19.3)
Moderate	19 (10.5)
Severe	13 (7.2)
Depression, n (%)	
None	109 (60.2)
Mild	45 (24.9)
Moderate	16 (8.8)
Severe	11 (6.1)

Participants who were 50 years and older were more likely to have metabolic syndrome. There was no association between metabolic syndrome and sex, race, or education. In comparing metabolic syndrome status, there was a statistically significant difference for age ($p < 0.001$), occupation ($p = 0.004$), and severity of anxiety ($p = 0.013$). However, there was no statistically significant difference for severity of depression ($p = 0.228$) based on metabolic syndrome status. Of patients who had metabolic syndrome, 30.8% of them had depression, whereas 42.2% of those who did not have metabolic syndrome had depression. Patients who had metabolic syndrome were less likely to have anxiety (15.4%) compared to those who did not have metabolic syndrome (43.0%). Interestingly, as severity of both anxiety and depression increased, participants had a lower likelihood of having metabolic syndrome. In fact, 100% of participants who had severe anxiety or depression were free from metabolic syndrome. In addition, the mean PHQ9 ($p = 0.027$) and the mean GAD7 ($p < 0.001$) scores were both significantly higher for those without metabolic syndrome when compared to those with metabolic syndrome. Results are shown in Table 2, and Figures 1 and 2.

Table 2. Metabolic syndrome, anxiety, and depression

Variables	MetS	No MetS	p values
Sex, n (%)			0.423
Women	20 (19.4)	83 (80.6)	
Men	19 (24.4)	59 (75.6)	
Age, n (%)			<0.001
18 – 30	1 (3.1)	31 (96.9)	
31 – 50	2 (4.8)	40 (95.2)	
51 – 70	20 (29.0)	49 (71.0)	
>70	16 (42.1)	22 (57.9)	
Race, n (%)			0.989
Hispanic	20 (21.5)	73 (78.5)	
Other	19 (21.6)	69 (78.4)	
Education, n (%)			0.066
High school	23 (24.2)	72 (75.8)	
Undergraduate	5 (13.2)	33 (86.8)	
Graduate	2 (8.7)	21 (91.3)	
Other	9 (36.0)	16 (64.0)	
Occupation, (%)			0.004
Professional	9 (18.0)	41 (82.0)	
Skilled	6 (12.2)	43 (87.9)	
Unemployed	7 (17.1)	34 (82.9)	
Retired	17 (41.5)	24 (58.5)	
Exercise, n (%)			0.728
No regular exercise	15 (25.0)	45 (75.0)	
1 - 2 hours/ week	11 (20.0)	44 (80.0)	
> 2 hours/ week	13 (19.7)	53 (80.3)	
Smoking, n (%)			0.764
Never	35 (21.3)	129 (78.7)	
Current	4 (23.5)	13 (76.5)	
Alcohol, n (%)			0.204
Never	18 (17.8)	83 (82.2)	
Current	21 (26.3)	59 (73.8)	
Depression, n (%)			0.228
None	27 (24.8)	82 (75.2)	
Mild	10 (22.2)	35 (77.8)	
Moderate	2 (12.5)	14 (87.5)	
Severe	0 (0.0)	11 (100.0)	
Anxiety, n (%)			0.013
None	33 (28.9)	81 (71.1)	
Mild	4 (11.4)	31 (88.6)	
Moderate	2 (10.5)	17 (89.5)	
Severe	0 (0.0)	13 (100.0)	
PHQ9, mean (± SD)	3.41 (3.52)	5.05 (5.52)	0.027
GAD7, mean (± SD)	2.38 (2.70)	5.35 (5.62)	<0.001

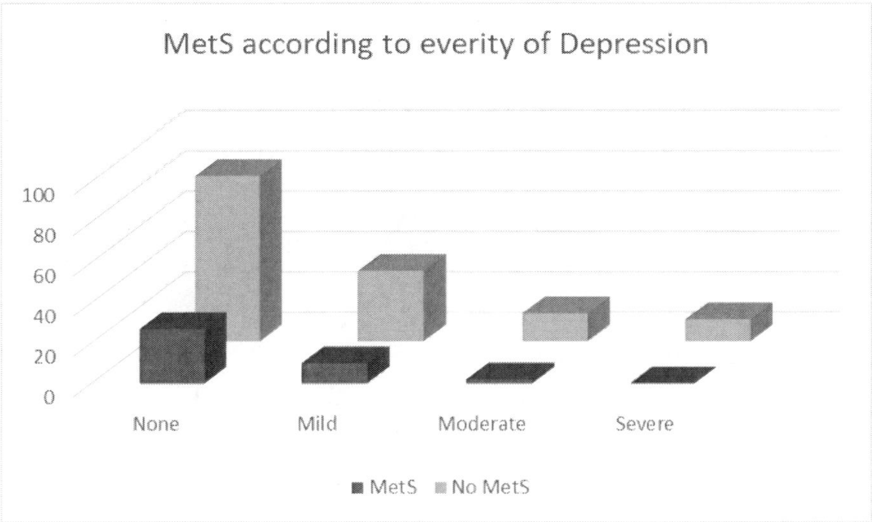

Figure 1. Prevalence of metabolic syndrome according to severity of depression.

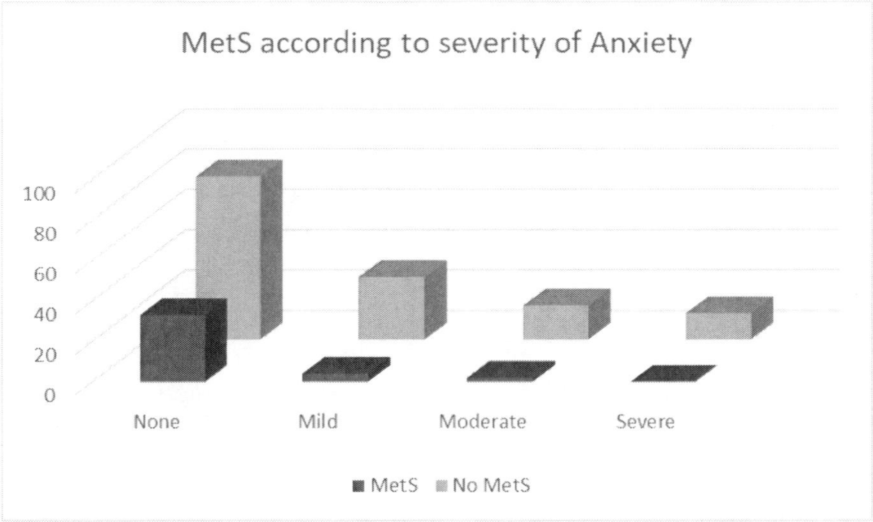

Figure 2. Prevalence of metabolic syndrome according to severity of anxiety.

DISCUSSION

To the best of our knowledge, this is the first study in Aruba to investigate the association between metabolic syndrome and anxiety or depression. Our results showed that anxiety and depression were both associated with metabolic syndrome reciprocally, contrary to expectation, wherein we hypothesized that there is a positive association.

In contrast to previous studies (14, 15), we found that anxiety and depression were more prevalent in participants without metabolic syndrome. Our results were similar to those of Glaus et al. (16), Herva et al. (17) and García-Toro et al. (18), even though their study samples were comprised of different demographics. A meta-analysis of eighteen cross-sectional studies showed that there was a slight increase in anxiety in patients with metabolic syndrome, with a pooled odds ratio of 1.07 (95% CI 1.01-1.12) (4). Of significance, in this study, we screened participants for anxiety with the GAD-7 questionnaire (10) and for depression with the PHQ-9 questionnaire (11). Both of these scales assess for anxiety or depression within two weeks of presentation. However, most of the studies in the meta-analysis (4) utilized the Spielberger Trait Anxiety Inventory (STAI) (19) and the Hospital Anxiety and Depression Scale (HADS)(20) for assessing anxiety. Nevertheless, there were inconsistent findings with these scales, even though both the STAI and HADS have more items compared to the GAD-7 or PHQ-9.

Our study showed that 37.0% of the participants had some level of anxiety, and 38.9% of participants had some level of depression. These are relatively high rates when compared to other studies on anxiety (21) and depression (22) in Latin America and the Caribbean. Even though our study found no significant association between metabolic syndrome and symptoms of depression, this might be accounted for by the lack of distinction of depression subtypes. Previous research emphasizes the importance of subtyping depression. Specifically, there have been significant findings with atypical depression and substance misuse (16).

The reciprocal association for metabolic syndrome and anxiety or depression in our study is not clearly understood. We suggest conducting large-scale longitudinal studies to investigate these relationships. However, one possible explanation for the positive association of metabolic syndrome and anxiety is the increase in sympathetic firing which, in turn, leads to an increase of metabolic syndrome components, such as hypertension and insulin resistance (23). In interpreting the contradictory findings between metabolic syndrome and anxiety or depression, we should consider the varying diagnostic criteria for metabolic syndrome, and the different instruments utilized to measure the symptoms of anxiety and depression. Unlike the other studies, we used the Harmonized criteria (1) to establish the presence of metabolic syndrome. Furthermore, the varying demographics of sample populations in the different studies should also be taken into consideration.

An important strength of this study is seen in the reliability and reproducibility through use of the GAD-7(24) and PHQ-9 (25). Recruitment of the sample via media announcements and flyers in catchment areas optimized a randomly diverse group. The cross-sectional design eliminated the common obstacle of diminished participant retention. However, our study has constraints due to limitations of statistical power and the possibility of self-selection bias, as our data was collected at a health fair. In addition, the GAD-7 and PHQ-9 are not intended to reflect a diagnosis but were used as screening tools to detect symptoms of anxiety or depression within a narrow window. Moreover, the dynamics of our cross-sectional study design does not allow for elucidation on cause and outcome for our study variables, notably metabolic syndrome and anxiety or depression.

In conclusion, the prevalence of anxiety and depression in Aruba is relatively high. Participants with metabolic syndrome had decreased levels of anxiety and depression. However, only anxiety and metabolic syndrome showed a significant statistical association. Future research should concentrate on comprehensive measures within large populations, thus allowing for isolation of variables, specifically anxiety/depression comorbidity as well as subtypes for both disorders. Conducting a longitudinal study would prove beneficial to explore the bidirectional association between metabolic syndrome and anxiety or depression. In addition, screening for depression and anxiety disorders is recommended in

Aruba, which can lead to improved clinical care and implications for public health.

ACKNOWLEDGMENTS

We gratefully acknowledge the following persons who have contributed immensely to data collection and data entry: Srishti Arya, Waleed Khan, Junea N Chowdhury, Biruk Gote, Joseph Sarra, Jonathan Rebibo, Devina Chintaman, and Saud Qureshi.

REFERENCES

[1] Alberti KG, Eckel RH, Grundy SM, Zimmet PZ, Cleeman JI, Donato KA, et al. Harmonizing the metabolic syndrome: a joint interim statement of the International Diabetes Federation Task Force on Epidemiology and Prevention; National Heart, Lung, and Blood Institute; American Heart Association; World Heart Federation; International Atherosclerosis Society; and International Association for the Study of Obesity. Circulation 2009;120(16):1640-5.

[2] Mottillo S, Filion KB, Genest J, Joseph L, Pilote L, Poirier P, et al. The metabolic syndrome and cardiovascular risk: A systematic review and meta-analysis. J Am Coll Cardiol 2010;56(14):1113–32.

[3] Meigs JB, Wilson PWF, Fox CS, Vasan RS, Nathan DM, Sullivan LM, et al. Body mass index, metabolic syndrome, and risk of type 2 diabetes or cardiovascular disease. J Clin Endocrinol Metab 2006;91(8):2906–12.

[4] Tang F, Wang G, Lian Y. Association between anxiety and metabolic syndrome: A systematic review and meta-analysis of epidemiological studies. Psychoneuroendocrinology 2017;77:112-21.

[5] Wiltink J, Michal M, Jünger C, Münzel T, Wild PS, Lackner KJ, et al. Associations between degree and sub-dimensions of depression and metabolic syndrome (MetS) in the community: Results from the Gutenberg Health Study (GHS). BMC Psychiatry 2018;18(1):1–10.

[6] Mattei G, Padula MS, Rioli G, Arginelli L, Bursi R, Bursi S, et al. Metabolic syndrome, anxiety and depression in a sample of Italian primary care patients. J Nerv Ment Dis 2018; 206(5):316-24.

[7] Capuron L, Lasselin J, Castanon N. Role of Adiposity-Driven Inflammation in Depressive Morbidity. Neuropsychopharmacology 2017;42(1):115–28.

[8] Luppino FS, van Reedt Dortland AK, Wardenaar KJ, et al. Symptom dimensions of depression and anxiety and the metabolic syndrome. Psychosom Med 2011;73(3):257–64.

[9] Ellouze F, Damak R, El Karoui M, et al. Depression in Tunisian type 2 diabetic patients: prevalence and association to glycemic control and to treatment compliance. Tunis Med 2017;95(3):210–14.

[10] Spitzer RL, Kroenke K, Williams JBW, Löwe B. A brief measure for assessing generalized anxiety disorder: The GAD-7. Arch Intern Med 2006;166(10):1092–7.

[11] Kroenke K, Spitzer RL, Williams JB. The PHQ-9: validity of a brief depression severity measure. J Gen Intern Med 2001;16(9):606–13.

[12] International Labor Organization. Resolution concerning updating the International Standard Classification of Occupations. International Standard Classification of Occupations, 2008 (ISCO-08). URL: https://www.stat.si/skp/Docs/resol08.pdf.

[13] Grundy SM, Cleeman JI, Daniels SR, Donato KA, Eckel RH, Franklin BA, et al. Diagnosis and management of the metabolic syndrome: An American Heart Association/National Heart, Lung, and Blood Institute scientific statement. Circulation 2005;112(17):2735–52.

[14] Kahl KG, Schweiger U, Correll C, Müller C, Busch ML, Bauer M, et al. Depression, anxiety disorders, and metabolic syndrome in a population at risk for type 2 diabetes mellitus. Brain Behav 2015;5(3):7.

[15] Carroll D, Phillips AC, Thomas GN, Gale CR, Deary I, Batty GD. Generalized anxiety disorder is associated with metabolic syndrome in the Vietnam Experience Study. Biol Psychiatry 2009;66(1):91–3.

[16] Glaus J, Vandeleur C, Gholam-Rezaee M, Castelao E, Perrin M, Rothen S, et al. Atypical depression and alcohol misuse are related to the cardiovascular risk in the general population. Acta Psychiatr Scand 2013;128(4):282-93.

[17] Herva A, Räsänen P, Miettunen J, Timonen M, Läksy K, Veijola J, et al. Co-occurrence of metabolic syndrome with depression and anxiety in young adults: the Northern Finland 1966 birth cohort study. Psychosom Med 2006;8(2):213-6.

[18] García-toro M, Vicens-pons E, Gili M, Roca M, Serrano-ripoll MJ, Vives M, et al. Obesity, metabolic syndrome and Mediterranean diet: Impact on depression outcome. J Affect Disord 2016;194:105–8.

[19] Spielberger CD, Gorsuch RL, Lushene R, Vagg PR, Jacobs GA. Manual for the State Trait Anxiety Inventory (Form Y). Palo Alto, CA: Consulting Psychologists Press, 1983.

[20] Zigmond AS, Snaith RP. The hospital anxiety and depression scale. Acta Psychiatrica Scandinavica 1983;67(6):361-70.

[21] Prina AM, Ferri CP, Guerra M, Brayne C, Prince M. Prevalence of anxiety and its correlates among older adults in Latin America, India and China: cross-cultural study. Br J Psychiatry 2011;199(6): 485–91.

[22] Alvarado BE, Zunzunegui MV, Beland F, Sicotte M, Tellechea L. Social and gender inequalities in depressive symptoms among urban older adults of Latin America and the Caribbean. Gerontol Ser B Psychol Sci Soc Sci 2007;62(4):S226–36.

[23] Lambert E, Dawood T, Straznicky N, Sari C, Schlaich M, Esler M, et al. Association between the sympathetic firing pattern and anxiety level in patients with the metabolic syndrome and elevated blood pressure. J Hypertens 2010; 28(3), 543-50.

[24] Löwe B, Decker O, Müller S, Brähler E, Schellberg D, Herzog W, et al. Validation and standardization of the Generalized Anxiety Disorder Screener (GAD-7) in the general population. Med Care 2008;46(3):266–74.

[25] Ann R, Zhang L, Lix LM, Gra LA, Walker JR, Fisk JD, et al. The validity and reliability of screening measures for depression and anxiety disorders in multiple sclerosis. Mult Scler Relat Disord 2018;20;9-15.

In: Public Health Themes in Grenada … ISBN: 978-1-53618-118-0
Editors: J. Merrick and L. Glasgow

Chapter 15

PREVALENCE OF METABOLIC SYNDROME AND OBESITY AMONG ADULTS IN ARUBA

Prakash VAK Ramdass*, MD, MPH, Taisha Ford, BSc, Rita Alexander, AS, Tanveer Sidhu, BSc, Chigozie F Ogbonnia, MSc and Angela Gomez, PhD
Department of Public Health and Preventive Medicine,
St George's University School of Medicine, St George's, Grenada

ABSTRACT

According to global data, the estimated prevalence of metabolic syndrome (MetS) in adults ranges from 11.9% in the Philippines to 43.3% in Puerto Rico. This study investigated the prevalence of MetS and obesity in Aruba. We hypothesized that there would be a relatively high prevalence of MetS and obesity in Aruba. We conducted a cross-sectional study in 2016. Data were collected on adults between the ages of 18 and 91 years during a Free Health Fair. Data collection methods included taking anthropometric measurements, blood pressure, and fasting blood glucose from the

---

* Correspondence: Dr. Prakash VAK Ramdass, Associate Professor of Clinical Epidemiology, St George's University School of Medicine, Department of Public Health and Preventive Medicine, St. George's, Grenada, West Indies. Email: prakash.ramdass@gmail.com.

participants. Descriptive statistics were computed for socio-demographic variables, clinical characteristics, and the prevalence of MetS and obesity. The independent samples *t*-test was used to compare continuous variables, and the χ^2 test was used to compare proportions between groups. The overall prevalence rate of MetS in our sample was 21.5%, with men (24.4%) having a slightly higher prevalence rate than women (19.4%). Notably, 40.9% of the participants had pre-obesity (BMI: 25–29.9) and 32.6% were obese (BMI ≥30), giving rise to 73.5% of the sample having a BMI ≥25. Our results have shown that metabolic syndrome and obesity are highly prevalent among adults in Aruba. Preventive measures should be taken to curtail these chronic conditions. In addition, patients with a body mass index higher than 25 should be screened for metabolic syndrome.

INTRODUCTION

Metabolic syndrome (MetS) is defined as a cluster of metabolic disorders with features of visceral obesity, elevated blood pressure, hyperglycemia/ insulin resistance, and atherogenic dyslipidemia (elevated triglycerides and decreased high density lipoprotein cholesterol levels (1). According to global data, the estimated prevalence of metabolic syndrome in adults ranges from 11.9% in the Philippines (2) to 43.3% in Puerto Rico (3).

In the United States (US) the prevalence of MetS in adults has substantially increased in the past decade, averaging approximately 34% between 2007–2012 (4). In the Caribbean region, the prevalence is estimated to be 21.1% in Jamaican adults (5) and 20.5% in adults of Saint Croix, US Virgin Islands (6). To date, there is no published data on the prevalence of MetS in Aruba. However, recent studies on the prevalence rates for MetS in cities in nearby countries were reported as 34.8% in Bucaramanga, Colombia (7), and 35.3% in Zulia, Venezuela (8). The prevalence rates reported above were based on the definition of MetS according to the National Cholesterol Education Program's Adult Treatment Panel III criteria (NCEP ATP III) (9), one of several definitions of MetS.

MetS has become a significant worldwide problem and it is associated with increased risk of cardiovascular disorders and all-cause mortality (10, 11) type 2 diabetes mellitus (12) and the most common types of cancers (13). Risk factors for developing MetS include obesity, visceral adiposity (14), and insulin resistance (15). With the increasing pandemic of obesity (16), there is a parallel increase in MetS (17).

The primary aim of this study is to determine the prevalence of MetS and obesity in Aruba. We hypothesized that there will be a high prevalence of MetS and obesity in the country.

OUR STUDY

We conducted a cross-sectional study during a one-day free health fair in Oranjestad, Aruba, in November 2016. The main purpose of this study was to assess the prevalence of metabolic syndrome and obesity among adults in Aruba.

Assessment of metabolic syndrome

We used the harmonized clinical criteria (1) to define metabolic syndrome, which requires that at least three of the following five criteria have to be met: fasting plasma glucose (≥100 mg/dL and or diabetes medication), triglycerides (≥150 mg/dL and or drug treatment for elevated triglycerides), HDL cholesterol (<40 mg/dL in males and <50 mg/dL in females and or drug treatment for reducing HDL cholesterol), blood pressure (systolic ≥130 mm Hg and or diastolic ≥85 mm Hg and or use of antihypertensive medication), and waist circumference (ethnicity and country-specific cut-off; we used the International Diabetes Federation (18) cut-offs for Europid: 94 cm for men and 80 cm for women). Patients who had abnormal laboratory results were contacted by the laboratory and were recommended to visit their health care provider.

Study population and setting

The health fair was publicized on local radio and television, and on flyers at popular supermarkets four weeks before the event. The health fair was held at Xavier University School of Medicine from 7 AM to 11 AM. The study was approved by the institutional review board of Xavier University School of Medicine, Aruba, and all participants provided written informed consent.

Adults who attended the health fair were eligible to participate in the study. A structured questionnaire was used to collect data on age, sex, race, occupation, education, marital status, and self-rated health of the participants. Other questions included diagnosis of diabetes, hypertension, and hypercholesterolemia, family history of known metabolic syndrome in at least one first-degree relative (father, mother, or sibling). Interviews were conducted in English, Papiamento, and Spanish.

Measurements and biochemical analyses

The three criteria used for the assessment according to the harmonized clinical criteria (1) were: measurement of waist circumference, measurement of blood pressure, and blood samples.

Waist circumference was measured with a soft tape, on standing subjects, at the level of the umbilicus. Bodyweight and height were measured with subjects in light clothing and without shoes. Body mass index (BMI) was calculated as the weight in kilograms divided by the height in meters squared (kg/m^2) and grouped according to the World Health Organization (WHO) international classification (19).

Blood pressure was measured on the right arm using a manual mercury sphygmomanometer after the subject had rested for 10 minutes. Systolic and diastolic blood pressures were recorded as the first and last Korotkoff sounds, respectively.

Venous blood samples were taken from the antecubital vein after overnight fast, and serum total cholesterol was measured by standard enzymatic assays within four hours of collection. Blood glucose level was measured using a glucometer (ACCU-CHEK® Active strips in Accu-Chek® Active test meter, Roche Diagnostics, Germany).

Statistical analyses

Due to a small sample size, race was grouped into Hispanic and Other (which included Caucasians, people of African ancestry, mixed-race, and other races).

Occupation was based on the International Standard for Classification of Occupations (ISCO-08) (20) and was grouped as professionals, skilled workers, unemployed, and retired. Professionals included groups 1-4 of ISCO-08 (managers; professionals; technicians and associate professionals; and clerical support workers) and skilled workers included groups 5-9 of ISCO-08 (service and sales workers; skilled agricultural, forestry and fishery workers; craft and related trades workers; plant and machine operators, and assemblers; and elementary occupations).

Descriptive statistics (mean ± standard deviation [SD] or percentages) were computed for socio-demographic variables, clinical characteristics, and the prevalence of MetS and obesity. We used the independent samples *t*-test to compare continuous variables and the $\chi 2$ test to compare proportions between groups. All variables were reported as statistically significant at the 0.05 significance level. Analyses were performed using SPSS version 24 (IBM Corp, Armonk, NY, US).

FINDINGS

Detailed demographic and clinical characteristics are summarized in Table 1. A total of 181 participants were evaluated, in which there were 78 (43.1%) men and 103 (56.9%) women. There was a statistically significant difference between men and women regarding occupation ($p < 0.001$), exercise ($p = 0.019$), and alcohol consumption ($p = 0.01$). There was also a significant difference (p = 0.01) in waist circumference for men (100.1 cm [SD ± 17.8]) compared to women (93.8 cm [SD ± 14.4]).

Table 1. Demographic characteristics of the study participants (N = 181)

Variables	Men	Women	Values
Age, years, mean (SD)	55.7 (18.3)	50.8 (19.2)	0.086
Race, n (%)			0.150
Hispanic	32 (34.4)	61 (65.6)	
Other	46 (52.3)	42 (47.7)	
Occupation, n (%)			< 0.001
Professional	21 (42.0)	29 (58.0)	
Skilled	26 (53.1)	23 (46.9)	
Unemployed	6 (14.6)	35 (85.4)	
Retired	25 (61.0)	16 (39.0)	
Education, n (%)			0.609
High school	45 (47.4)	50 (52.6)	
Undergraduate	14 (36.8)	24 (63.2)	
Graduate	10 (43.5)	13 (56.5)	
Other	9 (36.0)	16 (64.0)	
Diabetes, n (%)			0.293
Yes	16 (51.6)	15 (48.4)	
No	62 (41.3)	88 (58.7)	
Hypertension, n (%)			0.390
Yes	53 (41.1)	76 (58.9)	
No	25 (48.1)	27 (51.9)	
Hypercholesterolemia, n (%)			0.173
Yes	21 (52.5)	19 (47.5)	
No	57 (40.4)	84 (59.6)	
Exercise, n (%)			0.019
No regular exercise	26 (43.3)	34 (56.7)	
1-2 hours/week	16 (29.1)	39 (70.9)	
>2 hours/week	36 (54.5)	30 (45.5)	
Alcohol consumption, n (%)			0.010
Never	33 (32.7)	68 (67.3)	
Current	45 (56.3)	35 (43.8)	
Smoking, n (%)			0.729
Never	70 (42.7)	94 (57.3)	
Current	8 (47.1)	9 (52.9)	
Variables	Men	Women	Values

Family history of obesity, n (%)			0.845
Yes	23 (44.2)	29 (55.8)	
No	55 (42.6)	74 (57.4)	
Metabolic syndrome, n (%)			0.423
Yes	19 (48.7)	20 (51.3)	
No	59 (41.5)	83 (58.5)	
Body mass index, kg/m^2	28.8 (5.2)	28.0 (5.7)	0.350
Body mass index, kg/m^2, n (%)			0.266
18 – 24	20 (41.7)	28 (58.3)	
25 – 29	29 (39.2)	45 (60.8)	
30 – 34	17 (50.0)	17 (50.0)	
35 – 39	10 (62.5)	6 (37.5)	
> 40	2 (22.2)	7 (77.8)	
Waist circumference, cm	100.1 (17.8)	93.8 (14.4)	0.010
Waist-hip-ratio	0.982 (0.152)	0.998 (0.724)	0.866
FBG	106.9 (62.2)	98.7 (30.4)	0.273
Blood pressure, mmHg			
Systolic	129.0 (9.8)	125.5 (14.6	0.098
Diastolic	81.3 (9.9)	80.6 (9.7)	0.641

The overall prevalence rate of MetS in our sample was 21.5%, with men (24.4%) having a slightly higher prevalence rate than women (19.4%). Notably, 40.9% of the participants had pre-obesity (BMI 25–29.9) and 32.6% were obese (BMI ≥ 30), giving rise to 73.5% of the sample having a higher than normal body mass index (BMI ≥ 25).

The prevalence of MetS in the different BMI categories according to WHO's classification (19) are presented in Table 2. Our data showed that there was a statistical difference in the prevalence rates of MetS among the different BMI categories regarding age ($p < 0.001$), occupation ($p = 0.008$), and the presence of diabetes ($p < 0.001$) and hypertension ($p < 0.001$).

Figure 1 shows that the prevalence of MetS is higher for both men and women who have a BMI greater than 25. However, even though there is no linear trend with prevalence of MetS and increasing BMI levels, there is an increased prevalence of MetS with increased severity of obesity for men. This pattern was not observed for women. Interestingly though, half of the men and half of the women with moderate obesity (BMI 35.0 – 39.9) had

MetS and 100% of the men and 42.9% of the women with severe obesity had MetS.

Table 2. Prevalence of metabolic syndrome according to BMI categories

Variables	Normal Weight	Pre-obesity	Obesity	P values
Sex				0.468
Men	5.0	31.0	31.0	
Women	3.6	15.6	40.0	
Age				
18 – 30	5.6	0.0	0.0	< 0.001
31 – 50	0.0	5.0	8.3	
51 – 70	7.7	30.8	36.7	
>70	0.0	36.8	75.0	
Race				1.000
Hispanic	6.9	20.0	41.7	
Other	0.0	23.5	31.4	
Education				0.066
High school	4.5	25.0	36.4	
Undergraduate	0.0	5.9	28.6	
Graduate	0.0	12.5	25.0	
Other	12.5	44.4	50.0	
Occupation				0.008
Professional	0.0	19.0	33.3	
Skilled	0.0	0.0	35.3	
Unemployed	14.3	23.5	10.0	
Retired	0.0	50.0	52.9	
Diabetes				< 0.001
Yes	20.0	41.7	85.7	
No	2.3	17.7	20.0	
Hypertension				< 0.001
Yes	16.7	21.1	66.7	
No	2.4	21.8	9.4	
Hypercholesterolemia				0.190
Yes	0.0	18.8	45.0	
No	4.5	22.4	30.8	
Exercise				0.766
No regular exercise	7.1	22.2	42.1	
1 - 2 hours/ week	0.0	24.0	27.8	
> 2 hours/ week	4.5	18.2	36.4	

Variables	Normal Weight	Pre-obesity	Obesity	P values
Smoking				0.764
Never	2.4	19.7	36.8	
Current	14.3	37.5	0.0	
lcohol				0.204
Never	5.9	16.7	32.3	
Current	0.0	26.3	39.3	

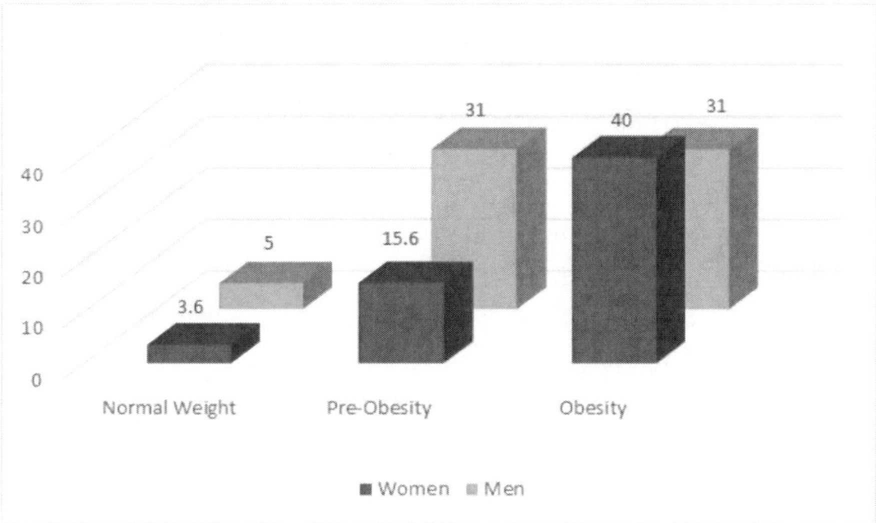

Figure 1. Prevalence of metabolic syndrome in BMI categories.

Discussion

To our knowledge, this is the first study to assess the prevalence rate of metabolic syndrome (MetS) in Aruba. Results from this study confirmed our hypothesis that Aruba has a high prevalence of MetS and obesity among adults. This high prevalence of MetS in Aruba is supported by data from previous studies with similar demographics (21). In addition, findings from our study corroborated with the prevalence rates of obesity from global data, especially those of the United States and countries in Latin America (22). We found that the prevalence of MetS was slightly higher among men. However, among the obese, women had a higher prevalence of MetS. Our results also showed that increasing age was a significant predisposing factor for developing MetS. Individuals over the age of 70 years showed a drastic increase in risk. However, our results differed from a study by Florez et al. (8), which showed that the 50-59 years old age group had the highest proportion of MetS.

The prevalence of MetS was disproportionate among the different occupational groups. Of particular interest, those who were retired and having a BMI greater than 25 were more likely to have MetS. Thus, a sedentary lifestyle may have contributed to having an increased prevalence of both obesity and MetS. However, a study by Browne et al. (23) showed that those who have a sedentary occupation but have met the requirements for physical activity have a reduced risk of developing MetS. However, on closer examination, we did not find a significant association between occupation and exercise.

Our results clearly show that the prevalence of MetS was independently associated with pre-obesity and obesity, hypertension, and diabetes. Thus, these findings suggest the importance of screening patients with diabetes, hypertension, and BMI greater than 25 for metabolic syndrome. Ärnlöv et al. showed that insulin resistance, higher BMI levels, and MetS had higher incidence rates of cardiovascular events (24).

The following methodological considerations have to be taken into account when interpreting our findings: firstly, the sampling approach was self-selection and, therefore, may not be representative of the entire population. Thus, the prevalence rate obtained in our study may not reflect the true prevalence rate for MetS in Aruba. However, our study may have underestimated the actual prevalence of MetS in Aruba because of the following reasons: we used the International Diabetes Federation cut-offs of waist circumference for Europid: 94 cm for men, instead of 90 cm, which is the suggested value for Ethnic Central and South American. Our sample comprised of 17.8% Hispanic men. In addition, biological measurements were obtained for fasting total cholesterol only, and not for triglycerides or HDL cholesterol levels. Thus, these criteria were not assessed in our diagnosis of MetS. Moreover, a study by Tull et al. (6) showed that Hispanic ethnicity was associated with an increased risk of MetS, high triglycerides, and low HDL-C. Secondly, our sample size was relatively small and may not have adequate statistical power.

We recommend that a population-based study with a larger sample size should be conducted to confirm our findings and to determine the country-wide prevalence of MetS in Aruba. The 51-70 years and >70 years age categories reported the highest level of MetS. In addition, those who were retired, had diabetes, and hypertension were at increased risk of MetS. Therefore, we suggest that people with these demographics should be screened for MetS. We also recommend having more health fairs and health-outreach programs for the people of Aruba. One of the benefits of health fairs is the increased likelihood of screening for chronic conditions, such as MetS, in individuals who may not otherwise get tested, due to their occupation or socioeconomic status.

CONCLUSION

In conclusion, our results have shown that metabolic syndrome and obesity are highly prevalent in the Aruban adult population. Preventive measures should be taken to curb these chronic and debilitating conditions. In addition, patients with a body mass index higher than 25 should be screened for metabolic syndrome.

ACKNOWLEDGMENTS

We would like to sincerely thank the following persons for their valuable contributions to data collection and data entry: Srishti Arya, Junea N Chowdhury, Biruk Gote, Jonathan Rebibo, Saud Qureshi, Joseph Sarra, and Devina Chintaman.

References

[1] Alberti KGMM, Eckel RH, Grundy SM, Zimmet PZ, Cleeman JI, Donato KA, et al. Harmonizing the metabolic syndrome: A joint interim statement of the International Diabetes Federation Task Force on Epidemiology and Prevention; National Heart, Lung, and Blood Institute; American Heart Association; World Heart Federation; International Atherosclerosis Society; and International Association for the Study of Obesity. Circulation 2009;120(16):1640-5.

[2] Morales DD, Punzalan FER, Paz-pacheco E, Sy RG, Duante CA. Metabolic syndrome in the Philippine general population: Prevalence and risk for atherosclerotic cardiovascular disease and diabetes mellitus. Diab Vasc Dis Res 2008;5(1): 6–43.

[3] Pérez CM, Guzmán M, Ortiz AP, Estrella M, Valle Y, Pérez N, et al. Prevalence of the metabolic syndrome in San Juan, Puerto Rico. Ethn Dis 2008;18(4):434–41.

[4] Xavier Moore J, Chaudhary N, Akinyemiju T. Metabolic syndrome prevalence by race/ethnicity and sex in the United States, National Health and Nutrition Examination Survey, 1988-2012. Natl Health Nutr Exam Surv Prev Chronic Dis 2017;14:1–16.

[5] Ferguson TS, Younger N, Tulloch-reid MK, Forrester TE, Cooper RS, Broeck J Van Den, et al. Prevalence of the metabolic syndrome in Jamaican adults and its relationship to income and education levels. West Indian Med J 2010;59(3):265-73.

[6] Tull ES, Thurland A, Laporte RE. Metabolic syndrome among Caribbean-born persons living in the US Virgin Islands. Rev Panam Salud Publica 2005;18(6): 418-26.

[7] Pinzón JB, Serrano NC, Díaz LA, Mantilla G, Velasco HM, Martínez LX, et al. [Impacto de las nuevas definiciones en la prevalencia del síndrome metabólico en una población adulta de Bucaramanga, Columbia]. Biomedica 2007;27(2):172–9. [Spanish].

[8] Florez H, Silva E, Fernanddez V, Ryder E, Sulbaran T, Campos G, et al. Prevalence and risk factors associated with the metabolic syndrome and dyslipidemia in white, black, Amerindian and mixed Hispanics in Zulia State, Venezuela. Diabetes Res Clin Pract 2005;69(1):63–77.

[9] INCEP-ATPIII. Executive Summary of the Third Report (NCEP) Expert Panel on Detection, Evaluation, and Treatment of High Blood Cholesterol in Adults (Adult Treatment Panel III). JAMA 2001;285(19):2486–97.

[10] Kastorini CM, Panagiotakos DB, Georgousopoulou EN, Laskaris A, Skourlis N, Zana A, Chrysohoou C, et al. Metabolic syndrome and 10-year cardiovascular disease incidence: The ATTICA Study. Nutr Metab Cardiovasc Dis 2016;26(3): 223-31.

[11] Liu L, Miura K, Fujiyoshi A, Kadota A, Miyagawa N, Nakamura Y, et al. Impact of metabolic syndrome on the risk of cardiovascular disease mortality in the United States and in Japan. Am J Cardiol 2014;113(1):84–9.

[12] Meigs JB, Wilson PWF, Fox CS, Vasan RS, Nathan DM, Sullivan LM, et al. Body mass index, metabolic syndrome, and risk of Type 2 diabetes or cardiovascular disease. J Clin Endocrinol Metab 2006;91(8):2906–12.

[13] Esposito K, Chiodini P, Colao A, Lenzi A, Giugliano D. Metabolic syndrome and risk of cancer: A systematic review and meta-analysis. Diabetes Care 2012;35(11):2402–11.

[14] Shah RV, Murthy VL, Abbasi SA, Blankstein R, Kwong RY, Goldfine AB, et al. Visceral adiposity and the risk of metabolic syndrome across body mass index: The MESA study. JACC Cardiovasc Imaging 2014;7(12):1221–35.

[15] McKeown NM, Meigs JB, Liu S, Saltzman E, Wilson PW, Kacques PF. Carbohydrate nutrition, insulin resistance, and the prevalence of the metabolic syndrome in the Framingham Offspring Cohort. Diabetes Care 2004;27(2):538-46.

[16] NCD Risk Factor Collaboration (NCD-RisC). Trends in adult body-mass index in 200 countries from 1975 to 2014: A pooled analysis of 1698 population-based measurement studies with 19•2 million participants. Lancet 2016;387(10026): 1377–96.

[17] Ansarimoghaddam A, Adineh HA, Zareban I, Iranpour S, HosseinZadeh A, Kh F. Prevalence of metabolic syndrome in Middle-East countries: Meta-analysis of cross-sectional studies. Diabetes Metab Syndr 2017;12(2):195-201.

[18] Grundy SM, Cleeman JI, Daniels SR, Donato KA, Eckel RH, Franklin BA, et al. Diagnosis and management of the metabolic syndrome: An American Heart Association/National Heart, Lung, and Blood Institute scientific statement. Circulation 2005;112(17):2735–52.

[19] Body mass index - BMI. URL: http://www.euro.who.int/en/health-topics/disease-prevention/nutrition/a-healthy-lifestyle/body-mass-index-bmi.

[20] ISCO. Resolution concerning updating the International Standard Classification of Occupations. Geneva: ISCO, 2010:1–34.

[21] Márquez-Sandoval F, Macedo-Ojeda G, Viramontes-Hörner D, Fernández Ballart JD, Salas Salvadó J, Vizmanos B. The prevalence of metabolic syndrome in Latin America: A systematic review. Public Health Nutr 2011;14(10):1702–13.

[22] Blüher M. Obesity: Global epidemiology and pathogenesis. Nat Rev Endocrinol 2019;15(5): 288–98.

[23] Browne RAV, Farias-Junior LF, Freire YA, Schwade D, Macedo GAD, Montenegro VB, et al. Sedentary occupation workers who meet the physical activity recommendations have a reduced risk for metabolic syndrome: A cross-sectional study. J Occup Environ Med 2017;59(11):1029-33.

[24] Arnlöv J, Ingelsson E, Sundström J, Lind L. Impact of body mass index and the metabolic syndrome on the risk of cardiovascular disease and death in middle-aged men. Circulation 2010;121(2):230-6.

In: Public Health Themes in Grenada ... ISBN: 978-1-53618-118-0
Editors: J. Merrick and L. Glasgow

Chapter 16

OVERWEIGHT AND OBESITY AMONG GRENADIAN ADOLESCENTS

Richard Scribner[1,*], MD, MPH, Roger Radix[1], MD, MPH, Trevor Noel[1], PhD MPH, Rebecca Andal[1], MD, Naomi Andal[1], MD, Christal Radix[1], BSc, Rhoda Frank[1], MBA, Jonell Benjamin[1], MPH, Jennifer James[1], MPH, Romero Benjamin[1], BSc, Claudia Leonardi[2], PhDH and Melinda Sothern[2], PhD

[1]Windward Island Research and Education Foundation, St Georges, Grenada, West Indies
[2]Louisiana State University School of Public Health, New Orleans, United States of America

---

[*] Correspondence: Richard Scribner, Professor, Department of Public Health and Preventive Medicine, St. Georges University, Grenada WI. Email: rscribne@sgu.edu.

Abstract

In this chapter, we examine the prevalence of overweight and obesity among a representative sample of Grenadian adolescents. Recent studies have been equivocal on the degree to which the obesity epidemic has affected Grenada with high rates of overweight and obesity among Grenadian adults. A nationally representative sample of first-year students (i.e., Form 1) (n = 689) aged 11 to 14 years old from the twenty-three secondary schools in Grenada was assessed as part of the Grenada School Nutrition Study (GSNS). Height and weight were objectively assessed using standard measures. Standardized BMI percentile (BMIz score) was calculated using the Centers for Disease Control and Prevention (CDC) criteria. BMIz scores above the 85th percentile were classified as overweight and BMIz scores above the 95th percentile were classified as obese. Overall Grenadian adolescents have low rates of overweight (17.6%) and obesity (7.6%). Girls had nearly twice the rates of overweight compared to boys (i.e., 22.7% versus 12.2%) but similar rates of obesity (i.e., 8.2% versus 6.8%). Grenadian adolescents demonstrate low rates of obesity compared to both Grenadian adults and their US counterparts. This discrepancy in overweight and obesity between Grenadian adults and adolescents suggest Grenada is undergoing an epidemiologic transition with regard to the obesity epidemic.

Introduction

The two overarching goals of the Healthy People 2010 initiative are to 1) increase quality and years of healthy life and 2) eliminate health disparities. The rising prevalence of overweight and obesity (OW/OB) represents the primary threat to the achievement of these goals in the coming years (1-4). Despite the growing awareness of the negative health impact of poor diet, physical inactivity, and excess weight, the prevalence of OW/OB has continued to increase in the United States (US) (2, 5). During the last three decades, according to national surveys (i.e., NHANES), the US obesity rate has doubled in adults and tripled in children and adolescents and is leading to growing disparities in obesity risk among poor and minority populations (6-9). The consensus among public health experts is that human genetic changes are not responsible for the rapid rise in obesity, and the explanation must lie in broad social determinants resulting in local environmental exposures that influence diet and physical activity (10-13).

Despite researchers having literally watched the epidemic of obesity unfold over the past three decades, not only in the US but across the globe, identification of the "drivers" of the epidemic remains contentious (14-16). The effort to characterize the "drivers" of the epidemic involves the identification of the factors responsible for upsetting the balance in the "energy intake/energy expenditure" equation over the past four decades. On the energy intake side, the global food system that provides a "Westernized" diet of cheap, palatable, energy dense-foods is implicated (14, 16, 17). On the expenditure side, the transition to sedentary occupations with low energy expenditure is implicated (18, 19). The inability to arrive at a consensus is attributed to the lack of research with designs sufficient to link local obesogenic environments - created by the societal drivers - with individual obesity-related behaviors (20-22).

The chance for characterizing the factors that "drove" the epidemic in the US over the past decades is gone. Even retrospective studies of dietary trends raise more questions than they answer, and they do not get at the role of obesogenic environments (23). Consequently, research on the drivers of the pandemic of obesity requires a study among a population that has not yet undergone the epidemiologic transition. According to the World Health Organization's (WHO) "Burden of disease" (GBD) approach, it is projected that non-communicable diseases (NCDs) will represent the greatest disease burden in low- and middle-income countries (LMIC) by 2030 (24, 25). The onset of NCDs, including cardiovascular disease, diabetes, and cancer represents an epidemiologic transition that is attributed to the emergence of local obesogenic environments (26-28). In addition, the epidemiologic transition in LMIC is believed to be occurring at a much faster rate due to the globalization of the corporate food infrastructure.

The current study was organized to determine the degree to which the epidemiologic transition with regard to obesity has affected Grenadian adolescents. A recent study by the CDC indicated the obesity epidemic has already impacted Grenadian adults. Consequently, it could be assumed that Grenadian adolescents were already also affected by the epidemic.

OUR STUDY

The current study is part of a project titled the Grenada School Nutrition Study (GSNS). The GSNS goal is to identify behavioral and environmental factors that might be intervened on to prevent the development of obesity among Grenadian adolescents.

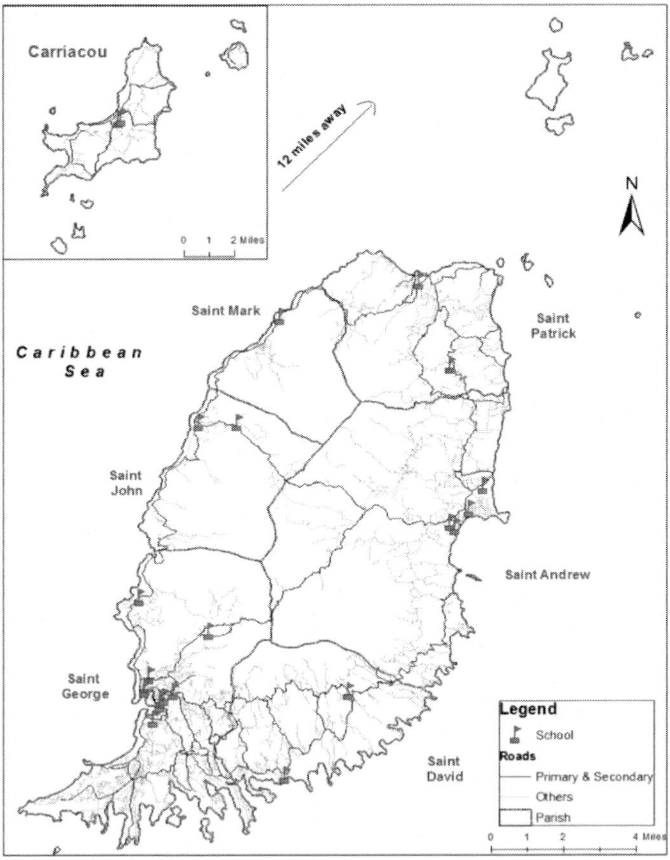

Figure 1. Map of Grenada demonstrating location of the 23 GNS schools.

Study sample

The GSNS was designed to be a representative sample of all first-year secondary students (i.e., Form 1) drawn from the 23 public and private secondary schools across the tri-island nation of Grenada. Form 1 students range in age from 11 to 14 years. Randomization was performed at the classroom level resulting in an eligible sample of 1,004 students in 35 classrooms (i.e., in schools with only one Form 1 class all students were included) making up roughly 55% of all Form 1 students in Grenada. Parental refusals (n= 276) and students who were absent on the day or did not complete all the assessments or surveys (n=39) resulted in an effective sample of 689 students in the cohort. All students were assigned a unique identifier linked to their informed consent signed by their parents. Personal identifiers in the form of parents' names, phone numbers, and school identification were collected for possible followup.

Study measures

Height, weight, and waist circumference were directly measured for each student in a privatized setting (e.g., trifold blind booth) in normal school clothing. Measurements using a portable stadiometer and electronic scale standardized before each session were repeated three times, and the average score reported.

Body mass index (BMI), calculated by dividing weight in kilograms by their height in meters squared, was used to assess excess body fat. Due to the greater sensitivity of the CDC classification system compared with the International Obesity Task Force (IOTF) classification system for characterizing excess body fat in a Caribbean adolescent population, the CDC age- and sex-specific cutoffs were used to characterize overweight (i.e., BMI≥85th percentile) and obese (i.e., BMI≥95th percentile) adolescents in terms of their standardized percentile (29).

Rural and urban designations were defined at the school level. Students attending school in the two largest towns in Grenada (i.e., St Georges and Grenville) were defined as urban students.

Statistical analysis

Multilevel models of students nested within schools were developed to characterize the overall and between school prevalence of overweight and obesity across Grenada. For this descriptive analysis, demographic measures including age, and gender were included in the analyses.

The basic multilevel models used a random coefficient for the intercept. Thus, at student level, we have the following model,

$$Y_{ij} = \pi_{0j} + \pi_1(\text{Gender})_{1ij} + \pi_2(\text{Age})_{2ij} + \varepsilon_{ij} \qquad \text{Level 1}$$

where Y_{ij} is the outcome (e.g., obesity related behavior measurements or BMI z-score) for student *i* in school *j*. π_{0j} is the intercept, which we allowed to randomly vary across schools, which also is the estimated mean response for school j. We assume fixed effects for a vector of student level risk factors. ε_{ij} is the random effect of student *i* in school *j,* which is assumed to have normal distribution mean 0 and constant variance σ^2 for i = 1,.....,n_j and j=1,......,23.

Table 1. BMIz scores for Grenadian adolescents by gender in the GSNS

	BMIz ≥ 95th	**BMIz ≥ 85th**
All	7.4%	16.6%
Male	6.8%	**12.2%**
Female	8.1%	**21.4%**

Note: Bolded prevalences are significantly different at $p < 0.05$.

The intercept π_{0j}, is allowed to randomly vary across all schools. Therefore, at the school level, we have the following model:

$$\pi_{0j} = \beta_{00} + u_{0j} \qquad \text{Level 2 (random intercept)}$$

FINDINGS

The overall rate of overweight and obesity among Grenadian adolescents in the first year of secondary schools was 16.6% and obesity 7.4%, respectively (see Table 1). There was significant sexual dimorphism in the rate of overweight Grenadians with females at greater risk than males (i.e., 21.4% versus 12.2%). The differences in obesity were not significantly different.

Table 2. Descriptive statistics for adolescents in GSNS schools by rural and urban areas

	N	Overall	Rural (N=283)	Urban (N=406)
Demographics				
Age, years	689	12.67	12.81	12.57
Race-Afro Caribbean, %	689	83.31	**89.05**	**79.31**
Gender, male%	689	48.91	**55.83**	**44.09**
Outcomes				
BMIz > 85th, %	689	17.56	**13.43**	**20.44**

Note: Bolded prevalences are significantly different at $p < 0.05$.

With regard to the difference in rates of OW/OB between adolescents attending rural versus urban schools there appeared to be significant differences in obesity rates such that urban students evidenced significantly higher rates of OW/OB compared with rural students (20.44% versus 13.43%) (see Table 2).

An empty multilevel model (i.e., Model 1, see Table 3) with obesity risk as the outcome yielded an intraclass correlation coefficient of 0.037, indicating that 3.73% of the variance in obesity rates was between schools. Adding age and gender into the model explained most of the school level effect (see Table 3, Model 2). Adding whether or not the school was in an urban or rural area did not significantly predict obesity risk and only explained a small amount of the school level effect (see Table 3, Model 3). Finally, including age and gender in the model explained most of the urban-rural effect suggesting the greater risk of obesity in urban schools was primarily due to the greater number of female students, who are at higher risk for obesity, in urban schools.

Table 3. Parameters estimates from multilevel models predicting obesity risk among 689 students nested within 23 schools

	Model 1	Model 2	Model 3	Model 4
Individual level Measures				
Age		**-0.1234**		**-0.1142**
Male		**-0.3229**		**-0.3159**
School level Measures				
Urban School			0.1861	0.1168
Random Effects				
School level effect u_{0j}	0.0511	0.0208	0.0475	0.0212
Individual level effect r_{ij}	1.3241	1.3116	1.3237	1.3112
Fit Statistics				
AIC	2172.2	2162.5	2172.5	2164.4

Note: Bolded coefficients are significantly different from 0 at $p < 0.05$.

DISCUSSION

The results document a low risk of overweight (i.e., 16.6%) and obesity among Grenadian adolescents despite significant sexual dimorphism in the rate of overweight Grenadian adolescents. Female adolescents have far greater risk of obesity compared to their male counterparts. Furthermore, it appears that the greater risk of obesity among the urban students is primarily due to the greater presence of female students in urban schools.

Since the study used the same growth curve cutoffs and procedures used for US adolescents in the NHANES, these rates of OW/OB can be compared with US adolescents. US black female and male adolescents of the same age had three (26.1% versus 8.1%) and four (25.4% versus 6.8%) times the rates of obesity (i.e., BMIz > 95th percentile) compared to their Grenadian counterparts, respectively (30). With regard to overweight (i.e., BMIz > 85th percentile), US females and male adolescents had two (44.7% versus 21.4%) and three (38.8% versus 12.2%) times the rates compared with their Grenadian counterparts, respectively.

These findings are significant in that they seem to contradict a recent study by the CDC indicating the obesity epidemic has already impacted Grenadian adults. In the CDC study, Block and colleagues (31) found that among Grenadian adults, 42% of women and 17% of men were obese, and across all adult age groups the rate of OW/OB reached as high as 72%. These findings suggest that adolescents in Grenada will undergo a dramatic transition in their rates of OW/OB, such that prevalence among the current female adolescent group has the potential to rise from a current rate of OW/OB of 21% to nearly 72% as they transition to adulthood.

ACKNOWLEDGMENT

The project, titled the Grenada school Nutrition Study (GNS), is funded by the International Research Development Center (IRDC) (Grant #106884).

REFERENCES

[1] Burke JP, Williams KL, Gaskill SP, Hazuda HP, Haffner SM, Stern MP. Rapid rise in the incidence of type 2 diabetes from 1987 to 1996: results from the San Antonio Heart Study. Arch Intern Med 1999;159(13):1450-6.

[2] Kanjilal S, Gregg EW, Cheng YJ, Zhang P, Nelson DE, Mensah G, et al. Socioeconomic status and trends in disparities in 4 major risk factors for cardiovascular disease among US adults, 1971-2002. Arch Intern Med 2006; 166(21):2348-55.

[3] Mensah GA, Mokdad AH, Ford ES, Greenlund KJ, Croft JB. State of disparities in cardiovascular health in the United States. Circulation 2005;111(10):1233-41.

[4] Romero CX, Romero TE, Shlay JC, Ogden LG, Dabelea D. Changing trends in the prevalence and disparities of obesity and other cardiovascular disease risk factors in three racial/ethnic groups of USA adults. Adv Prev Med 2012;2012:172423.

[5] Jeffery RW, Utter J. The changing environment and population obesity in the United States. Obes Res 2003;11(Suppl):12S-22S.

[6] Ogden CL, Carroll MD, Curtin LR, McDowell MA, Tabak CJ, Flegal KM. Prevalence of overweight and obesity in the United States, 1999-2004. JAMA 2006;295(13):1549-55.

[7] Flegal KM, Carroll MD, Ogden CL, Curtin LR. Prevalence and trends in obesity among US adults, 1999-2008. JAMA 2010;303(3):235-41.

[8] Devaux M, Sassi F. Social inequalities in obesity and overweight in 11 OECD countries. Eur J Public Health 2013;23(3):464-9.

[9] Beauchamp A, Backholer K, Magliano D, Peeters A. The effect of obesity prevention interventions according to socioeconomic position: A systematic review. Obes Rev 2014;15(7):541-54.

[10] Kumanyika S, Jeffery R, Morabia A, Kumanyika, Antipatis VJ. Obesity prevention: the case for action. Int J Obes Relat Metab Disord 2002;26(3):425-36.

[11] Hill JO, Wyatt HR, Reed GW, Peters JC. Obesity and the environment: where do we go from here? Science 2003;299(5608):853-5.

[12] Koplan JP, Liverman CT, Kraak VI, Committee on Prevention of Obesity in Children and Youth. Preventing childhood obesity: Health in the balance: executive summary. J Am Diet Assoc 2005;105(1):131-8.

[13] Sallis J F, Glanz K. Physical activity and food environments: solutions to the obesity epidemic. Milbank Q 2009;87(1):123-54.

[14] Swinburn BA, Sacks G, Hall KD, McPherson K, Finegood DF, Moodie ML. The global obesity pandemic: Shaped by global drivers and local environments. Lancet 2011;378(9793):804-14.

[15] Blair SN, Archer E, Hand GA. Commentary: Luke and Cooper are wrong: physical activity has a crucial role in weight management and determinants of obesity. Int J Epidemiol 2013;42(6):1836-8.

[16] Luke A, Cooper RS. Physical activity does not influence obesity risk: time to clarify the public health message. Int J Epidemiol 2013;42(6):1831-6.

[17] Popkin BM, Adair LS, Ng SW. Global nutrition transition and the pandemic of obesity in developing countries. Nutr Rev 2012;70(1):3-21.

[18] Franco M, Orduñez P, Caballero B, Granados JAT, Lazo M, Bernal JL. Impact of energy intake, physical activity, and population-wide weight loss on cardiovascular disease and diabetes mortality in Cuba, 1980-2005. Am J Epidemiol 2007;166(12):1374-80.

[19] Church TS, Thomas DM, Tudor-Locke C, Katzmarzyk T, Earnest CP, Rodarte QR. Trends over 5 decades in US occupation-related physical activity and their associations with obesity. PLoS One 2011;6(5):e19657.

[20] Wang Y, Beydoun MA. The obesity epidemic in the United States-gender, age, socioeconomic, racial/ethnic, and geographic characteristics: a systematic review and meta-regression analysis. Epidemiol Rev 2007;29:6-28.

[21] Popkin BM. Global changes in diet and activity patterns as drivers of the nutrition transition. Nestle Nutr Workshop Ser Pediatr Program 2009;63:1-14,259-68.

[22] Bleich SN, Ku R. Relative contribution of energy intake and energy expenditure to childhood obesity: a review of the literature and directions for future research. Int J Obes (Lond) 2011;35(1):1-15.

[23] Popkin BM, Siega-Riz AM, Haines PS, Jahns L. Where's the fat? Trends in US diets 1965-1996. Prev Med 2001;32(3):245-54.

[24] Murray CJ, Lopez AD. Alternative projections of mortality and disability by cause 1990-2020: Global Burden of Disease Study. Lancet 1997;349(9064): 1498-504.

[25] Mathers CD, Loncar D. Projections of global mortality and burden of disease from 2002 to 2030. PLoS Med 2006;3(11):e442.

[26] Monteiro CA, Conde WL, Popkin BM. The burden of disease from undernutrition and overnutrition in countries undergoing rapid nutrition transition: A view from Brazil. Am J Public Health 2004;94(3):433-4.

[27] World Health Organization. Preventing chronic disease: A vital investment. Geneva: WHO, 2005.

[28] Strong K, Mathers C, Epping-Jordan J, Beaglehole R. Preventing chronic disease: a priority for global health. Int J Epidemiol 2006;35(2):492-4.

[29] Nichols SD, Cadogan F. BMI-based obesity cutoffs and excess adiposity in a Caribbean adolescent population of African origin. Eur J Clin Nutr 2009;63(2): 253-8.

[30] Kuczmarski RJ, Ogden CL, Guo SS, Grummer-Strawn LM, Flegal KM, Mei Z. 2000 CDC Growth Charts for the United States: methods and development. Vital Health Stat 2002;11(246):1-190.

[31] Block RC, Dozier AM, Hazel-Fernandez L, Guido JJ, Pearson TA. An epidemiologic transition of cardiovascular disease risk in Carriacou and Petite Martinique, Grenada: the Grenada Heart Project, 2005-2007. Prev Chronic Dis 2012;9:E90.

In: Public Health Themes in Grenada … ISBN: 978-1-53618-118-0
Editors: J. Merrick and L. Glasgow © 2020 Nova Science Publishers, Inc.

Chapter 17

ACTIVE AGING: WINDREF'S SPORTS FOR HEALTH PROGRAM AMONG THE ELDERLY IN GRENADA, WEST INDIES

Satesh Bidaisee*, MSPH, Christina Wilson, BSC and Calum NL Macpherson, PhD
School of Graduate Studies, St George's University, Grenada, Windward Islands Research and Education Foundation, Grenada and School of Medicine, St George's University, St George's, Grenada, West Indies

ABSTRACT

Life expectancy in Grenada is expected to increase by 10% in the coming decade and, with it, a simultaneous increase in the demand on the healthcare system. Supportive environments and services need to be

* Correspondence: Satesh Bidaisee, , Professor, , Department of Public Health and Preventive Medicine, St George's University, St George's, Grenada, West Indies. Email: sbidaisee@sgu.edu.

provided for the aging population and those with chronic diseases. In this chapter, we assess the impact of the Windward Island Research and Education Foundation (WINDREF) Sports for Health program on the physical, social, and mental well-being of the aging population in Grenada. A total of 23 participants aged 65 years and older (22 females, 1 male) were included in this cross-sectional study. A survey was administered at baseline in July 2017 and again after being enrolled in the Sports for Health program for a minimum of seven months and at the end of one year in July 2018. An adapted version of the RAND Health Survey was used. A statistically significant correlation was found between the following quality of life scales among participants: health vs. pain ($p = 0.013$), emotion vs. pain ($p = 0.009$), emotion vs. health ($p = 0.008$) and emotion vs. energy ($p = 0.022$). WINDREF's Sports for Health program has demonstrated that the quality of life characteristics for the aging population improved after participating. Although the sample size was small, the results showed important outcomes that indicate a benefit in community-based programs for the aging population. It also demonstrated the need to encourage more men to participate in such community-based programs.

INTRODUCTION

Internationally, average life expectancy at birth in 1960 was about 52 years, and today, it is over 70 years (1). There are over one billion people aged 60 years and older in low- and middle-income countries around the world (2). Countries vary in their life expectancies based on many factors, but this is a massive accomplishment. It is evidence of previous decades of success in coordinated research and practice implemented by leading medical, academic, and public health communities. The public health system has been a guiding force in improving health outcomes resulting in prolonged life and reduced disease burden. It has largely been accomplished by enhancing knowledge through research and establishing public health values around the world. But, with this success has come new challenges, including non-communicable or chronic diseases and the increasing incidence of health issues more closely related to human behavior.

Each decade, a broad theme emerges among the international community, which prioritizes specific challenges to populations on a global scale. Setting agendas in this way is important in order to maintain a coordinated and global effort to achieve new population health goals. The World Health Organization (WHO) has declared the decade 2020-2030 as the international decade for healthy aging, which the organization defines as *the process of developing and maintaining the functional ability that enables well-being in older age* (3). Simply, every person should have an opportunity to live a long life with the ability to participate to the fullest extent in what they value.

Unfortunately, aging is often equated with an increasing burden of disease and a poor quality of life (4, 5). It is important to better understand this population and its unique needs. Chronic disease and health-related behaviors are only two of the many factors that influence a person's ability to live a full life as they age. These factors greatly affect the quality of life and are important focus of many interventions. Chronic disease also represents a massive portion of health care expenditure and is likely to gain acceptance among a wide range of organizations as an area of focused intervention.

Influencing human behavior is complex and uniquely challenging, particularly in an age where everything that might be considered "unhealthy" is readily accessible. The ecological approach has been applied successfully in public health intervention planning and implementation aimed at health promotion and changing health-related behaviors (6). This is a broad theory, but many of its principles focus on the influence of the environment on behavior and the importance of social process and collaborative effort (7). Contemporary models apply the ecological model in more focused ways and have suggested variations in its application, including comprehensive guidelines on program planning (8, 9). In general, community-based programs for health promotion have been shown to be effective and sustainable approaches in targeting risk factors of chronic disease and improving health education (10). This framework may also be applied to programs specifically targeting the aging population.

Sports for health, Grenada

In Grenada, life expectancy was estimated at 73 years between 2003 and 2005. It is estimated that life expectancy will increase by 10% in the coming decade, which will place an increasing demand on the healthcare system (11). A recent Pan American Health Organization (PAHO) report stated the need for the Grenadian health system to develop supportive environments and appropriate services, specifically for the aging population (11). Chronic disease is also an important target for health promotion and intervention among all age groups in Grenada. According to the Ministry of Health, in Grenada, 37% of deaths are due to cardiovascular diseases, 21% due to diabetes, and 26% are due to hypertension (11). An increase in deaths due to complications of diabetes, along with deaths due to complications from cardiovascular diseases, has also been noted.

Access to health care and services plays a central role in health and well-being. In an effort to address health inequalities in the Caribbean, WINDREF recently established the Caribbean Center for Health Equity (CCHE) at St George's University (SGU) in Grenada. The goal of this center is to coordinate regional efforts and establish a network of partners across the Caribbean in support of education, research, and service in health equity. Among the ongoing projects at the CCHE is the Sport for Health program, which focuses on providing health and nutrition education, as well as a place where members of the community can participate in fitness activities and training. The program is available to all Grenadians, having locations across 5 sporting fields in the parishes of St George, St John, St Andrew, and St David. The implementation of the Sports for Health program appears to follow an ecological approach in its focus on community engagement and creating environments for health promotion activities.

Current study

The purpose of this study is to assess the impact of Sports for Health on participants over the age of 65 years. While the program provides services to all ages among the Grenadian community, this study seeks to better understand its efficacy in the aging population. The information presented reflected the participant's quality of life and their performance in the program. Although multiple studies have been conducted on the positive impact of participation in health promotion activities in the aging population, there is a need for such studies in developing countries.

The study assessed whether the sports for health program improved the physical, mental, and social well-being of the participants after having completed 12 months in the program. This was determined by comparing baseline survey responses with responses gathered after 12 months. The anticipated primary outcome of the study is that the "Sports for Health Program" will have a positive impact on the physical health and quality of life from baseline to the 12-month time point. The outcomes should show, which scales of quality of life, such as physical functioning, energy, pain, social and emotional well-being will be improved by participating in this program.

Study design

This was a cross-sectional study that collected survey responses from participants at baseline in July 2017 and after being enrolled in the study for one year, who are henceforth referred to as the 12-month point population in July 2018. The WINDREF Sports for Health program is located across five sporting fields in the parishes of St George, St John, St Andrew, and St David.

OUR STUDY

The survey used in this study was a combination of the RAND Health Survey, along with questions regarding demographic characteristics. The RAND Health Survey is a composition of questions from the RAND 36-

Item Health Survey (Version 1.0), which targets the overall well-being of an individual. The validity and reliability of the RAND health survey were demonstrated through the usage of the survey in the Wilson, Hutson, and VanStry study comparing the quality of life amongst breast cancer patients.

The survey in this study was administered to the participants that met the inclusion criteria both at baseline and after one year of participation. These same participants that filled out the first set of surveys also completed the same surveys after one year of participating in the study.

Participants were enrolled for seven months to a year for 11 of the participants (43.5%), and over a year for 12 of the participants (56.5%). A total of 20 (87%) of the participants attend 3-5 exercise sections per week.

Inclusion criteria

Inclusion criteria for the baseline population was having an age of 65 years or more at the time of enrollment in the Sports for Health program. Participants were expected to continuously attend the fitness sessions at least three days per week for a year. There were no exclusion criteria for the baseline information.

Study population

The sample population was taken from the whole target population. A total of 23 participants, comprising 22 females and one male, met the inclusion criteria and were evaluated in this study. The average age of the participants was 67.6, with a standard deviation of 1.9. The ages of the participants ranged from 65 to 73 years.

Variables

The dependent variables are the scales for well-being from the RAND health survey and current health indicators found on the demographics survey. The independent variables are the rest of the questions in the demographic survey such as age, length of enrollment, attendance rate, and level of education.

Data analysis

Descriptive narrative characteristics, such as mean, standard deviation, 95% confidence interval for the mean, upper limit, and lower limit for the continuous variables have been and will continue to be assessed by comparing the baseline and 12-month time point, the males and females, and other variables of interest, in order to visualize the distribution. SPSS was utilized to evaluate the results. Results were charted in Excel.

Questionnaire Part 2, RAND Health Survey, was analyzed using a two-step scoring method designed by Hays, Shermbourne, and Mazel (11). Step 1 in scoring the results was to recode the answer. Each answer was scored according to a range of 0 to 100, with 100 being the most favorable health state. The questions were organized into scales representing the dependent variables of the study. Step 2 was to organize the questions according to their specific scale, and then the scores of the answers in each scale were averaged. The answers that were left blank were not represented in the average score for each scale. Using this method of determining the average (mean), standard deviation, and p-values helped to determine the reliability, central tendency, and variability of the scales. Statistical significance was considered when the p-value was less than 0.05. The null hypothesis can be rejected for the specific statistical test. All the required statistical tests were analyzed according to a 95% confidence interval, with statistical significance noted as a p-value of less than 0.05.

Table 1. RAND health survey

Characteristic	Mean	SD
Physical functioning	91.3	15.9
The following items are about activities you might do during a typical day. Does your health now limit you in these activities? If so, how much?		
Vigorous activities	67.4	35.7
Moderate Activity	95.7	14.4
Lifting or carrying groceries	95.7	14.4
Climbing several flights of stairs	89.1	21.1
Climbing one flight of stairs	100.0	0.0
Bending, kneeling, or stooping	82.6	24.3
Walking more than a mile	97.8	10.4
Walking less than a mile	93.5	22.9
Bathing or dressing yourself	100.0	0.0
Pain	82.2	22.9
How much bodily pain have you had during the past 4 weeks?	70.4	24.0
During the past 4 weeks, how much did the pain interfere with your normal work?	86.9	22.4
During the past 4 weeks, to what extent has your physical health or emotional problems interfered with your normal social activities with family, friends, neighbors, or groups?	89.1	22.3
General health	77.9	18.8
I seem to get sick a little easier than other people	83.7	17.9
I am as healthy as anybody I know	70.7	25.7
I expect my health to get worse	94.6	10.5
In general would you say your health is?	63.0	21.1
Emotional well-being	77.4	13.1
Have you felt calm and peaceful?	75.7	13.4
Have you felt so down that nothing could cheer you up?	74.8	8.98
Have you been a happy person?	81.7	17.0
Energy and fatigue	74.8	12.4
Did you have a lot of energy?	49.6	13.3
Did you feel worn out?	62.2	12.8

FINDINGS

The mean and standard deviation are depicted for the participant's answers from the survey in Table 1. The questions are grouped into four categories; physical functioning, pain, general health, emotional well-being, and energy, and fatigue. Answers to the survey questions have been scored according to a range of 0 to 100, with 100 being *the most favorable health state*. The mean and standard deviation are also included.

Table 2. Analysis of quality of life scales

Scales	Age	
Physical	Pearson Correlation	-.194
	Sig. (2-tailed)	.375
	N	23
Pain	Pearson Correlation	.248
	Sig. (2-tailed)	.253
	N	23
Health	Pearson Correlation	.426*
	Sig. (2-tailed)	.042
	N	23
Age	Pearson Correlation	1
	Sig. (2-tailed)	
	N	23
Emotion	Pearson Correlation	.543**
	Sig. (2-tailed)	.007
	N	23
Energy	Pearson Correlation	-.004
	Sig. (2-tailed)	.984
	N	23

* Correlation is significant at the p = 0.05 level (2-tailed).
** Correlation is significant at the p = 0.01 level (2-tailed).

Table 3. Analysis of participant's attendance rates and quality of life scales

Spearman's rho	Enrollment Length	
Physical	Correlation Coefficient	.117
	Sig. (2-tailed)	.595
Pain	Correlation Coefficient	.156
	Sig. (2-tailed)	.477
Health	Correlation Coefficient	.245
	Sig. (2-tailed)	.259
Age	Correlation Coefficient	.020
	Sig. (2-tailed)	.926
Emotion	Correlation Coefficient	.172
	Sig. (2-tailed)	.434
Energy	Correlation Coefficient	.117
	Sig. (2-tailed)	.595

The participant's health vs. pain (p = 0.013), emotion vs. pain (p = 0.009), emotion vs. health (p = 0.008), and emotion vs. energy (p = 0.022) are found to be significantly significant, hence, a relationship could exist between these variables. Physical functioning compared to energy and fatigue are not statistically significant.

A Pearson's correlation test was utilized to determine if age had a statistically significant relationship with the quality of life scales. According to Table 2, there is only one statistically significant relationship that can be assumed, which is age and emotion.

A Spearman's correlation test was applied to determine if participant's attendance rates are associated with their quality of life scales and no significant associations were found between these factors; hence, conclusions cannot be made about their relationships (see Table 3). A graph of these results can be seen in figure 1. To confirm that attendance rates do not act as confounding variables for quality of life scales, an ordinal regression test was performed. The test of parallel lines in the ordinal regression test failed to reject the null hypothesis that the slope coefficients are the same across the response categories. An ordinal regression test assumed that pain, physical functioning, health, and emotion are not significantly affected by the participant's attendance rate.

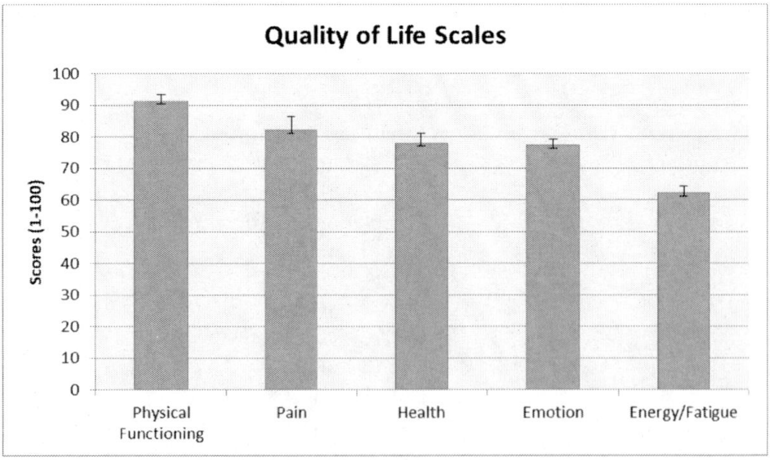

Figure 1. Quality of life scales.

A Spearman's correlation test was also used to determine if the participant's enrollment length had a significant association with their health scales. Conclusions cannot be made about the relationship between quality of life scales and enrollment length.

Discussion

Community-based exercise interventions have become a growing theme for helping elderly persons improve their health. After the completion of this cross-sectional study, there is hope that this study will continue to recruit more male participants and persons aged 65 years and older, in order to form generalizations about the target aging population and improve validity. It is recognized that there are more females in Grenada's aging population than males, but the difference is not as extreme as shown in this study.

The quality of life and well-being of the participants were determined utilizing a RAND health survey, which categorized the responses according to five health scales. The responses to the survey were scored from 0 to 100, with 100 representing the *most favorable health state*. The highest scale was the participant's physical functioning with a mean score of 91.3, and the lowest score was found in the participant's energy and fatigue with a mean score of 74.8. Since the majority of these participants had been active members of the Sports for Health program for over seven months, additional reasoning behind these results could be that the Sports for Health program has quickly improved the participant's physical functioning.

The age of the participants is also an important independent variable, which is why a Pearson's correlation test was conducted to ensure that age did not act as an effective modifier of the health indicators. According to the test, the health scale for emotion can be assumed to have a statistically significant positive association with emotion ($p = 0.007$). Although the participants in the study might have been attending the exercise sessions in different quantities and at different rates, this shows that their participation appeared to be beneficial to their mental well-being when analyzing their health scales.

Increased knowledge about the effectiveness of community-based interventions can promote the expansion of the Sports for Health program as well as the implementation of programs specific to the aging population. It is an important area of research as Grenada's aging population is expected to increase significantly in the coming decade and will require effective health and well-being programs such as Sports for Health. WINDREF's Sports for Health program has demonstrated that quality of life characteristics for the aging population can be improved with a community-based exercise intervention. Lessons learned and best practices will be shared with other countries through publication of the results.

Acknowledgments

The authors thank the Royal Grenada Police Force for assisting in the implementation of this community-based service, and the participants in this study. The name for the WINDREF Sports for Health Program was changed to the Baroness Howells Sports for Health Program in 2018 in honor of Baroness Howells, the President of WINDREF, who has a great interest in this program and its outcomes. Funding for this program comes from the Baroness Howells Sports for Health Fund.

References

[1] World Bank. Life expectancy at birth (total years). URL: https://data.worldbank.org/indicator/sp.dyn.le00.in.

[2] World Health Organization. Decade of healthy aging 2020-2030. Geneva: World Health Organization, 2019. URL: https://www.who.int/ageing/decade-of-healthy-ageing.

[3] Institute of Medicine. Committee for the Study of the Future of Public Health. The future of public health. A history of the public health. Washington, DC: National Academies Press, 1988. URL: https://www.ncbi.nlm.nih.gov/books/NBK218224/.

[4] Levy B, Banaji M. Implicit ageism. In: Nelson TD, editor. Ageism: stereotyping and prejudice against older persons. Cambridge, MA: MIT Press, 2002:127–8.

[5] Richard L, Gauvin L, Raine K. Ecological models revisited: their uses and evolution in health promotion over two decades. Annu Rev Public Health 2011;32:307-26.

[6] Best A, Stokols D, Green LW, Leischow S, Holmes B, Buchholz K. An integrative framework for community partnering to translate theory into effective health promotion strategy. Am J Health Promot 2003;18:168–76.

[7] Bunnell R, O'Neil D, Soler R, Payne R, Giles WH, Collins J, et al. Fifty communities putting prevention to work: accelerating chronic disease prevention through policy, systems and environmental change. J Commun Health 2012;37(5):1081-90.

[8] World Health Organization. Integrated chronic prevention and control. Geneva: World Health Organization, 2014. URL: http://www.who.int/chp/about/integrated_cd/en/.

[9] Wilson RW, Hutson LM, VanStry D. Comparison of two quality-of-life questionnaires in women treated for breast cancer: The RAND 36-item health survey and the Functional Living Index–Cancer. Phys Ther 2005;85(9):851-60.

[10] Pan American Health Organization. Grenada. URL: http://www.paho.org/hq/index.php?option = com_docman&task = doc_view&gid = 25229&Itemid =

[11] Hays RD, Sherbourne CD, Mazel RM. The Rand 36-item health survey 1.0. Health Economics 1993;2(3):217-27.

In: Public Health Themes in Grenada … ISBN: 978-1-53618-118-0
Editors: J. Merrick and L. Glasgow © 2020 Nova Science Publishers, Inc.

Chapter 18

DIFFERENTIAL EXPOSURE TO SOCIAL DETERMINANTS OF OBESITY AMONG RURAL AND URBAN GRENADIAN ADOLESCENTS

Roger Radix*[1]*, MD, MPH,
Richard Scribner*[1,*]*, MD, MPH, Jerry Mitchell*[1]*, MPH,
Trevor Noel*[1]*, PhD, MPH, Rebecca Andal*[1]*, MD,
Naomi Andal*[1]*, MD, Christal Radix*[1]*, BSc,
Rhoda Frank*[1]*, MBA, Jonell Benjamin*[1]*, MPH,
Jennifer James*[1]*, MPH, Romero Benjamin*[1]*, BSc,
Claudia Leonardi*[2]*, PhDH and Melinda Sothern*[2]*, PhD
[1]Windward Island Research and Education Foundation,
St Georges, Grenada
[2]Louisiana State University School of Public Health,
New Orleans, United States of America

[*] Correspondence: Richard Scribner, Professor, Department of Public Health and Preventive Medicine, St. Georges University, Grenada WI. Email: rscribne@sgu.edu.

Abstract

In this chapter, we examine rural and urban differences in exposure to social and environmental factors believed to be social determinants of obesity among Grenadian adolescents. A nationally representative sample of first-year students (i.e., Form 1) (n = 689) from the twenty-three secondary schools in Grenada was assessed as part of the Grenada School Nutrition Study (GSNS). Various measures of social and environmental determinants of obesity were obtained both at the individual and school levels using surveys or field observations, respectively. Urban (n = 13) and rural (n = 10) schools were determined by school location in relation to the two largest towns in Grenada. Exposure to unhealthy food outlets (i.e., shops selling sugar-sweetened beverages, candy, or highly processed foods) was determined by the density of either snack shops (i.e., bakeries, snack shops, markets, vending zones, tuck shops) or franchise fast food outlets (i.e., KFC, Subway) within a .75 km buffer around each school. Rural students were more likely to be Afro Caribbean (89.1% versus 79.3%) and male (55.8% versus 44.1%). Significant differences between rural and urban students were noted for car access (40.7% versus 53.3%), computer access (61.6% versus 73.5%), and snacking after school (83.6% versus 90.5%), respectively. Rural students' school environment had a lower mean density of snack shops (1.53 versus 3.39 shops/square km) and mean fast food outlet density (0 versus 1.17 outlets/square km) than urban students' school environment. For a number of measures, rural students in Grenada had significantly lower exposure to social and environmental factors believed to associated with overweight and obesity.

Introduction

The consensus among public health experts is that human genetic changes are not responsible for the rapid rise in obesity, and the explanation must lie in broad social determinants resulting in local environmental exposures that influence diet and physical activity (1-4). A consequence of this new understanding is evidenced in a new overarching goal in Healthy People 2020 (5). In addition to increasing years of healthy life and eliminating health disparities, the goal of – "creating social and physical environments that promote health" - has been added.

Despite the acknowledged importance of "obesogenic" environments in the epidemic there is little consensus on the aspects of the environment that have driven the epidemic as well as the factors that have given rise to the growing disparities in obesity-related outcomes by race and socioeconomic status (6, 7). Although researchers have watched the epidemic of obesity unfold over the past three decades, not only in the US but across the globe, identification of the "drivers" of the epidemic remains contentious (8-10). The effort to characterize the "drivers" of the epidemic involves the identification of the factors responsible for upsetting the balance in the "energy intake/energy expenditure" equation over the past four decades. On the energy intake side, the global food system that provides a "Westernized" diet of cheap, palatable, energy-dense foods is implicated (8, 10, 11). On the expenditure side, the transition to sedentary occupations with low energy expenditure is implicated (12, 13). The inability to arrive at a consensus is attributed to the lack of research with designs sufficient to link local obesogenic environments - created by the societal drivers - with individual obesity-related behaviors (6, 14, 15).

The current study is designed to begin to identify these drivers of the global epidemic of obesity in a country that has not yet been affected. The study was designed to identify modifiable factors in the school and local environment that were thought to lead to obesity among adolescents. The study targets adolescents entering secondary school because it is a critical developmental stage when adolescents exercise greater autonomy in their decisions regarding diet and physical activity (4). Consequently, it is a period when the effects of the school and local environments will begin to have an impact on obesity-related behaviors.

OUR STUDY

The current study is part of a project titled the Grenada School Nutrition Study (GSNS). The GSNS goal is to identify behavioral and environmental factors that might be intervened on to prevent the development of obesity among Grenadian adolescents.

Table 1. Descriptive statistics for demographic, outcome, behavioral, and school environment variables by urban school status for GSNS schools

	N	Overall	Rural Schools (N = 283)	Urban Schools (N = 406)
Demographics				
Age, years	689	12.67	**12.81**	**12.57**
Race-Afro Caribbean, %	689	83.31	**89.05**	**79.31**
Gender, male	689	48.91	**55.83**	**44.09**
Outcomes				
BMIz > 85th, %	689	17.56	**13.43**	**20.44**
Behaviors				
Car Access, %	687	47.89	**40.07**	**53.33**
TV Access, %	666	79.43	76.84	81.22
Computer, %	664	68.67	**61.62**	**73.54**
Snack after school, %	626	87.70	**83.59**	**90.54**
Junk snack, %	676	41.86	40.07	43.11
Walk to school, %	687	15.14	17.44	13.55
MVPA, % wear time	126	8.10	8.77	7.62
Sedentary, % wear time	126	58.90	57.86	59.63
School Environment				
Snack Store Density	23	8.24	1.53	3.39
Fast Food Density	23	0.664	0	1.17

Note: Bolded prevalences are significantly different at $p < 0.05$.

Study sample

The GSNS was designed to be a representative sample of all first-year secondary students (i.e., Form 1) drawn from the 23 public and private secondary schools across the tri-island nation of Grenada. Form 1 students ranged in age from 11 to 14 years. Randomization was performed at the classroom level resulting in an eligible sample of 1,004 students in 35 classrooms (i.e., in schools with only one Form 1 class all students were included) making up roughly 55% of all Form 1 students in Grenada.

Parental refusals (n= 276) and students who were absent on the day or did not complete all the assessments or surveys (n=39) resulted in an effective sample of 689 students in the cohort. All students were assigned a unique identifier linked to their informed consent signed by their parents. Personal identifiers in the form of parents' names, phone numbers, and school identification were collected for possible follow up.

Data collection

Throughout the academic school year, one school was assessed each week. Three formal visits were scheduled at each school during the week. The first day (i.e., Tuesday) involved the collection of anthropometric data: height, weight, and waist circumference. On the second day (i.e., Wednesday), the student survey and the principal survey were conducted. On the third day (i.e., Thursday), the students were instructed on the wearing of accelerometers. They were instructed to wear the device for four days from Thursday through Sunday.

The school food environment assessments were coordinated with the aid of a Geographic Information System (GIS) developed for the GSNS. The extent of the school environment was defined by a .75 km buffer around each school. Within each school environment, project field staff visited each food outlet and conducted a Store Assessment. The location of each school and store was recorded using a Garmin GPSMAO 76CSx. The reading was taken at the most central location within the school or store. The accuracy varied by 3 to 7 feet.

Study measures

Height, weight, and waist circumference were directly measured for each student in a privatized setting (e.g., trifold blind booth) in normal school clothing. Measurements using a portable stadiometer and electronic scale standardized before each session were repeated three times, and the average score reported.

Body Mass Index (BMI), calculated by dividing weight in kilograms by height in meters squared, was used to assess excess body fat. Due to the greater sensitivity of the Centers for Disease Control and Prevention (CDC) classification system compared with the International Obesity Task Force (IOTF) classification system for characterizing excess body fat in a Caribbean adolescent population, the CDC age- and sex-specific cutoffs were used to characterize overweight (i.e., BMI≥85th percentile) and obese (i.e., BMI≥95th percentile) adolescents in terms of their standardized percentile (16). Rural and urban designations were defined at the school level. Students attending school in the two largest towns in Grenada (i.e., St Georges and Grenville) were defined as urban students.

Percent time in moderate or vigorous physical activity (MVPA) was assessed using Actigraph GT3X+ accelerometers (ActiGraph, Pensacola, FL). A subsample of adolescents wore the accelerometer at their waist on an elasticized belt for two school days and two weekend days. Non-wearing time and cumulative time spent within specific intensity ranges were calculated using SAS (SAS Institute, Inc, Cary, North Carolina) syntax developed by the National Cancer Institute (http://appliedresearch.cancer.gov/nhanes_pam/). Non-wear time was defined as any sequence of at least 60 consecutive minutes of zero activity counts. The cut points of Evenson and Terry (17) for the various physical activity levels were used, as recommended by Trost and colleagues (18). A valid day was defined as 8 hours or more of wear, and participants had to have a minimum of 2 valid days to be included in the analysis. Total time spent in sedentary and moderate-to-vigorous intensity physical activity was expressed as a percentage of wearing time.

Measures of the school food environment were developed using the GSNS Geographic Information System (GIS). In the GIS, data for each Store Assessment was linked to the location of the respective food outlet georeferenced relative to the school environments. Consequently, measures reflect the density of specific aggregated store conditions from the Store Assessments in the school environment. The measures included: 1) density of fast food outlets, 2) density of unhealthy food outlets (snack shop density), and 3) density of outlets with healthy foods. Density items were based on outlets per square kilometer in the school buffer area (see Figure 1).

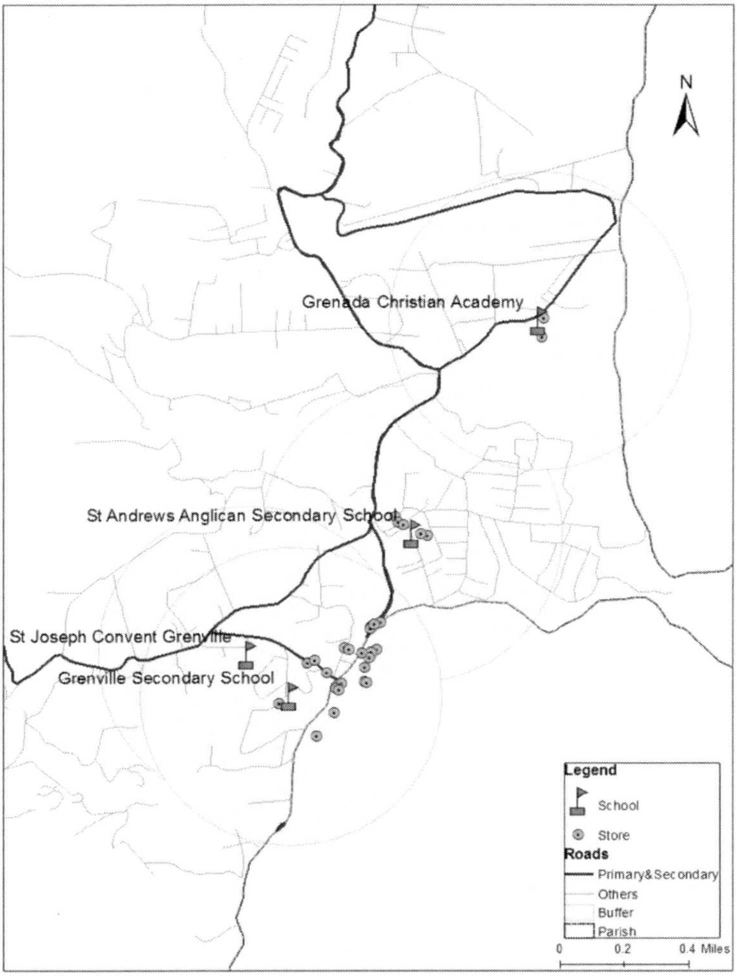

Figure 1. Map demonstrating school environments for the four schools with food stores.

Statistical analysis

Multilevel models of students nested within schools were developed to characterize the overall and between school prevalence of overweight and obesity across Grenada. For this descriptive analysis, demographic measures including age, and gender were included in the analyses. The basic multilevel models used a random coefficient for the intercept. Thus at student level, we have the following model,

$$Y_{ij} = \pi_{0j} + \pi_1(\text{Gender})_{1ij} + \pi_2(\text{Age})_{2ij} + \varepsilon_{ij} \qquad \text{Level 1}$$

where Y_{ij} is the outcome (e.g., obesity related behavior measurements or BMI z-score) for student *i* in school *j*. π_{0j} is the intercept, which we allowed to randomly vary across schools, which also is the estimated mean response for school j. We assume fixed effects for a vector of student level risk factors. ε_{ij} is the random effect of student *i* in school *j,* which is assumed to have normal distribution mean 0 and constant variance σ^2 for i = 1,.....,n_j and j=1,......,23.

The intercept π_{0j}, is allowed to randomly vary across all schools. Therefore, at the school level, we have the following model:

$$\pi_{0j} = \beta_{00} + \beta_{01}W(\text{Urban School})_{1j} + u_{0j} \qquad \text{Level 2 (random intercept)}$$

FINDINGS

Rural students were more likely to be Afro Caribbean (89.1% versus 79.3%) and male (55.8% versus 44.1%). Rural students were also less likely to be overweight or obese (i.e., BMIz >85th percentile).

With regard to obesity-related behaviors, significant differences between rural and urban students were noted for car access (40.7% versus 53.3%), computer access (61.6% versus 73.5%), and snacking after school (83.6% versus 90.5%), respectively. In addition, the rural students' school environment had a lower mean density of snack shops (1.53 versus 3.39 shops/square km) and mean fast food outlet density (0 versus 1.17 outlets/square km) than urban students' school environment.

Table 2. Parameters estimates (95% CI) from multilevel models for obesity related behaviors

	Model 1	Model 2	Model 3	Model 4	Model 5
Individual level Measures					
Computer		0.153 (-.041,0.347)		0.143 (-0.052,0.337)	0.154 (-0.052,0.337)
Male					**-0.3279 (-0.524,-0.132)**
School level Measures					
Urban School			0.1861 (-0.441,0.103)	0.169 (-0.103,0.441)	0.128 (-0.116,0.372)
Random Effects					
School level effect	0.0511	0.0450	0.0475	0.04334	0.0248
Individual level effect	1.3241	1.3258	1.3237	1.3253	1.3148
Fit Statistics					
AIC	2172.2	2095.2	2172.5	2095.7	2087.8

Multi-level analyses were run to try and explain the urban-rural differences in obesity rates in terms of either individual or school environment level factors. In multilevel analysis predicting the risk of obesity, none of the individual behaviors or school food environment measures was observed to explain the urban-rural differences in obesity risk (see Table 2). For example, when access to computers was added to the model, the factor did not significantly predict obesity risk, although greater access to computers was positively associated with obesity risk. In addition, the inclusion of computer access to the model slightly reduced the effect of urban school status on obesity risk, but neither factor was significant (see Table 2, Model 3).

Table 3. Odds ratios (OR) and 95% CI from multilevel logistic models on individual nested within school level measures, predicting obesity (BMI ≥ 85^{pctl})

	Model 1	Model 2	Model 3	Model 4	Model 5	Model 6
Individual level Measures						
Male		**0.52 (0.33, 0.80)**		**0.53 (0.34, 0.82)**	**0.53 (0.35, 0.81)**	**0.55 (0.36, 0.84)**
Age, years		0.77 (0.57, 1.05)		0.79 (0.58, 1.08)	0.77 (0.57, 1.05)	0.80 (0.58, 1.09)
Computer					**1.67 (1.04, 2.70)**	1.61 (1.00, 2.60)
School level Measures						
Urban School			1.69 (0.96, 2.96)	1.49 (0.93, 2.40)		1.41 (0.90, 2.19)
Random Effects						
Tract level effect	0.2204	0.0699	0.1738	0.0500	0	0
Change from Model 1	--	-68.3%	-21.1%	-77.3%	-100.0%	-100.0%
Fit Statistics						
-2Res Log Pseudo-						

Note: Bolded OR are significantly different from 1 at $p < 0.05$.

DISCUSSION

For several individual behaviors and school environment characteristics, rural students in Grenada had significantly lower exposure to social and environmental factors believed to be associated with overweight and obesity. However, in multilevel modeling controlling for demographic factors, the individual behaviors, and the school environment characteristics, individual behaviors did not explain the effect of urban school status on obesity risk.

While it is clear that students attending schools in rural parishes of Grenada have a lower risk profile with regard to presumed behavioral factors associated with obesity, explaining the rural versus urban differences were not explained by the individual behaviors measured in this study. Of note is the lack of a difference in MVPA level between the two groups. Consequently, it is unclear why the reported measures - computer use and car access - were significantly different between rural and urban students, given they imply differences in physical activity. Furthermore, the results suggest the difference in unmeasured factors associated with junk food consumption may be implicated. While the school level differences in the availability of junk food were not significant, the large difference in effect does appear to represent a trend given the sample size of only seven.

There were several weaknesses in the study. First, the gender difference related to urban and rural schools is an issue. The fact that females were more represented in urban schools may account for the urban-rural difference in overweight students in urban schools. However, higher socioeconomic status (SES) and high SES is related to car, computer, and junk food access in other studies. It may be that there is an interaction between rural versus urban school attendance and SES where overweight urban females attend rural schools and normal weight rural females attend urban schools, which were considered elite, thus biasing the results to the null. In addition, the accelerometer data was not ideal. In the analysis, students that did not complete the entire program were included in the analysis. Consequently, the lack of difference between rural and urban areas could be due to measurement error.

Finally, there appeared to be urban-rural differences in rates of overweight adolescents. While individual behaviors did not explain the differences there appeared to be confounding by individual SES. For example, computer access, the one behavior associated with overweight status, was significant across all schools but controlling for school status resulted in an insignificant finding. Future studies of rural versus urban differences in overweight and obesity should acknowledge the role of SES interaction biasing results to the null.

ACKNOWLEDGMENT

The project, titled the Grenada school Nutrition Study (GNS), is funded by the International Research Development Center (IRDC) (Grant #106884).

REFERENCES

[1] Kumanyika S, Jeffery R, Morabia A, Kumanyika, Antipatis VJ. Obesity prevention: the case for action. Int J Obes Relat Metab Disord 2002;26(3):425-36.

[2] Hill JO, Wyatt HR, Reed GW, Peters JC. Obesity and the environment: where do we go from here? Science 2003;299(5608):853-5.

[3] Koplan JP, Liverman CT, Kraak VI, Committee on Prevention of Obesity in Children and Youth. Preventing childhood obesity: health in the balance: executive summary. J Am Diet Assoc 2005;105(1):131-8.

[4] Sallis J F, Glanz K. Physical activity and food environments: Solutions to the obesity epidemic. Milbank Q 2009;87(1):123-154.

[5] US Department of Health and Human Services. Healthy people adolescents health, 2014. URL: https://www.healthypeople.gov/2020/topics-objectives/topic/Adolescent-Health.

[6] Bleich SN, Ku R. Relative contribution of energy intake and energy expenditure to childhood obesity: a review of the literature and directions for future research. Int J Obes (Lond) 2011;35(1):1-15.

[7] Ding D, Gebel K. Built environment, physical activity, and obesity: what have we learned from reviewing the literature? Health Place 2012;18(1):100–5.

[8] Swinburn BA, Sacks G, Hall KD, McPherson K, Finegood DF, Moodie ML. The global obesity pandemic: shaped by global drivers and local environments. Lancet 2011; 378(9793):804-14.

[9] Blair SN, Archer E, Hand GA. Commentary: Luke and Cooper are wrong: physical activity has a crucial role in weight management and determinants of obesity. Int J Epidemiol 2013;42(6):1836-8.

[10] Luke A, Cooper RS. Physical activity does not influence obesity risk: time to clarify the public health message. Int J Epidemiol 2013;42(6):1831-6.

[11] Popkin BM, Adair LS, Ng SW. Global nutrition transition and the pandemic of obesity in developing countries. Nutr Rev 2012;70(1):3-21.

[12] Franco M, Orduñez P, Caballero B, Granados JAT, Lazo M, Bernal JL. Impact of energy intake, physical activity, and population-wide weight loss on cardiovascular disease and diabetes mortality in Cuba, 1980-2005. Am J Epidemiol 2007;166(12):1374-80.

[13] Church TS, Thomas DM, Tudor-Locke C, Katzmarzyk T, Earnest CP, Rodarte QR. Trends over 5 decades in U.S. occupation-related physical activity and their associations with obesity. PLoS One 2011;6(5):e19657.

[14] Wang Y, Beydoun MA. The obesity epidemic in the United States-gender, age, socioeconomic, racial/ethnic, and geographic characteristics: A systematic review and meta-regression analysis. Epidemiol Rev 2007;29:6-28.

[15] Popkin BM, Siega-Riz AM, Haines PS, Jahns L. Where's the fat? Trends in US diets 1965-1996. Prev Med 2001;32(3):245-54.

[16] Nichols SD, Cadogan F. BMI-based obesity cutoffs and excess adiposity in a Caribbean adolescent population of African origin. Eur J Clin Nutr 2009;63(2):253-8.

[17] Evenson KR, Terry JW Jr. Assessment of differing definitions of accelerometer nonwear time. Res Q Exerc Sport 2009;80(2):355-62.

[18] Trost SG, Loprinzi PD, Moore R, Pfeiffer KA. Comparison of accelerometer cut points for predicting activity intensity in youth. Med Sci Sports Exerc 2011;43(7):1360–8.

In: Public Health Themes in Grenada … ISBN: 978-1-53618-118-0
Editors: J. Merrick and L. Glasgow © 2020 Nova Science Publishers, Inc.

Chapter 19

ANALYSIS OF URINE SAMPLES FOR ANTIMICROBIAL RESISTANCE PROFILES IN GRENADA, 2015-2018

Michael J. Montalbano*[1,*]*, MD,
Shawn Charles*[2]*, MD, MPH and
Lindonne Glasgow*[3]*, MSPH, DrPH
[1]Department of Anatomical Sciences, St George's University, St George's, Grenada
[2]Ministry of Health, St George's, Grenada
[3]Department of Public Health and Preventive Medicine, St George's University, St George's, Grenada

ABSTRACT

Antimicrobial resistance (AMR) is a serious global public health problem. Worldwide, annual mortality is half-a-million people from AMR

---

[*] Correspondence: Michael Montalbano, Instructor, Anatomical Sciences, School of Medicine, St George's University, St George's, Grenada, West Indies. Email: mmontal1@sgu.edu.

infections. AMR also results in additional healthcare spending for non-fatal cases. In the presence of growing levels of AMR, further use of antibiotics should conform to relevant current empirical findings. A retrospective secondary analysis was performed on data collected from 2018 for catheter and clean void urine specimens collected at the Grenada General Hospital for uropathogens. The data were compared to the average of the preceding three years, as reported in published literature, to determine their susceptibility to different antimicrobials. The data were submitted after the Institutional Review Board (IRB) approval and redaction of identifiable patient information. A total of 9,054 urine collections were tested and reported for 2018. There were 583 catheter specimens and 8,471 clean void specimens. Those microbes that met inclusion criteria for both specimen types were Klebsiella pneumoniae, Proteus mirabilis, and Pseudomonas aeruginosa. Klebsiella pneumonia and Proteus mirabilis were shown to have statistically significant differences in resistance patterns between the published average of the preceding three years (2015-2017) and the 2018 collection. This study provides information on bacterial antibiotic susceptibility profiles of isolates from urine specimens from the Grenadian population. The findings of a trend towards increasing resistance emphasize the necessity of continued surveillance as part of the multimodal strategies recommended in infection prevention control programs. The findings in this study can be extremely useful to assist healthcare providers in planning treatment regimes for patients with urinary tract infections (UTI) in Grenada. Further, the Ministry of Health in Grenada can use the evidence from this study to support framing its response to the World Health Organization's (WHO) call to countries to address AMR and to improve antibiotic stewardship.

INTRODUCTION

Modern use of antibiotics began with the development of penicillin by Alexander Fleming (1881-1955) in 1928. Almost immediately, however, there were concerns that the capacity of these drugs to combat infections would not last. By 1946, Fleming said, "the public will demand [penicillin]... then will begin an era...of abuses. The microbes are educated to resist penicillin and a host of penicillin-fast organisms is bred out which can be passed to other individuals... I hope the evil can be averted." By 1962 methicillin-resistant staphylococcus aureus (MSRA) had developed in the

United Kingdom (1). Now, the WHO claims that, "without urgent action, we are heading for a post-antibiotic era, in which common infections and minor injuries can once again kill" (2).

There is substantial evidence that antimicrobial resistance (AMR) is a serious health issue. There is presently an annual worldwide mortality of half-a-million people from infections due to AMR (3). If the situation is left unabated, it is estimated that mortality due to AMR will rise to 10 million people annually by the year 2050 (4). There is also substantial morbidity in non-fatal cases that contribute to the environmental "resistome," viz. collection of AMR genes that are cultivated and transmitted among pathogenic microbes. In turn, more robust resistomes require longer durations of treatment for infections. In the United States alone, this leads to an additional $35 billion, or $18,000 to $29,000 per patient, per year (1, 3). In addition, as the world becomes a global community, there is concern that AMR pathogens will spread to more places and in a shorter time. There is now evidence to suggest that even short durations in transit create more robust resistomes in places such as airplane sewage (5).

To control AMR related impacts, antibiotic stewardship is prudent. However, it has been found that the antibiotic choice for treatment is inappropriate in at least 30% of cases (6). In Trinidad, it has been shown that at least 62% of surgical prescriptions were inappropriate (7). To counter this problem, an evidence-based approach should be used to increase the effectiveness of antimicrobial interventions. However, information on AMR for the human population in Grenada is limited. Analyzed data for UTI antimicrobial patterns and other types of infections are very limited. Specifically, there are no data publicly available for uropathogens after 2017 either from private institutions or the global reporting systems such as the Global Antimicrobial Resistance Surveillance System (GLASS) of the World Health Organization (2, 8). This study was performed to provide evidence of uropathogen AMR prevalence in the population of Grenada from 2018. This information can be extremely useful to assist healthcare providers in planning treatment regimes for UTI in Grenada. The Ministry of Health in Grenada can also use the evidence generated in this study to inform its response to the WHO's call to countries to address AMR and to improve antibiotic stewardship.

OUR STUDY

A retrospective secondary data analysis was performed for urine samples collected over a one-year period, January 2018 to December 2018, at Grenada General Hospital Laboratory. The data received from the Ministry of Health for the analysis was anonymized. The IRB at St. George's University (SGU) granted approval for the study (St. George's University IRB Ref 19030).

The information provided was WHONET compatible antibiogram data including the year of collection, host, number of samples, type of specimen collected, as well as microbial organism cultured, antibiotic(s) used for susceptibility testing, and the results. Urine clean void and urine catheter specimens were included from both inpatients and outpatients. The microbial organisms isolated from the specimens and reported were *Escherichia coli*, *Klebsiella pneumoniae, Proteus mirabilis, Raoultella terrigena, Pseudomonas aeruginosa, Staphylococcus aureus, Staphylococcus epidermidis, Enterococcus* sp., and *Streptococcus* sp. The antibiotics used for susceptibility testing were amoxicillin/clavulanate i.e., augmentin, ampicillin, trimethoprim/sulfamethoxazole, ciprofloxacin, levofloxacin, norfloxacin, gentamicin, amikacin, cefazolin, cefuroxime, cefoxitin, cefotaxime, ceftazidime, ceftriaxone, imipenem, and vancomycin.

Inclusion criteria consisted of urine specimens from the Grenada General Hospital Laboratory in the year 2018. Data were excluded if they contained incomplete or unclear documentation, or if the total number of samples collected for a category was limited ($n < 30$). Data that did not meet the criteria nor were included in the publication of the selected preceding years were not used in the analysis. A chi-square analysis was done to assess the level of change in AMR as of 2018 in comparison to published average uropathogen findings in Grenada from 2015 to 2017 (8). The data were extracted into Microsoft Excel and analyzed using Statistical Package for Social Sciences (SPSS) software.

FINDINGS

A total of 9,054 urine collections were tested, reported, and met minimum inclusion criteria over the 2018 period. Out of the total, there were 583 catheter specimens and 8,471 clean void specimens. Microbes meeting criteria for both specimen types were *Klebsiella pneumoniae, Proteus mirabilis, Pseudomonas aeruginosa*, and streptococci (see Table 1, Table 2). Of these microbial specimens, a chi-square analysis was performed of the 2018 antibiotic profiles that were of sufficient size (n>30) and had existing data for comparison from the three years prior in the published literature (8, 9). After implementing these criteria, *Klebsiella pneumoniae* with ampicillin, *Proteus mirabilis* with augmentin, as well as *Proteus mirabilis* with cefuroxime were available for statistical analysis. *Klebsiella pneumoniae* isolates showed a statistically significant increase in resistance against ampicillin, X^2 (1, N = 152) = 11.52, $p < .05$. *Proteus mirabilis* isolates showed a statistically significant increase against augmentin, X^2 (1, N = 280) = 188.45, $p < .05$. *Proteus mirabilis* isolates also showed a statistically significant increase against cefuroxime, X^2 (1, N= 146) = 100.03, $p < .05$.

Table 1. Uropathogens and select resistances (2015-2017)

	Total number from all urine samples (as reported by (8))	Resistant to Augmentin	Resistant to Ampicillin	Resistant to Cefuroxime
Klebsiella pneumoniae	186	36%	80%	27%
Proteus mirabilis	96	36%	48%	24%

Table 2. Uropathogens and select resistances (2018)

	Total number from all urine samples	Resistant to Augmentin	Resistant to Ampicillin	Resistant to Cefuroxime
Klebsiella pneumoniae	271	55%	3%	54%
Proteus mirabilis	4321	92%	40%	84%

DISCUSSION

The data collected in this study show *Klebsiella pneumoniae* resistant to augmentin and cefuroxime, which is the same as reported in a prior analysis of uropathogens in Grenada analyzed from 2015 to 2017 (8). The current findings shows that since then there has also been a statistically significant increase in *Klebsiella pneumoniae* against ampicillin. Additionally, the current analysis show a statistically significant increase in *Proteus mirabilis* resistance against augmentin and cefuroxime.

There were several limiting factors in this study. It is possible that high levels of AMR over the short time period of analysis were due to low statistical power for certain subsets of specimens. However, the period under investigation may have been of sufficient duration as it has been documented that up to 70% of *Staphylococcus aureus* strains can become resistant to antibiotics, such as erythromycin, within six months of exposure onset (3, 10). Additionally, as this study used secondary data, there was no way to control factors such as whether there was a lack of refrigeration of the samples, broth contamination, use of a non-sterile container for collection, and less than the minimum recommended volume of urine being submitted for analysis. While the current study had a higher number of total samples, there was also no ability to remove repeated specimen testing or polymicrobial samples. Prior studies from the same population with more stringent criteria of non-repeat monobacterial clinical isolates have yielded fewer samples (11). Future analyses can better parse patient information by accounting for subsections and collecting demographic data, such as age and gender. This would allow for comparisons to other Caribbean countries for prevalence rates of UTI as well as reported cases of AMR genes such as metallo-beta-lactamases (12).

Findings from this investigation, and similar studies, can support evidence-based prescribing of antibiotics. Constant exposure to antibiotics at low levels promotes virulence through hormesis since the factors that contribute to pathogenicity also act as chemical communication with other microbes when present at concentrations below the threshold of inhibition (13). Imipenem at sub-inhibitory concentration levels induces beta-lactamase production in pseudomonas strains, ampicillin at sub-inhibitory concentration levels induce pathogenicity in *Escherichia coli*, and ciprofloxacin at sub-inhibitory concentration levels increase the transfer of pathogenicity factors to *Staphylococcus aureus* (6). Due to hormesis, it would be ideal to reduce the amount of constant low-level exposure to antimicrobials (1). With sufficient recent AMR data, there can be shorter courses of antibiotic treatment that do not negatively affect mortality can be encouraged (14).

Novel, more cost-effective search methods, are on the horizon for discovering new antimicrobials. However, they are not yet fully integrated into business models and the effects are not fully understood (15). Alternative treatment methods are pending but are not yet proven to be clinically or financially effective (16,17). The use of biomarkers, such as procalcitonin, and non-antibiotics that demonstrate antimicrobial activity, such as ticagrelor, have not been shown to work independently of antibiotics, rather than augment them (18,19). It has thus become increasingly ineffective to financially subsidize private industry as compared to enhancing public health measures, directly (20). As such, it is more prudent for small island states like Grenada to apply intermediate steps to protect and prolong health through antibiotic stewardship and associated public health interventions.

The data on AMR collected here can work in tandem with extending antibiotic stewardship into agricultural use as well. In the United States, 80% of antibiotics sold are for agricultural and farm use and up to 70% of administered antibiotics exit the body unmetabolized through urine, leading to at least 10% of pharmacologically active compounds being retained even after conventional water treatment (21, 22, 23). In Grenada, specifically, antibiotic stewardship for poultry farmers can be an important point of intervention (24). Additionally, effective public health measures, such as vaccinations, should be extended as well. AMR of *Streptococcus pneumoniae* serotype 19A, which is prevalent after introduction of the seven valent vaccine, is decreasing in children under five years in the Latin American and Caribbean region (25). Implementing vaccinations in aquaculture would not only prevent AMR in water sources but also produce greater yield for farmers (23). Public health policies should support these measures to protect the health of Grenadian citizens.

In conclusion, AMR is a growing problem and the solution lies in a multidisciplinary approach to intervention as well as generating strong evidence on which to premise actions. The use of data can support the development of measures to promote the physical and fiscal wellbeing of the public, through infection control that reduces the cost and morbidity of infections. This study documents antimicrobial resistance profiles from uropathogens in Grenada collected in 2018. In comparison to published data for the three years prior, 2018 uropathogens showed statistically significant increases in AMR among *Klebsiella pneumoniae* to ampicillin, and *Proteus mirabilis* to augmentin as well as cefuroxime. Although the conclusions of this study should be taken with some caution until further confirmatory studies are performed, other studies have shown there is an overall trend towards increased AMR. This trend highlights the need for continued surveillance in order to adjust future antimicrobial guidelines. With other reported findings, the results from this study can be stored in a database that can be used for AMR reporting and to inform education campaigns for medical professionals and the public, and promoting evidence-based clinical guidelines as well as antibiotic stewardship in Grenada and, more widely, in the Caribbean.

REFERENCES

[1] Bartlett JG, Gilbert DN, Spellberg B. Seven ways to preserve the miracle of antibiotics. Clin Infect Dis 2013;56(10) 1445-50.

[2] World Health Organization. Global antimicrobial resistance surveillance system (GLASS) report: early implementation 2017-2018. Geneva: World Health Organization, 2018.

[3] Kraemer SA, Ramachandran A, Perron GG. Antibiotic pollution in the environment: from microbial ecology to public policy. Microorganisms 2019;7(6):180.

[4] O'Neill J. Tackling drug-resistant infections globally: Final report and recommendations. URL: https://amr-review.org/sites/default/files/160518_Final%20paper_with%20cover.pdf.

[5] Heß S, Kneis D, Österlund T, Li B, Kristiansson E, Berendonk TU. Sewage from airplanes exhibits high abundance and diversity of antibiotic resistance genes. Environ Sci Technol 2019;52(23):13898-905.

[6] Ventola CL. The antibiotic resistance crisis part 1: Causes and threats. P&T 2015; 40(4):277-83.

[7] Pinto Pereira LM, Philips M, Ramlal H, Teemul K, Prabhakar P. Third generation cephalosporin use in a tertiary hospital in Port of Spain, Trinidad: Need for an antibiotic policy. BMC Infect Dis 2004;4(1):59.

[8] Sharma D, Preson SE, Hage R. Emerging antibiotic resistance to bacterial isolates from human urinary tract infections in Grenada. Cureus 2019;11(9):e5752.

[9] Perla RJ, Carifio J. Use of the chi-square test to determine significance of cumulative antibiogram data. Am J Infect Dis 2005;1(4):162-7.

[10] Podnecky NL, Fredheim EGA, Kloos J, Sørum V, Primicerio R, Roberts AP, et al. Conserved collateral antibiotic susceptibility networks in diverse clinical strains of Escherichia coli. Nat Commun 2018;9(1):3673.

[11] High DP, Joshi R, Lambert GA, Ross ZM. Aetiology and antibiotic susceptibility profiles of blood culture isolates from Grenada General Hospital (2009-2013). Poster session presented at: Phi Zeta Research Emphasis and Research Day; St George's University, Grenada, West Indies. URL: https://mycampus.sgu.edu/c/document_library/get_file?uuid=fb030db5-6f36-4c7f-80d5-a4989e009321&groupId=246297.

[12] Bastian S, Nordmann P, Creton E, Malpote E, Thiery G, Martino F, et al. First case of NDM-1 producing klebsiella pneumoniae in Caribbean islands. Int J Infect Dis 2015;34:53-4.

[13] Vishwanathan VK. Off-label abuse of antibiotics by bacteria. Gut Microbes 2014; 5(1):3-5.

[14] Jones BE, Ying J, Stevens V. Empirical anti-MRSA vs. standard antibiotic therapy and risk of 30-day mortality in patients hospitalized for pneumonia. JAMA Intern Med 2020. doi:10.1001/jamainternmed.2019.7495.

[15] Stokes JM, Yang K, Swanson K, Jin W, Cubillos-Ruiz A, Donghia NM, et al. A deep learning approach to antibiotic discovery. Cell 2020;180:688-702.

[16] McDaniel CT, Panmanee W, Winsor GL, Gill E, Bertelli C, Schurr MJ, et al. AB569, a nontoxic chemical tandem that kills major human pathogenic bacteria. Proc Natl Acad Sci USA 2020;117 (9):4921-30.

[17] Domenech A, Brochado AR, Sender V, Hentrich K, Henriques-Normark B, Typas A, et al. Proton motive force disruptors block bacterial competence and horizontal gene transfer. Cell Host Microbe 2020;S1931-3128(20)30073-1.

[18] Lancellotti P, Musumeci L, Jacques N, Servais L, Goffin E, Pirotte B, et al. Antibacterial activity of ticagrelor in conventional antiplatelet dosages against antibiotic-resistant gram-positive bacteria. JAMA Cardiol 2019;4(6):596-9.

[19] Rhee C. Using procalcitonin to guide antibiotic therapy. Open Forum Infect Dis 2016; 4(1):ofw249.

[20] Zintzaras E, Ioannidis JP. Modelling of escalating outpatient antibiotic expenditures. J Antimicrob Chemother 2003;52:1001-4.

[21] Oldenkamp R, Beusen AHW, Huijbregts MAJ. Aquatic risks from human pharmaceuticals-modelling temporal trends of carbamazapine and ciprofloxacin at the global scale. Environ Res Lett 2019;14(3):034003.

[22] Watts JEM, Schreier HJ, Lanska L, Hale MS. The rising tide of antibiotic resistance in aquaculture: sources, sinks and solutions. Mar Drugs 2017;15(6):158.

[23] World Health Organization. The evolving threat of antimicrobial resistance: Options for action. Geneva: World Health Organization, 2012.

[24] Glasgow L, Forde M, Brow D, Mahoney C, Fletcher S, Rodrigo S. Antibiotic use in poultry production in Grenada. Veterinary Medicine International 2019; 2019:6785195.

[25] Agudelo CI, DeAntonio R, Castañeda E. Streptococcus pneumoniae serotype 19A in Latin America and the Caribbean 2010-2015: A systematic review and a time series analysis. Vaccine 2018;36:4861-74.

In: Public Health Themes in Grenada … ISBN: 978-1-53618-118-0
Editors: J. Merrick and L. Glasgow © 2020 Nova Science Publishers, Inc.

Chapter 20

TRENDS IN MORBIDITY AND MORTALITY OF COMMUNITY-ACQUIRED PNEUMONIA IN GRENADA DURING 2015-2019

Shawn Charles[1], MD, MPH, Lindonne Glasgow[2,*], MSPH, DrPH, Joel Maruthanal[2], MD and Prakash Ramdass[2], MD, MPH

[1]Ministry of Health, St George's, Grenada, West Indies and [2]School of Medicine, Department of Public Health and Preventive Medicine, St George's University, St George's, Grenada, West Indies

ABSTRACT

Lower respiratory infection is a leading cause of morbidity and mortality worldwide. Pneumonia is an acute form of lower respiratory infection that is characterized by inflammation of the lung parenchyma and ranks as the

* Correspondence: Dr. Lindonne Glasgow, Assistant Professor, Department of Public Health and Preventive Medicine, St George's University, PO Box 7, True Blue, St George's, Grenada, West Indies. Email: lglasgow@sgu.com.

4th leading cause of death in Grenada. Pneumonia is categorized either as community-acquired pneumonia or as hospital-acquired pneumonia and can be caused by many pathogens, including streptococcus pneumoniae, hemophilus influenzae, mycoplasma pneumoniae, chlamydophila pneumoniae, influenza virus, coronavirus, and respiratory syncytial virus. The main objective of this study was to describe patterns of morbidity and mortality for community-acquired pneumonia in Grenada during 2015-2019. We retrospectively analyzed the morbidity and mortality of community-acquired pneumonia in Grenada during 2015-2019. Extracted data included the total number of admissions for each month and year; demographic data, including age, and sex; and patient outcomes (survived/died) for those admitted with community-acquired pneumonia. A total of 1,165 patients with community-acquired pneumonia were admitted during 2015-2019. There were 606 (52.0%) women, 557 (47.8%) men, and 2 (0.2%) of unknown gender. The number of cases of community-acquired pneumonia admitted increased significantly over the 5-year period, with 2019 reporting the highest number of cases. The overall case fatality ratio for the 5-year period was 20.5%, with 2015 reporting the highest proportion (29.1%). The proportion of hospital admissions for community-acquired pneumonia increased significantly during 2015-2019 in Grenada. There is an exceedingly high case fatality ratio for community-acquired pneumonia.

INTRODUCTION

Lower respiratory infection is a leading cause of morbidity and mortality worldwide (1). Pneumonia is an acute form of lower respiratory infection that is characterized by inflammation of the lung parenchyma. Pneumonia can be caused by many pathogens, including streptococcus pneumoniae, hemophilus influenzae, staphylococcus aureus, klebsiella pneumoniae, pseudomonas aeruginosa, mycoplasma pneumoniae, chlamydophila pneumoniae, rhinovirus, influenza, parainfluenza virus, coronavirus, and respiratory syncytial virus (2). Pneumonia is categorized either as community-acquired pneumonia (CAP), in which infection is acquired outside of the hospital setting, or as hospital-acquired pneumonia (HAP), in which infection is acquired after 48 hours of being admitted to the hospital (3).

Data shows that lower respiratory infection is the 4th leading cause of death worldwide (4). This statistic is mirrored by reported mortality data for Grenada (5). However, recent data shows that the global mortality rate of pneumonia is on the decline, despite more people above age 70 years dying from pneumonia (6). Healthcare utilization and cost of hospitalization relating to the treatment of pneumonia is also substantial (7).

The main objective of this study was to describe patterns of morbidity and mortality for community-acquired pneumonia in Grenada during 2015-2019. Our primary hypothesis was that there would be an observable decline in hospital admissions for community-acquired pneumonia in Grenada during this 5-year period.

Our study

We retrospectively analyzed the morbidity and mortality of community-acquired pneumonia in Grenada during 2015-2019. Data for this analysis were obtained from the Grenada General Hospital medical records department. Grenada General Hospital is the main referral hospital for all public and private health care providers in Grenada. It is a 198-bed secondary/tertiary hospital that includes the only intensive care unit (ICU) on the island and several specialist services. In this study, data were extracted from January 1, 2015 to December 31, 2019. All data obtained from the medical records were de-identified and uploaded in an Excel® sheet. Extracted data included the total number of admissions for each month and year; demographic data, including age and sex; and patient outcomes (survived/died) for those admitted with community-acquired pneumonia. The International Classification of Diseases 10th revision (ICD10) (8) coding system was used to categorize acute respiratory infections. Specifically, we analyzed data for Code J18 (pneumonia, unspecified organism). We compared the admission rates of pneumonia regarding age, sex, and month of admission, and examined the trends over the 5-year period. The case fatality ratio for pneumonia was compared for this time period.

Table 1. Number of cases of pneumonia admitted by year and sex

Year	Women	Men	Unknown	Total
2015	76 (51.4)	72 (48.6)	0 (0.0)	148
2016	127 (53.8)	108 (45.8)	1 (0.4)	236
2017	105 (52.8)	93 (46.7)	1 (0.5)	199
2018	147 (52.9)	131 (47.1)	0 (0.0)	278
2019	151 (49.7)	153 (50.3)	0 (0.0)	304
Total	606 (52.0)	557 (47.8)	2 (0.2)	1165

OUR FINDINGS

A total of 1,165 cases of community-acquired pneumonia were admitted during 2015-2019. There were 606 (52.0%) women, 557 (47.8%) men, and 2 (0.2%) of unknown gender. Details are shown in Table 1. The number of cases of community-acquired pneumonia admitted increased significantly over the 5-year period, with 2019 reporting the highest number of cases. In 2019 the number of admissions for community-acquired pneumonia doubled that for 2015. With the exception of 2019, more women were admitted for community-acquired pneumonia during the 5-year period.

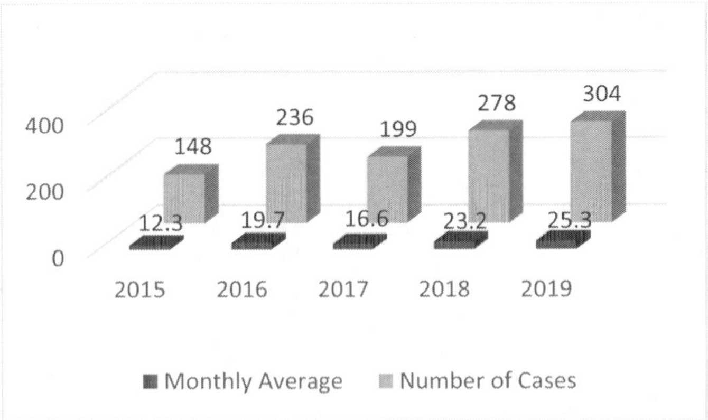

Figure 1. Number of cases of pneumonia admitted by year and monthly average.

There was a seasonal variation of hospital admissions for community-acquired pneumonia, with higher numbers being reported during the period of December to March. The annual total and average monthly number of admissions of community-acquired pneumonia cases are shown in Figure 1. The number of admissions for community-acquired pneumonia recorded in 2019 was 9.4% higher than in 2018. The average monthly number of cases has also increased over the same period. Additionally, the number of cases in December 2019 was 61.5% higher than the average over the previous three years (see Figure 2).

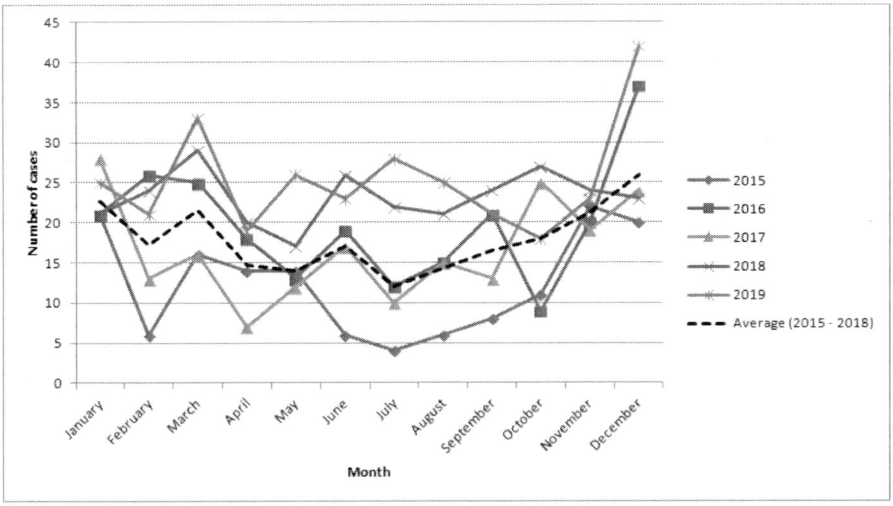

Figure 2. Number of cases of pneumonia admitted by year and month.

The 65-years and older age group consistently had the most hospitalizations for community-acquired pneumonia during 2015-2019 (with an average of 48.6% over this period). In 2019, 54.6% of all admissions for pneumonia were 65 years and older. The 45-to-64-years age group reported the second highest proportion of hospitalization for community-acquired pneumonia, averaging 24.8% over the 5-year period. An increasing trend in hospitalizations was also observed in this age group (see Figure 3).

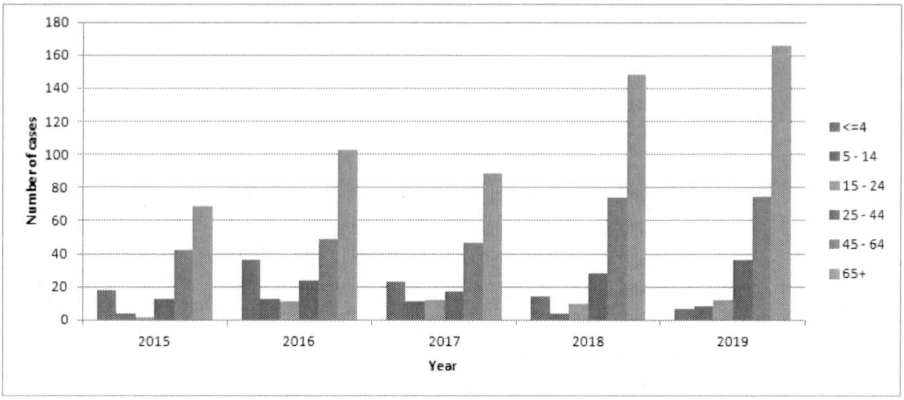

Figure 3. Number of cases of pneumonia admitted by year and age.

The distribution of patients who died from according to year and age is shown in Figure 4. The total number of deaths recorded for the 5-year period was 239, with a yearly average of 48. The highest number of fatalities, 58, was recorded in 2019, in which 20.3% of the deaths were recorded occurred in December. Most of the patients who died from community-acquired pneumonia were 65 years or older, contributing to an average of 70.6% of deaths. The proportion of deaths in this age group ranged from 62.8% in 2015 to 74.6% in 2019.

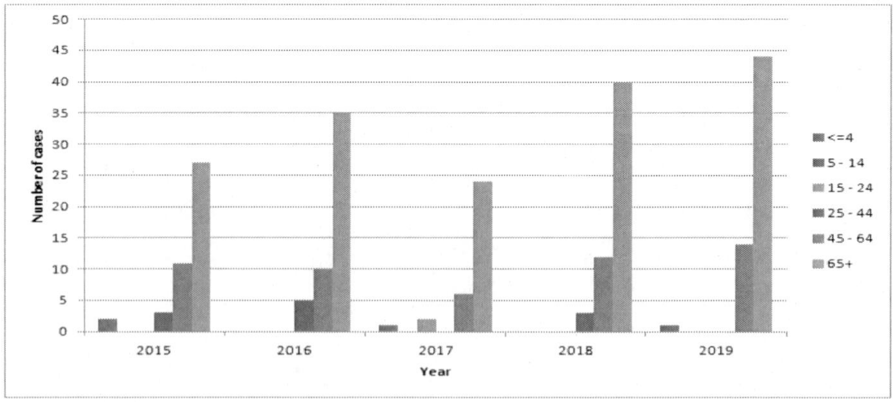

Figure 4. Number of cases died from pneumonia by year and age.

Table 2. Case fatality ratio for pneumonia during 2015-2019

Year	# Cases (% deaths)		Total
	Women	Men	
2015	76 (31.6)	72 (26.4)	148 (29.1)
2016	127 (22.8)	108 (19.4)	235 (21.3)
2017	105 (13.3)	93 (20.4)	198 (16.7)
2018	147 (16.3)	131 (22.7)	278 (19.9)
2019	151 (14.6)	153 (23.5)	304 (19.1)
Total	606 (18.6%)	557 (22.6)	1163 (20.5)

The case fatality ratio for community-acquired pneumonia during 2015-2019 is shown in Table 2. The overall case fatality ratio for the 5-year period was 20.5%, with 2015 reporting the highest proportion (29.1%). With the exception of 2015 and 2016, men had a higher case fatality rate compared to women. The case fatality rate for each year hovered around 20%, with the exception of 2015.

Discussion

Over the study period, the frequency of community-acquired pneumonia increased significantly, rejecting our hypothesis that there would be an observable decline in hospital admissions in Grenada. Our results are in contrast to global data, which shows that there is a decreasing trend in the incidence of lower respiratory infections (1). The reasons for this upward trend in incidence are unclear. One possible reason may be the underutilization of vaccination for streptococcus pneumoniae, hemophilus influenzae and the influenza virus. However, a recent report shows that Grenada has 95% immunization coverage (9), but the data did not specify for which diseases. Currently, pneumococcal vaccine is not included in Grenada's national vaccination program. Thus, the immunization data should be closely examined to decipher whether this is a contributory factor for the increased incidence of community-acquired pneumonia.

Another possible reason for the increased incidence of community-acquired pneumonia may be as a result of increased infection by atypical pathogens (10). However, our report lacks data regarding the specific pathogens causing community-acquired pneumonia in Grenada. This is because there is minimal testing for the causative agent of community-acquired pneumonia. Grenada has one state-owned clinical laboratory that performs public health functions. This laboratory does not have the capacity to test for and identify viral respiratory pathogens.

Similar to other data (11), our results showed that elderly persons were more likely to be diagnosed with community-acquired pneumonia. Thus, this demographic should be the target of interventions aimed at preventing the disease and its complications. Our results also showed a seasonal variation in the hospitalizations of community-acquired pneumonia, mirroring other studies (12, 6). Grenada depends heavily on tourism as a pillar of its economy and increasing numbers of tourists visit the island each year. Moreover, the "flu season" in North America coincides with the winter tourist season and thousands of visitors travel to Grenada by air and sea. Thus, this increases the risk of importation of respiratory pathogens into Grenada, which can even initiate an epidemic. In addition, our report had similar findings to a study by Choi et al. (13) regarding gender differences in hospitalized for community-acquired pneumonia, in which men had increased risk.

Our results showed that pneumonia has a high fatality rate, particularly in the elderly. On average, about a fifth of patients admitted for pneumonia during 2015-2019 has died. The Ministry of Health, being the custodian of the healthcare system in Grenada, should consider the lessons of 2019 in preparing for future "flu seasons". It is imperative that The Ministry of Health intensify its preventive efforts in order to curb the incidence of respiratory infections. Public service announcements should be released in the media outlining measures that can be taken to prevent the disease. Currently, hand hygiene and cough hygiene are being recommended as preventive measures. The influenza vaccine should also be promoted, targeting the groups at increased risk. There is also a need for effective surveillance at ports of entry so that respiratory infections can be rapidly and easily identified, and persons quarantined, if necessary. In this "flu season" and with the advent of COVID-19, surveillance has dramatically increased in Grenada and around the world. However, this initiative should continue in the years to come.

Even though there are challenges in detecting the cause-specific pathogen for pneumonia, with comprehensive molecular testing, pathogen detection can be significantly improved. However, adequate and appropriate treatment should be readily available for patients diagnosed with lower respiratory infections. Presently, there is no antiviral treatment available to treat patients requiring medication. Additionally, no antiviral influenza medication was available in Grenada in 2019, both in the private and public sectors. Seasonal influenza vaccines are usually made available to groups at risk.

This study had several limitations. Firstly, this study was conducted using secondary data from Grenada's main public hospital. The study only represents cases with severe enough disease to require hospitalization and does not include cases treated ambulatorily. As such, morbidity and mortality due to community-acquired pneumonia in the state of Grenada cannot be generalized from these results. Secondly, data on comorbidities, laboratory confirmation information on cases and, apart from age and sex, data on other risk factors were not available for this study. Underlying health issues and the pathogen causing disease may have had a great impact on the outcomes observed in the study. Lastly, information on the adequacy of the treatment regimens was not analyzed; this too may have provided further insight into the outcomes observed. Further research is therefore suggested to identify the factors associated with admission and mortality due to community-acquired pneumonia in Grenada.

In conclusion, the proportion of hospital admissions for community-acquired pneumonia increased significantly during 2015-2019 in Grenada, and the case fatality rate of community-acquired pneumonia is exceedingly high. Measures have to be taken to improve vaccination in order to prevent lower respiratory infections. In addition, comprehensive molecular testing should be done to accurately identify causative pathogens of lower respiratory infections. Finally, there is a dire need for medications to treat lower respiratory infections caused by viruses.

REFERENCES

[1] Troeger C, Blacker B, Khalil IA, Rao PC, Cao J, Zimsen SRM, et al. Estimates of the global, regional, and national morbidity, mortality, and aetiologies of lower respiratory infections in 195 countries, 1990–2016: A systematic analysis for the Global Burden of Disease Study 2016. Lancet Infect Dis 2018;18(11):1191–210.

[2] Centers for Disease Control and Prevention. Causes of pneumonia, 2020. URL: https://www.cdc.gov/pneumonia/causes.html.

[3] Lanks CW, Musani AI, Hsia DW. Community-acquired pneumonia and hospital-acquired pneumonia. Med Clin North Am 2019;103:487–501.

[4] World Health Organization. Top 10 causes of death. URL: https://www.who.int/gho/mortality_burden_disease/causes_death/top_10/en/.

[5] Institute for Health Metrics and Evaluation. Grenada 2017. Seattle, WA: University of Washington, 2019. URL: http://www.healthdata.org/grenada.

[6] Naghavi M, Abajobir AA, Abbafati C, Abbas KM, Abd-Allah F, Abera SF, et al. Global, regional, and national age-sex specifc mortality for 264 causes of death, 1980-2016: A systematic analysis for the Global Burden of Disease Study 2016. Lancet 2017;390(10100):1151–210.

[7] Tong S, Amand C, Kieffer A, Kyaw MH. Trends in healthcare utilization and costs associated with acute otitis media in the United States during 2008-2014. BMC Health Serv Res 2018;18(1):318.

[8] Center for Disease Control and Prevention. International classification of diseases, Tenth revision, Clinical modification. URL: https://www.cdc.gov/nchs/icd/icd10cm.htm.

[9] Pan American Health Organization. Vaccination week 2017 in Grenada. URL: https://www.paho.org/ecc/index.php?option=com_content&view=article&id=560:vaccination-week-2017-in-grenada&Itemid=264.

[10] Zubairi ABS, Zafar A, Salahuddin N, Haque AS, Waheed S, Khan JA. Atypical Pathogens causing community-acquired pneumonia in adults. J Pak Med Assoc 2012;62(7):653-6.

[11] Hughes MM, Carmack AE, McCaffrey K, Spencer M, Reed GM, Hill M, et al. Estimating the incidence of influenza at the state level: Utah, 2016–17 and 2017–18 influenza seasons. MMWR 2019;68(50):1158–61.

[12] Cilloniz C, Ewig S, Gabarrus A, Ferrer M, Puig de la Bella Casa J, Mensa J, et al. Seasonality of pathogens causing community-acquired pneumonia. Respirology 2017;22(4):778–85.

[13] Choi W Il, Rho BH, Lee MY. Male predominance of pneumonia and hospitalization in pandemic influenza A (H1N1) 2009 infection. BMC Res Notes 2011;4:351.

In: Public Health Themes in Grenada … ISBN: 978-1-53618-118-0
Editors: J. Merrick and L. Glasgow

Chapter 21

HEALTH IMPACT AND MULTISECTORAL RESPONSE TO A MAJOR FLOODING EVENT IN TRINIDAD, OCTOBER 2018

Laura-Lee G Boodram[1,*], PhD, MSc, Corey Dillon[2], DHV, Sharis Garcia[1], BSc, Hannah H Covert[3], PhD, Maureen Y Lichtveld[3], MD, MPH and Carl J Hospedales[1], MBBS, MSc

[1]Caribbean Public Health Agency, Port of Spain, Trinidad and Tobago, [2]Southwest Regional Health Authority, San Fernando, Trinidad and Tobago and [3]Tulane University School of Public Health and Tropical Medicine, New Orleans, United States of America

ABSTRACT

In this chapter, we examine the effectiveness of the flood early warning system utilized by Trinidad and assess the multisectoral response to

---

* Correspondence: Dr. Laura-Lee G. Boodram, Caribbean Public Health Agency, Port of Spain, Trinidad and Tobago, West Indies. Email: boodrala@carpha.org.

mitigate the health impact of flooding. The work consisted of two components. Firstly, a qualitative, key informant interview process was conducted, examining factors related to timeliness of early warning alerts, multisectoral impact including health, emergency response efforts, and recommended mitigation actions. Interviewees sampled were purposively selected from different sectors and were directly involved in the flood response. Consent was obtained before proceeding with interviews and transcriptions were analyzed using thematic analysis. The second component, targeted at assessing health impacts of flooding, collected and descriptively analyzed syndromic disease surveillance data from health centers serving flood-affected areas. Seven key informants in total were recruited from three organizations, including two local government regional corporations, the Ministry of Health, and a local Non-Governmental Organization. Major factors that led to the flooding included a combination of poor urban planning and development and unusually heavy precipitation within a short period of time that led to severe riverine flooding in North Central Trinidad. Households, entire communities, businesses, schools, and the agricultural and health sector were impacted. Syndromic surveillance conducted at health centers in the north-central area described a post-flooding rise in respiratory and gastrointestinal disease cases. The October 2018, Trinidad flooding event tested several organizational emergency response systems within the country. Climate resilience must be considered in health sector planning to strengthen surveillance systems and appropriately respond to health disasters.

INTRODUCTION

The Caribbean Region is particularly vulnerable to natural disasters, such as hurricanes, flooding, and drought. Climate change, which influences hydrometeorological events, is driven by global warming and is of major concern for Small Island Developing States (SIDS) in the Caribbean. The Intergovernmental Panel on Climate Change (IPCC) 2007 report details an observed 0.2°C increase per decade in the Caribbean region over the last 30 years (1).

The period June 1 to November 30 each year marks the Atlantic Hurricane season (2). Over the past few years, the region has seen a rise in the frequency and severity of storms, including three Category 5 storms within the last two years (2), which heavily impacted human life and island economies. Over the last 30 years, climate variability, regional warming, and modifications in rainfall patterns have been recorded by Caribbean islands, however, climate change is responsible for a shift in the range and pattern of this variability (3).

Rainfall in Trinidad and Tobago varies across the two islands and within each island. Local and remote climate influencers such as El Niño and La Niña phases of the El Niño Southern Oscillation (ENSO) play important roles with respect to rainfall patterns. There also exists a strong relationship between local rainfall variability and the Inter Tropical Convergence Zone (ITCZ), which is linked to prolonged rainfall periods in Trinidad and Tobago (4).

On October 16, 2018 the Trinidad and Tobago Meteorological Service (TTMS) issued its first early warning message of a potential major flooding event in Trinidad, approximately 72 hours before the start of the event. This was followed by a yellow alert Common Alert Protocol (CAP) during the 17th – 19th October, which detailed an active ITCZ that would lead to flash flooding. On October 18, 2019 the TTMS upgraded their alert to the orange level, which was further escalated to the red level, projecting extensive riverine flooding along the Caroni River, and advising citizens to protect life, livelihood, and property (K. Kerr pers. comm. 11 February 2019).

Following this, a major flooding event occurred across the north-central and eastern parts of Trinidad, which resulted in the Trinidad and Tobago Government declaring a natural disaster and engaged all levels of response from national to local government, as well as civil society and community relief efforts. Communities along the Caroni flood basin were heavily impacted, with evacuations being necessary in some cases. Reports from the Trinidad Office of Disaster Preparedness and Management (ODPM) and the Caribbean Disaster Management Agency (CDEMA) indicated that flooding impacted 100,000 to 150,000 people, with 800 people being evacuated and 300 seeking shelter support (5).

This report aims to examine the effectiveness of the early warning system utilized by the Trinidadian authorities, assess the multisectoral response that evolved to mitigate the impacts of flooding, inclusive of the health outcomes, and make recommendations for future mitigation efforts.

Our Study

This study consisted of two components; the first utilized information gained through semi-structured, key informant interviews. The interview protocol sought information on various factors, including timelines of alerts issued by the relevant authorities, factors that contributed to the flooding event, impact on various sectors including health, success of the response efforts, and recommendations for future mitigation actions. Interviewees sampled were purposively selected, held key positions within their organizations, and were directly involved in the flood response process. Interviewees were selected from different sectors, including emergency and disaster response, public health, and civil society. Consent was obtained before recording and assurances were given that anonymity would be preserved. No personal identifying information was collected. Notes and audio transcriptions were manually reviewed and categorized using thematic analysis. The results were summarized and are presented in the section below.

The second component, targeted at assessing health impacts of the flooding, was based on collecting and analyzing syndromic disease surveillance data from health centers serving flood-affected areas. Syndromes/disease classifications examined included respiratory infections, acute viral illness, and gastroenteritis.

Findings

A total of seven key informant interviews were conducted, inclusive of four personnel from the local government regional corporations, two from the Ministry of Health, and one from a non-governmental organization (NGO). The local government corporations directly serviced the flood-affected areas.

Timeliness of alerts

Official warnings from the Office of Disaster Preparedness and Management, as well as the Meteorological Office were dispatched, however, the reach and timeliness of the messages were not consistent throughout the response community. In one instance, the local government office acted independently of these alerts based on community reports received. Other response offices indicated satisfaction with timely alerts. Messages to the general Trinidadian population were disseminated on local television, radio channels, the TTMS website, and social media beginning three days prior to the start of the flooding event.

Factors contributing to flooding

The main contributors to the major flood event of October 2018 were proposed to be a combination of poor urban planning and drainage development, as well as the timing of hydrometeorological events. Main areas affected included North Central Trinidad (primarily the Caroni river flood basin) and Sangre Grande on the Eastern side of the island and Mayaro in the south. Communities built close to the river flood zone were impacted first. Between 17-19 October 2018, Trinidad experienced one month's worth of rainfall. Some meteorological weather sub-stations reported between 6-10 inches of rainfall over the three days, with areas such as Sangre Grande, North Oropouche, San Rafael, Carapo, Talparo and Guaico Tamana receiving 12-14 inches. This unusually large amount of rainfall in such a short space of time, coupled with high tides, prevented riverine and land runoff, resulted in the Caroni River overflowing its banks at several points, leading to inundation of surrounding communities and farms. Other factors included blockage of riverine systems due to improper solid waste disposal practices by local communities living near the river.

Impact of flooding event

Within the private sector, several whole communities in the north-central area, including St. Helena, Kelly, Las Lomas, Greenvale, as well as Sangre Grande in the east, and Mayaro in the south of the island were inundated with floodwaters. Levels reached greater than four feet high in the community of Greenvale, which required evacuation. Personal items such as clothing, household items, and appliances, furniture, and electronics were lost. Homes and buildings suffered infrastructural damages, and vehicles were also damaged by floodwaters. In the agricultural sector, crops and livestock were lost, and many local businesses suffered losses. Major transportation routes, such as the Uriah Butler Highway, were impassable to regular traffic for two days, and roads in and around the aforementioned communities were also impassable. The main commercial airport, Piarco, was also closed due to runway flooding. Schools were in affected communities were closed.

Due to the impassable roads, some health facilities could not service the local population due to persons' inability to get to and from the health centers, more so in the Eastern region. Some of the facilities that were directly impacted were the Sangre Grande General Hospital, the Mayaro Emergency Health Services, and the St. Helena Health Centre. Health care staff servicing facilities were unable to commute and assist in response efforts.

Response efforts

As reports were received about the severity of flooding, response teams from the Trinidad and Tobago Regiment, the Trinidad and Tobago Police Service, the National Fire Service, and staff members of the Regional Corporations and NGOs, were mobilized to help communities. The ODPM, under the Ministry of National Security, coordinated the national level response, whereas, the Regional Corporations, which have local emergency and disaster response units, coordinated the community-level response. Areas first affected were Sangre Grande and Greenvale. Shelters were opened to accommodate those whose homes would have been affected by the floods. Rescue teams went out using boats and trucks to help rescue trapped persons in order to take them to the aforementioned shelters and health centers, where they could be assessed and treated as necessary. Some of the affected persons included vulnerable groups such as pregnant women, the disabled, and the elderly.

Mental health professionals were also deployed to shelters and health centers to provide counseling for persons who were traumatized by the event, however, the uptake of this service was limited, with affected persons focusing on accessing medical treatment services for illness and injuries. On the national level, citizens, faith-based organizations, businesses, schools, and NGOs mobilized resources from the population and supplied toiletries, food household items, and clothes to affected communities. The government of Trinidad and Tobago supplied monetary compensation to flood-affected victims to assist in the purchasing of clothing, furniture, and aid for small home repairs.

Syndromic disease surveillance

The flooding event occurred during epidemiological week 42. Limited syndromic surveillance data were available from health centers serving affected communities in the north-central area. Primarily respiratory and gastroenteritis data were collected. Health centers recorded no data recorded for undifferentiated fever syndrome. Increases were seen in acute respiratory infection in both the < and > 5-year age groups in the eight weeks following the flooding event (see Figures 1 and 2). A similar pattern was seen with gastroenteritis data in both the < and > 5-year age groups (see Figures 3 and 4). The local surveillance system also captures acute viral illness with the number of cases recorded higher during the eight weeks post-flooding (see Figure 5). No baseline or epidemic threshold data were obtained for the reviewed weeks.

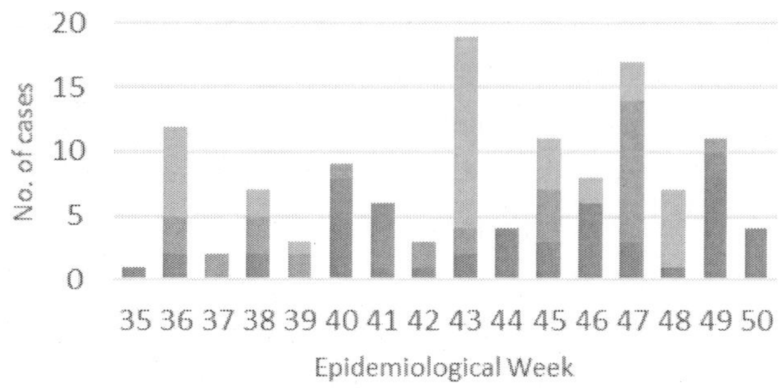

Figure 1. Cases of acute respiratory infection <5 years by epidemiological week, 2018, in North Central Trinidad Health Centres.

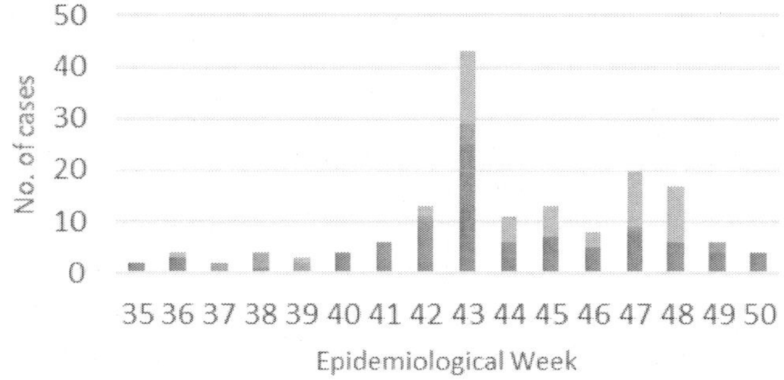

Figure 2. Cases of acute respiratory infection >5 years by epidemiological week, 2018, in North Central Trinidad Health Centres.

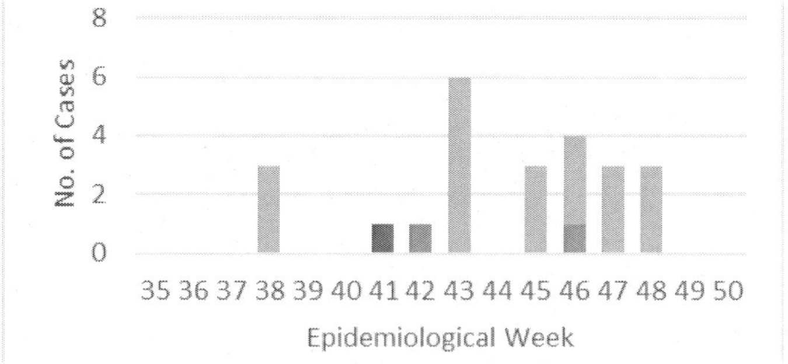

Figure 3. Cases of gastroenteritis <5 years by epidemiological week, 2018, in North Central Trinidad Health Centres.

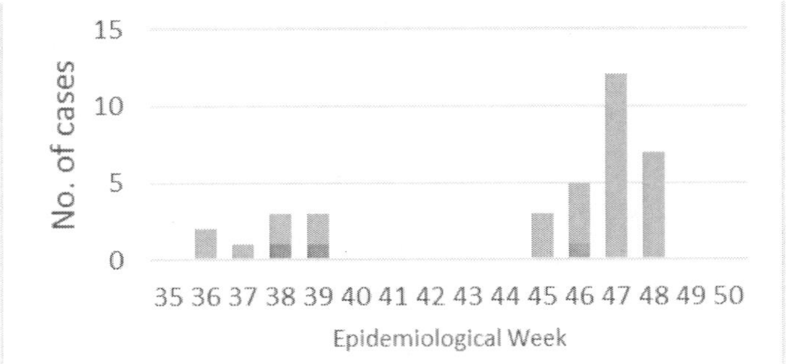

Figure 4. Cases of gastroenteritis >5 years by epidemiological week, 2018, in North Central Trinidad Health Centres.

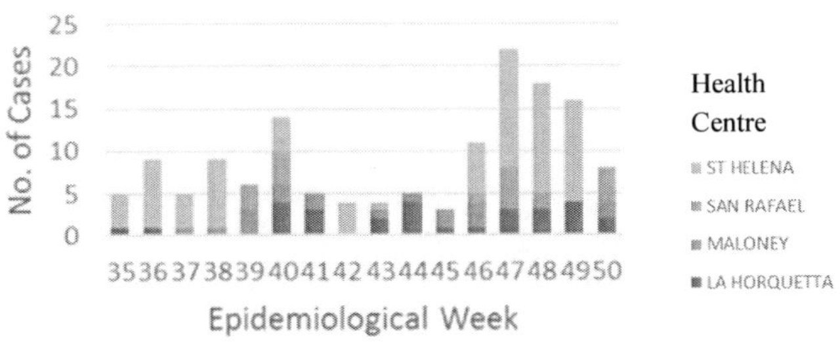

Figure 5. Cases of acute viral illness by epidemiological week, 2018, in North Central Trinidad Health Centres.

DISCUSSION

In Trinidad and Tobago, the highest rainfall and flood associated events are typically observed during November, however, over the last few years, a potential shift may be seen towards October (3, 4). Above-average rainfall during three days in October 2018 precipitated what has been termed as an unprecedented flooding event in Trinidad, which impacted on a large scale communities, transportation routes, the agriculture, business, education, and health sectors. Additionally, the destruction of vegetation through bush fires/farming activities along the Northern and Central range of Trinidad, impacts on watersheds, further worsening flood events.

The early warning alerts issued by the TTMS were provided to the public and response agencies allowed most communities to prepare for the potential flooding event. The color-coded nature of these alerts targeted attention to the gravity of the developing situation, allowing response agencies and citizens time for some level of preparation. Social media was noted as being heavily used in the dissemination of messages. In terms of the effectiveness of the response, a noted disparity was a certain degree of disconnect between the emergency/disaster response units of the Regional Corporations and the ODPM. The Corporations largely acted independently within their areas of responsibility with limited communication and coordination between the local and national level response systems.

Floodwaters pose immediate dangers to human health, and long-term effects result from displacement and worsened living conditions. Of particular concerns following flooding is the rise in communicable diseases, such as food and water-borne diseases, respiratory disease, and arboviral/mosquito-borne diseases (7). While mosquito breeding sites may be washed away during flooding events, residual pooling post-flooding creates new breeding sites, increasing the transmission potential of viruses, such as Dengue, Chikungunya, and Zika (7). Injuries during flood incidents are quite common, and the stress levels and trauma experienced by both flood victims, as well as relief and aid workers, are well documented (8). Where flooding impacts transportation routes, this limits access to health services and medicinal supplies, which will also affect persons with chronic disease. In the October Trinidad flooding, access to health care was largely available, with the limitation more being seen in the inability of health care staff from flood-affected areas to commute and provide services at facilities. Future emergency response plans should describe mechanisms to mitigate the effects of major routes impacted by flooding.

Interpretation of the limited syndromic surveillance data available from health centers servicing affected communities was difficult. Baseline/threshold levels are not calculated at the local levels of the surveillance system and as records are paper-based, access to data to generate baselines is often not feasible. Data from local levels are aggregated and forwarded to the national level. Hence, for the weeks investigated, a determination cannot be made as to whether the rise in cases of acute respiratory infection and gastroenteritis was unusual for the period observed. The majority of health centers did not collect disease-specific data, either due to lack of human resources, limited coordination among sentinel physicians, lack of training, or limited collection of specimens to facilitate diagnostic testing confirmation. Of note, is that the St. Helena health center reported the highest number of cases across all syndromes (see Figures 1-5), however, a determination cannot be made about the reliability of this data or whether the pattern seen is an artifact due to a higher level of focus on reporting in this center.

In Trinidad, the classification of disease under acute viral illness is broad/nonspecific. In many instances, if regional syndromic classification guidelines are adhered to, the majority of viral cases would be reallocated under respiratory or undifferentiated fever syndromes (9). This points to the need for continuous training and sensitization of physicians and surveillance personnel. Although no deaths resulted from the flooding event, the lack of continued post-disaster surveillance in the weeks/months that followed as services and lives were disrupted does not allow for an effective assessment of health impact. Post-disaster surveillance should also include shelter surveillance encompassing areas such as environmental health, food safety, water quality, and even pet/companion wellness. Syndromic, disease-specific surveillance, and mortality surveillance are critical.

Within the Caribbean, health systems need to rapidly increase their transition to climate resiliency to manage projected reductions in food quality and security, increases in water stress, increases in the magnitude and frequency of extreme weather and climate events, increases in the geographic range of mosquito-borne diseases, and changes in the burdens of other climate-sensitive health outcomes. Resilience strategies can include improvements in emergency flood notifications; improvements to infrastructure that accommodate river flow; community education and outreach campaigns; restoration of watersheds and stricter enforcement of urbanization and development. The October 2018 Trinidad flooding event tested several response systems within the country. While the efforts at the local and national governmental levels are to be commended, improvements are required in terms of having coordinated, integrated responses. There is also a strong need to improve disease surveillance capacity at the local health center/sentinel site level to generate accurate, detailed data for timely public health action and response.

Key informant interviews were conducted with persons from the Regional Corporations, the Ministry of Health and NGOs/Civil Society. Groups such as the ODPM, Ministry of Social Development, faith-based organizations, and schools were unable to be included during the project time allotted for the interview process. Also, as baseline and threshold health data were unavailable for the weeks investigated, it is unknown if the rise in cases of acute respiratory infection and gastroenteritis was unusual for the period of time observed.

Acknowledgments

This work was supported through a grant from the National Oceanic and Atmospheric Administration International Research and Applications Project (NA18OAR4310338).

References

[1] Intergovernmental Panel on Climate Change (IPCC). Climate change 2007 Synthesis report, 2008. URL: https://www.ipcc.ch/site/assets/uploads/2018/02/ar4_syr_full_report.pdf.

[2] National Hurricane Centre and Central Pacific Hurricane Centre. Tropical cyclone climatology, 2019. URL: https://www.nhc.noaa.gov/climo/.

[3] Trinidad and Tobago Guardian. Climate change shifting patterns, intensity of rain, 2018. URL: https://www.guardian.co.tt/news/climate-change-shifting-6.2.722875.f339d714de.

[4] Trinidad and Tobago Meteorological Service. Climate, 2019 URL: http://www.metoffice.gov.tt/Climate.

[5] CDEMA. CDEMA news situation reports. CDEMA situation report #1 - Adverse weather resulted in severe flooding in Trinidad and Tobago as of 10:00AM (AST) on October 22, 2018. 2018. Accessed 2019 Dec 04. URL: https://www.

humanitarianresponse.info/sites/www.humanitarianresponse.info/files/documents/files/cdema_situation_report_no1__severe_flooding_in_trinidad_tobago.pdf.

[6] Intergovernmental Panel on Climate Change (IPCC). Special report: Global warming of 1.5 deg °C. 2018. URL:https://www.ipcc.ch/sr15/chapter/chapter-1/.

[7] Caribbean Institute for Meteorology and Hydrology (CIMH). Caribbean Health Climatic Bulletin 2019. URL: http://rcc.cimh.edu.bb/caribbean-health-climatic-bulletin-vol-3-issue-3-september-2019/.

[8] WHO. Floods and health. Fact sheets for health professionals, 2014. URL: http://www.euro.who.int/__data/assets/pdf_file/0016/252601/Floods-and-health-Fact-sheets-for-health-professionals.pdf.

[9] CARPHA. Regional surveillance policy guidelines. 2011. URL: http://carpha.org/downloads/Regional-Surveillance-Guidelines-Interim-Policy%20(1)%20(1).pdf.

SECTION THREE: ACKNOWLEDGMENTS

In: Public Health Themes in Grenada … ISBN: 978-1-53618-118-0
Editors: J. Merrick and L. Glasgow © 2020 Nova Science Publishers, Inc.

Chapter 22

About the Editors

Lindonne Glasgow, MSPH, DrPH, was born in Grenada and educated in Grenada and the United States. She is an Assistant Professor and Deputy Chair in the Department of Public Health and Preventive Medicine at St George's University in St George's in Grenada, West Indies. For over 10 years, she developed, piloted and managed various projects for eight Caribbean countries, crosscutting social, health, and environmental issues. She holds a Master of Science in Public Health (MSPH) degree and a Doctor of Public Health (DrPH) degree. Some of her recent research focused on evaluating pesticide use and health risk, harvested rainwater quality, antibiotic use in animal food production and human health care, climate change and ecosystems. One of her most outstanding work, among other "first" studies in Grenada, was estimating the prevalence and burden of foodborne diseases in the country for which she received a Leaders Award in 2010 from the International Conference on Emerging Infectious Disease, Centers for Disease Control and Prevention and the US Department of Defense Armed Forces Health Surveillance Center. Email: lglasgow@sgu.com

Joav Merrick, MD, MMedSci, DMSc, born and educated in Denmark is professor of pediatrics, Division of Pediatrics, Hadassah Hebrew University Medical Center, Mt Scopus Campus, Jerusalem, Israel and Kentucky Children's Hospital, University of Kentucky, Lexington, Kentucky United States and professor of public health at the Center for Healthy Development, School of Public Health, Georgia State University, Atlanta, United States, the former medical director of the Health Services, Division for Intellectual and Developmental Disabilities, Ministry of Social Affairs and Social Services, Jerusalem, the founder and director of the National Institute of Child Health and Human Development in Israel. Numerous publications in the field of pediatrics, child health and human development, rehabilitation, intellectual disability, disability, health, welfare, abuse, advocacy, quality of life and prevention. Received the Peter Sabroe Child Award for outstanding work on behalf of Danish Children in 1985 and the International LEGO-Prize ("The Children's Nobel Prize") for an extraordinary contribution towards improvement in child welfare and well-being in 1987. In 2017 appointed a Kentucky Colonel by the Commonwealth of Kentucky, the highest honor the governor can bestow to a person. Email: jmerrick@zahav.net.il

In: Public Health Themes in Grenada … ISBN: 978-1-53618-118-0
Editors: J. Merrick and L. Glasgow

Chapter 23

About St George's University, Department of Public Health and Preventive Medicine (SGU-DPHPM), St George's, Grenada

The Department of Public Health and Preventive Medicine (SGU-DPHPM) was established in 1999 to develop and deliver its Master of Public Health (MPH) graduate program. As an international center of medical education, SGU welcomed the opportunity to train medical students and graduates in public health towards strengthening primary health care and serve for capacity building for the Caribbean international regions towards health systems strengthening. Since 1999, SGU-DPHPM has graduated over one thousand healthcare professionals that serve in over 50 countries. The mission of SGU-DPHPM is to provide an academic focal point for interdisciplinary education, research and service with a focus that is both globally relevant and locally applicable.

Education

SGU-DPHPM administers a Council on Education for Public Health (CEPH) accredited MPH program with areas of concentration in global health, preventive medicine, veterinary public health, epidemiology, environmental and occupational health and health policy and administration. SGU-DPHPM also coordinates public health education for the Doctor of Medicine (MD) program as well as collaborates in veterinary public health for the Doctor of Veterinary Medicine (DVM) program. Additionally, SGU-DPHPM provides graduate course for students in the School of Graduate Studies Masters and Doctoral programs, a Certificate in Public Health program for public health practitioners and supports workforce development and community health education through ongoing training initiatives. Students and graduates of SGU-DPHPM MPH program successfully enhance their graduate public health experience with a commitment to lifelong learning as Certified Public Health (CPH) professionals from the United States National Board of Public Health Examiners (NBPHE). SGU-DPHPM focus on inter-professional education, research and service is lead through the scholarship of its faculty and students collaborations and in partnership with international institutions and colleagues. Details of SGU-DPHPM's scholarship can be accessed from the website (sgu.edu).

Research

The affiliated faculty of SGU-DPHPM, over the years, have published work from projects and research activities thorough national and international collaborations. For the past 20 years, in collaboration with SGU's research institute, Windward Islands Research and Education Foundation (WINDREF), SGU-DPHPM faculty, students and project/research partners and collaborators have administered over 10 million USD in grant funding and over 250 publications across peer reviewed journals and national and international publications. WINDREF, established in 1994 is registered as a 501(c)3 in the United States, a Charitable Trust in the United Kingdom and

a Non-Governmental Organization in Grenada. Through WINDREF's coordination with administrative support, laboratory capacity, grants management, statistical
support and network of research fellows, SGU-DPHPM faculty and students are actively engaged in research activities. SGU-DPHPM research is also supported by SGU's Office of Research which includes access to institutional funding and support as well as Institutional Review Board (IRB) and Institutional Animal Care and Use Committee (IACUC) which serves to review research work for ethical clearance.

Service

Over the past 20 years of SGU-DPHPM, many activities became focused on collaboration with various local, regional and international initiatives, which has resulted in collaboration around the establishment of a World Health Organization (WHO) Collaborating Center in Environmental and Occupational Health. Also, in response to the disproportionate and adverse effects of the climate on health, a United Nations Frame Convention on Climate Change, Regional Collaborating Center (UNFCCC-RCC) was established for collaborations. Furthermore, SGU-DPHPM has partnered with local and regional governments and community based organizations in response to disasters, vector borne disease outbreaks and overall management of non-communicable diseases. Service activities are additionally conducted with SGU-DPHPM's active Public Health Students Association (PHSA). PHSA routinely partners with medical and veterinary students to conduct community health clinics as well as health education and environmental health management services across Grenada. SGU-DPHPM additionally contains the Gamma Kappa chapter of Delta Omega Honors Society, which is the oldest professional public health society. Delta Omega Honors Society prides itself in community service and informs community work in response to community assessment and identified community needs.

Partners and collaborations

SGU-DPHPM education, research and service are delivered in collaborations with the Schools of Medicine, Veterinary Medicine, Arts and Sciences and Graduate Studies at SGU. SGU-DPHPM also supports organizations in Grenada with their annual work plan, including the Grenada Public Health Association (PHSA), Grenada Diabetes Association (GDA) and the Grenada Cancer Society (GCS). Regionally, SGU-DPHPM supports the work of the Organization of Eastern Caribbean States (OECS), Caribbean Public Health Agency (CARPHA) and the Pan American Health Organization (PAHO). Through memberships and fellowships, SGU-DPHPM is also actively involved in the work of the American Public Health Association (APHA), Association of Schools and Programs in Public Health (ASPPH), Consortium on Universities in Public Health (CUGH), Royal Society of Public Health (RSPH), Royal Society of Tropical Medicine and Hygiene (RSTMH) and global agencies such as World Health Organization (WHO), World Bank and the United Nations (UN). Funding partnership and collaborations are engaged through agencies such as the National Institutes of Health (NIH), World Bank, World Diabetes Foundation (WDF), United Nations Development Program (UNDP) United Nations Global Environmental Facility (UN-GEF), Centers for Disease Control and Prevention (CDC), National Institutes for Occupational Safety and Health (NIOSH), United States Department of Agriculture (USDA), Public Health Canada, African Medical Research and Education Foundation (AMREF) and the Caribbean Community (CARICOM) and Caribbean Public Health Agency (CARPHA). SGU-DPHPM, with its interdisciplinary local to global focus, have also partnered with several institutions in the Caribbean: T.A. Marryshow Community College (TAMCC), University of the West Indies (UWI), University of Trinidad and Tobago, University of Technology, Jamaica, Pasteur Institute, Guadeloupe, Institute of Tropical Medicine, Cuba; North America: New York University (NYU), State University of New York (SUNY), Sanford University, John's Hopkins University Bloomberg School of Public Health (JHU), Colombia University, Mailman School of Public Health: South America: Universidad de Antioquia,

Colombia, University of Guyana, Guyana; Europe: Northumbria University (NU) and the Royal Veterinary College (RVC); United Kingdom; Switzerland: Swiss Tropical Medicine Institute; Africa: Juba Medical College, South Sudan, University of Kwa-Zulu, Natal, South Africa, Makerere University, Uganda: Asia: Mahidol University, Kasetsart University, Chitkara University, MS Ramaiah Medical College, Indian Institute of Health Management Research (IIHMR), Konkuk University and Polytechnic Institute in Singapore.

Contact

Lindonne Glasgow, DrPH
Assistant Professor, Public Health and Preventive Medicine,
St George's University
Grenada, West Indies
Email: lglasgow@sgu.edu

In: Public Health Themes in Grenada … ISBN: 978-1-53618-118-0
Editors: J. Merrick and L. Glasgow

Chapter 24

About the National Institute of Child Health and Human Development in Israel

The National Institute of Child Health and Human Development (NICHD) in Israel was established in 1998 as a virtual institute under the auspicies of the Medical Director, Ministry of Social Affairs and Social Services in order to function as the research arm for the Office of the Medical Director. In 1998 the National Council for Child Health and Pediatrics, Ministry of Health and in 1999 the Director General and Deputy Director General of the Ministry of Health endorsed the establishment of the NICHD.

Mission

The mission of a National Institute for Child Health and Human Development in Israel is to provide an academic focal point for the scholarly interdisciplinary study of child life, health, public health, welfare, disability, rehabilitation, intellectual disability and related aspects of human development. This mission includes research, teaching, clinical work, information and public service activities in the field of child health and human development.

Service and academic activities

Over the years many activities became focused in the south of Israel due to collaboration with various professionals at the Faculty of Health Sciences (FOHS) at the Ben Gurion University of the Negev (BGU). Since 2000 an affiliation with the Zusman Child Development Center at the Pediatric Division of Soroka University Medical Center has resulted in collaboration around the establishment of the Down Syndrome Clinic at that center. In 2002 a full course on "Disability" was established at the Recanati School for Allied Professions in the Community, FOHS, BGU and in 2005 collaboration was started with the Primary Care Unit of the faculty and disability became part of the master of public health course on "Children and society". In the academic year 2005-2006 a one semester course on "Aging with disability" was started as part of the master of science program in gerontology in our collaboration with the Center for Multidisciplinary Research in Aging. In 2010 collaborations with the Division of Pediatrics, Hadassah Hebrew University Medical Center, Jerusalem, Israel around the National Down Syndrome Center and teaching students and residents about intellectual and developmental disabilities as part of their training at this campus.

Research activities

The affiliated staff have over the years published work from projects and research activities in this national and international collaboration. In the year 2000 the International Journal of Adolescent Medicine and Health and in 2005 the International Journal on Disability and Human Development of De Gruyter Publishing House (Berlin and New York) were affiliated with the National Institute of Child Health and Human Development. From 2008 also the International Journal of Child Health and Human Development (Nova Science, New York), the International Journal of Child and Adolescent Health (Nova Science) and the Journal of Pain Management (Nova Science) affiliated and from 2009 the International Public Health Journal (Nova Science) and Journal of Alternative Medicine Research (Nova Science). All peer-reviewed international journals.

National collaborations

Nationally the NICHD works in collaboration with the Faculty of Health Sciences, Ben Gurion University of the Negev; Department of Physical Therapy, Sackler School of Medicine, Tel Aviv University; Autism Center, Assaf HaRofeh Medical Center; National Rett and PKU Centers at Chaim Sheba Medical Center, Tel HaShomer; Department of Physiotherapy, Haifa University; Department of Education, Bar Ilan University, Ramat Gan, Faculty of Social Sciences and Health Sciences; College of Judea and Samaria in Ariel and in 2011 affiliation with Center for Pediatric Chronic Diseases and National Center for Down Syndrome, Department of Pediatrics, Hadassah Hebrew University Medical Center, Mount Scopus Campus, Jerusalem.

International collaborations

Internationally with the Department of Disability and Human Development, College of Applied Health Sciences, University of Illinois at Chicago; Strong Center for Developmental Disabilities, Golisano Children's Hospital at Strong, University of Rochester School of Medicine and Dentistry, New York; Centre on Intellectual Disabilities, University of Albany, New York; Centre for Chronic Disease Prevention and Control, Health Canada, Ottawa; Chandler Medical Center and Children's Hospital, Kentucky Children's Hospital, Section of Adolescent Medicine, University of Kentucky, Lexington; Chronic Disease Prevention and Control Research Center,

Baylor College of Medicine, Houston, Texas; Division of Neuroscience, Department of Psychiatry, Columbia University, New York; Institute for the Study of Disadvantage and Disability, Atlanta; Center for Autism and Related Disorders, Department Psychiatry, Children's Hospital Boston, Boston; Department of Pediatric and Adolescent Medicine, Western Michigan University Homer Stryker MD School of Medicine, Kalamazoo, Michigan, United States; Department of Paediatrics, Child Health and Adolescent Medicine, Children's Hospital at Westmead, Westmead, Australia; International Centre for the Study of Occupational and Mental Health, Düsseldorf, Germany; Centre for Advanced Studies in Nursing, Department of General Practice and Primary Care, University of Aberdeen, Aberdeen, United Kingdom; Quality of Life Research Center, Copenhagen, Denmark; Nordic School of Public Health, Gottenburg, Sweden, Scandinavian Institute of Quality of Working Life, Oslo, Norway; The Department of Applied Social Sciences (APSS) of The Hong Kong Polytechnic University Hong Kong.

Targets

Our focus is on research, international collaborations, clinical work, teaching and policy in health, disability and human development and to establish the NICHD as a permanent institute in Israel in order to conduct model research and provide policy aspects in the field of interest.

Contact

Professor Joav Merrick, MD, MMedSci, DMSc
Director, National Institute of Child Health and Human Development, Jerusalem, Israel. E-mail: jmerrick@zahav.net.il

SECTION FOUR: INDEX

INDEX

A

B

C

D

E

F

G

L

M

N

O

P

Q

R

S

T

U

V

W

Z